This edition is dedicated to Imogen Rose Barker, who died tragically February 2007: a wonderful daughter and an inspiration to many.

Companion website

This book has an accompanying website at:

www.ataglanceseries.com/neuroscience

Features:
- Interactive multiple choice questions for each chapter
- Self-assessment case studies from the book and extra online case studies
- Chapter key points for revision
- Flashcards of key figures with interactive on/off labels
- Figures from the book in PowerPoint format
- Neuroscience and medical glossaries

Neuroanatomy and Neuroscience at a Glance

Roger A. Barker

BA, MBBS, MRCP, PhD
Cambridge Centre for Brain Repair and Department of Neurology
University of Cambridge
Cambridge, UK

Francesca Cicchetti

PhD
Centre de Recherche du CHUL (CHUQ)
Université Laval
Québec
Canada

and Neuropharmacology by

Michael J. Neal

DSc, PhD, MA, BPharm
Emeritus Professor of Pharmacology
Department of Pharmacology
King's College
London, UK

Fourth Edition

WILEY-BLACKWELL

A John Wiley & Sons, Ltd., Publication

This edition first published 2012 © 2012 by John Wiley & Sons, Ltd.
Previous editions © 1999, 2003, 2008 Roger Barker and Stephen Barasi

Wiley-Blackwell is an imprint of John Wiley & Sons, formed by the merger of Wiley's global Scientific, Technical and Medical business with Blackwell Publishing.

Registered office:	John Wiley & Sons, Ltd, The Atrium, Southern Gate, Chichester, West Sussex, PO19 8SQ, UK
Editorial offices:	9600 Garsington Road, Oxford, OX4 2DQ, UK
	The Atrium, Southern Gate, Chichester, West Sussex, PO19 8SQ, UK
	111 River Street, Hoboken, NJ 07030-5774, USA

For details of our global editorial offices, for customer services and for information about how to apply for permission to reuse the copyright material in this book please see our website at www.wiley.com/wiley-blackwell.

The right of the author to be identified as the author of this work has been asserted in accordance with the UK Copyright, Designs and Patents Act 1988.

Library of Congress Cataloging-in-Publication Data

Barker, Roger A., 1961–
  Neuroanatomy and neuroscience at a glance / Roger A. Barker, Francesca Cicchetti ; and neuropharmacology by Michael J. Neal. – 4th ed.
       p. ; cm. – (At a glance series)
  Rev. ed. of: Neuroscience at a glance / Roger A. Barker, Stephen Barasi ; and neuropharmacology by Michael J. Neal.. 3rd ed. 2008.
  Includes bibliographical references and index.
  ISBN 978-0-470-65768-3 (pbk. : alk. paper)
  I. Cicchetti, Francesca. II. Neal, M. J. III. Barker, Roger A., 1961– Neuroscience at a glance. IV. Title. V. Series: At a glance series (Oxford, England)
  [DNLM: 1. Nervous System Physiological Phenomena. 2. Nervous System–anatomy & histology. 3. Nervous System Diseases. WL 102]
  616.8–dc23
                                                                    2011042259

A catalogue record for this book is available from the British Library.

Set in 9/11.5 pt TimesNRMT by Toppan Best-set Premedia Limited
Printed and bound in Malaysia by Vivar Printing Sdn Bhd

1 2012

Contents

Introduction 6
Acknowledgements 7
List of abbreviations 8

Part 1 Anatomical and functional organization
1 Development of the nervous system 10
2 Organization of the nervous system 12
3 Autonomic nervous system 14
4 Enteric nervous system 16
5 Meninges and cerebrospinal fluid 18
6 Blood supply to the central nervous system 20
7 Cranial nerves 22
8 Anatomy of the brainstem 24
9 Organization of the spinal cord 26
10 Organization of the cerebral cortex and thalamus 28
11 Hypothalamus 30

Part 2 Cells and neurophysiology
12 Cells of the nervous system I: neurones 32
13 Cells of the nervous system II: neuroglial cells 34
14 Ion channels 36
15 Resting membrane and action potential 38
16 Neuromuscular junction (NMJ) and synapses 40
17 Nerve conduction and synaptic integration 42
18 Neurotransmitters, receptors and their pathways 44
19 Main CNS neurotransmitters and their function 46
20 Skeletal muscle structure 48
21 Skeletal muscle contraction 50

Part 3 Sensory systems
22 Sensory systems: an overview 52
23 Sensory transduction 54
24 Visual system I: the eye and retina 56
25 Visual system II: the visual pathways and
    subcortical visual areas 58
26 Visual system III: visual cortical areas 60
27 Auditory system I: the ear and cochlea 62
28 Auditory system II: the auditory pathways
    and language 64
29 Vestibular system 66
30 Olfaction and taste 68
31 Somatosensory system 70
32 Pain systems I: nociceptors and
    nociceptive pathways 72
33 Pain systems II: pharmacology and management 74
34 Association cortices: the posterior parietal and
    prefrontal cortex 76

Part 4 Motor systems
35 Organization of the motor systems 78
36 Muscle spindle and lower motor neurone 80
37 Spinal cord motor organization and locomotion 82
38 Cortical motor areas 84
39 Primary motor cortex 86
40 Cerebellum 88
41 Basal ganglia: anatomy and physiology 92
42 Basal ganglia diseases and their treatment 94

Part 5 Consciousness and higher brain function
43 Reticular formation and sleep 96
44 Consciousness and theory of mind 98
45 Limbic system and long-term potentiation 100
46 Memory 102
47 Emotion, motivation and drug addiction 104
48 Neural plasticity and neurotrophic factors I:
    the peripheral nervous system 106
49 Neural plasticity and neurotrophic factors II:
    the central nervous system 108

Part 6 Applied neurobiology: the principles of neurology and psychiatry
50 Approach to the patient with
    neurological problems 110
51 Examination of the nervous system 112
52 Investigation of the nervous system 114
53 Imaging of the central nervous system 116
54 Clinical disorders of the sensory systems 118
55 Clinical disorders of the motor system 120
56 Eye movements 122
57 Neurochemical disorders I: affective disorders 124
58 Neurochemical disorders II: schizophrenia 126
59 Neurochemical disorders III: anxiety 128
60 Neurodegenerative disorders 130
61 Neurophysiological disorders: epilepsy 132
62 Neuroimmunological disorders 134
63 Neurogenetic disorders 136
64 Cerebrovascular disease 138
65 Neuroradiological anatomy 140

Part 7 Self-assessment case studies
Case studies and questions 143
Answers 148

Index 153

A companion website is available for this book at: www.ataglanceseries.com/neuroscience

Introduction

Neuroanatomy and Neuroscience at a Glance is designed primarily for medical students as a revision text or review of basic neuroscience mechanisms, rather than a comprehensive account of the field of medical neuroscience. The book does not attempt to provide a systematic review of clinical neurology, although one of the new features of the fourth edition is the introduction of more clinical cases to illustrate how neurology builds on a good knowledge of basic neuroscience. In addition, the changing nature of medical training has meant that rather than teaching being discipline based (anatomy, physiology, pharmacology, etc.), the current approach is much more integrated with the focus on the entire system. Students pursuing a problem-based learning course will also benefit from the concise presentation of integrated material.

This book summarizes the rapidly expanding field of neuroscience with reference to clinical disorders, such that the material is set in a clinical context with the later chapters being more clinically oriented. However, learning about the organization of the nervous system purely from clinical disorders is short-sighted as the changing nature of medical neuroscience means that areas with little clinical relevance today may become more of an issue in the future. An example of this is ion channels and the recent burgeoning of a host of neurological disorders secondary to a channelopathy. For this reason, some chapters focus more on scientific mechanisms with less clinical emphasis.

Each chapter presents the bulk of its information in the form of an annotated figure, which is expanded in the accompanying text. It is recommended that the figure is worked through with the text rather than just viewed in isolation. The condensed nature of each chapter means that much of the information has to be given in a didactic fashion. Although the text focuses on core material, some additional important details are also included.

The book has been restructured beginning with the anatomical and functional organization of the nervous system (Chapters 1–11); the cells of the nervous system and how they work (Chapters 12–21); the sensory components of the nervous system (Chapters 22–34); the motor components of the nervous system (Chapters 35–42); the autonomic, limbic and brainstem systems underlying wakefulness and sleep along with neural plasticity (Chapters 43–49); and, finally, a section on the approach, investigation and range of clinical disorders of the nervous system (Chapters 50–65). We have included new chapters on the enteric nervous system, the major central nervous system (CNS) neurotransmitters and their function, language, stroke and the approach to the patients with a neurological problem.

Each section builds on the previous ones to some extent, and so reading the introductory chapter may give a greater understanding to later chapters in that section; for example, the somatosensory system chapter (Chapter 31) may be better read after the chapter on the general organization of sensory systems (Chapter 22).

In this latest edition of the book we have attempted to further integrate the clinical relevance of neurobiology into the text and website and brought in a new approach and author, Dr Francesca Cicchetti. This, coupled to the feedback we received from students, teachers and professors, accounts for the restructuring of the book and the addition of new chapters. We have also now included at the end of each chapter a 'Did you know?' section while Section 7 consists of relevant clinical scenarios for each chapter along with questions and answers. The companion website has key revision points and multiple choice questions relating to the content of each chapter.

We hope that you find this new book a useful accompaniment to your studies from undergraduate to post-graduate to clinical level.

Roger Barker
Cambridge
Francesca Cicchetti
Quebec

Acknowledgements

We would like to thank all the students that we have taught over the years who have helped us refine this book as well as the team at Wiley-Blackwell for all their help and innovative ideas in this new, more colourful edition of the book.

List of abbreviations

5-HIAA	5-hydroxy indole acetic acid	**EEG**	electroencephalography/electroencephalogram
5-HT	5-hydroxytryptamine (serotonin)	**EMG**	electromyography/electromyogram
A1	primary auditory cortex	**enk**	enkephalin
ACA	anterior cerebral artery	**ENS**	enteric nervous system
ACh	acetylcholine	**EP**	evoked potential
AChE	acetylcholinesterase	**epp**	end-plate potential
AChR	acetylcholine receptor	**EPSP**	excitatory postsynaptic potential
ACTH	adenocorticotrophic hormone	**FEF**	frontal eye field(s)
ADH	antidiuretic hormone (vasopressin)	**fMRI**	functional magnetic resonance imaging
ALS	amyotrophic lateral sclerosis	**FTD**	fronto-temporal dementia
AMPA-R	α-amino-3-hydroxy-5-methyl-4-isoxazole propionic acid glutamate receptor	**GABA**	γ-aminobutyric acid
		GABA-R	γ-aminobutyric acid receptor
ANS	autonomic nervous system	**GAD**	glutamic acid decarboxylase
APP	amyloid precursor protein	**GDNF**	glial cell line derived neurotrophic factor
ATP	adenosine triphosphate	**Glut-R**	glutamate receptor
AuD	autosomal dominant	**GoC**	Golgi cell
AuR	autosomal recessive	**Golf**	G-protein associated with olfactory receptors
BBB	blood–brain barrier	**GPe**	globus pallidus external segment
BM	basilar membrane	**GPi**	globus pallidus internal segment
BMP	bone morphogenic protein	**G-protein**	guanosine triphosphate-binding protein
cAMP	cyclic adenosine monophosphate	**GrC**	granule cell
CBM	cerebellum	**GTO**	Golgi tendon organ
CBP	calcium-binding protein	**GTP**	guanosine triphosphate
CCK	cholecystokinin	**HLA**	histocompatibility locus antigen
cf	climbing fibre	**HMM**	heavy meromyosin
cGMP	cyclic guanosine monophosphate	**HMSN**	hereditary motor sensory neuropathy
CMCT	central motor conduction time	**HTM**	high-threshold mechanoreceptor
CMUA	continuous motor unit activity	**Hz**	hertz
CNS	central nervous system	**IC**	inferior colliculus
CNTF	ciliary neurotrophic factor	**ICA**	internal carotid artery
COMT	catecholamine-*O*-methyltransferase	**IHC**	inner hair cell
CoST	corticospinal tract	**ILN**	intralaminar nuclei (of the thalamus)
COX	cyclo-oxygenase	**IN**	interneurone
CPG	central pattern generator	**IP3**	inositol triphosphate
CPK	creatine phosphokinase	**IPSP**	inhibitory postsynaptic potential
CRH	corticotrophin-releasing hormone	**JPS**	joint position sense
CRPS	complex regional pain syndrome	**LEMS**	Lambert–Eaton myasthenic syndrome
CSF	cerebrospinal fluid	**LGMD**	limb girdle muscular dystrophy
CT	computed tomography	**LGN**	lateral geniculate nucleus of the thalamus
CVA	cerebrovascular accident	**LMM**	light meromyosin
DA	dopamine	**LMN**	lower motor neurone
DAG	diacylglycerol	**LTD**	long-term depression
DAT	dementia of the Alzheimer type/dopamine transporter (scan)	**LTP**	long-term potentiation
		MAO	monoamine oxidase
dB	decibel	**MAO$_A$**	monoamine oxidase type A
DC	dorsal column	**MAO$_B$**	monoamine oxidase type B
DCN	dorsal column nuclei	**MAOI**	monoamine oxidase inhibitor
DCNN	deep cerebellar nuclei neurone	**MCA**	middle cerebral artery
DMD	Duchenne's muscular dystrophy	**MCS**	minimally conscious state
DNA	deoxyribonucleic acid	**MD**	mediodorsal nucleus of the thalamus
DRG	dorsal root ganglion	**mepp**	miniature end-plate potential
DSCT	dorsal spinocerebellar tract	**MGN**	medial geniculate nucleus of the thalamus
DSIP	delta sleep-inducing peptide	**MHC**	major histocompatibility complex
ECG	electrocardiography/electrocardiogram	**MLF**	medial longitudinal fasciculus
ECT	electroconvulsive therapy	**MN**	motor neurone

MND	motor neurone disease	**RuST**	rubrospinal tract
MRA	magnetic resonance angiography	**SA**	slowly adapting receptor
MRI	magnetic resonance imaging	**SCA**	spinocerebellar ataxia
MRV	magnetic resonance venography	**SMA**	supplementary motor area
MsI	primary motor cortex	**SmI**	primary somatosensory cortex
MUSK	muscle specific kinase	**SmII**	second somatosensory area
NA	noradrenaline (norepinephrine)	**SNAP**	soluble NSF attachment protein
NCS	nerve conduction studies	**SNARE**	SNAP receptor
NFT	neurofibrillary tangle	**SNc**	substantia nigra pars compacta
NGF	nerve growth factor	**SNP**	senile neuritic plaques
NMDA	N-methyl-D-aspartate	**SNr**	substantia nigra pars reticulata
NMDA-R	N-methyl-D-aspartate glutamate receptor	**SNS**	sympathetic nervous system
NMJ	neuromuscular junction	**SOC**	superior olivary complex
NO	nitric oxide	**SP**	substance P
NS	neostriatum	**SPECT**	single photon emission computed tomography
NSAID	non-steroidal anti-inflammatory drug	**SR**	sarcoplasmic reticulum
OD	ocular dominance	**SSRI**	selective serotonin reuptake inhibitor
OHC	outer hair cell	**STN**	subthalamic nucleus
PAG	periaqueductal grey matter	**STT**	spinothalamic tract
PCA	posterior cerebral artery	**SVZ**	subventricular zone
PDE	phosphodiesterase	**SWS**	slow-wave sleep
PET	positron emission tomography	**TENS**	transcutaneous nerve stimulation
pf	parallel fibre	**TeST**	tectospinal tract
PG	prostaglandin	**TIA**	transient ischaemic attack
PGO	pontine–geniculo-occipital	**TM**	tectorial membrane
PICA	posterior inferior cerebellar artery	**TNF**	tumour necrosis factor
PMC	premotor cortex	**TRH**	thyrotrophin-releasing hormone
PMN	polymodal nociceptors	**T-tubule**	transverse tubule
PMP	peripheral myelin protein	**UMN**	upper motor neurone
PNS	peripheral nervous system	**UPS**	ubiquitin–proteosome system
PPC	posterior parietal cortex	**V1**	primary visual cortex (Brodmann's area 17)
PPN	pedunculopontine nucleus	**VA–VL**	ventroanterior–ventrolateral nuclei of the thalamus
PPRF	paramedian pontine reticular formation	**VCN**	ventral cochlear nucleus
PuC	Purkinje cell	**VEP**	visual evoked potential
RA	rapidly adapting receptor	**VeST**	vestibulospinal tract
REM	rapid eye movement	**VLPA**	ventrolateral preoptic area
ReST	reticulospinal tract	**VOR**	vestibulo-ocular reflex
riMLF	rostral interstitial nucleus of the medial longitudinal fasciculus	**VP**	ventroposterior nucleus of the thalamus
RMS	rostral migratory stream	**VPL**	ventroposterior nucleus of the thalamus, lateral part
RN	raphé nucleus	**VPM**	ventroposterior nucleus of the thalamus, medial part
RNA	ribonucleic acid	**VPT**	vibration perception threshold
		VSCT	ventral spinocerebellar tract

1 Development of the nervous system

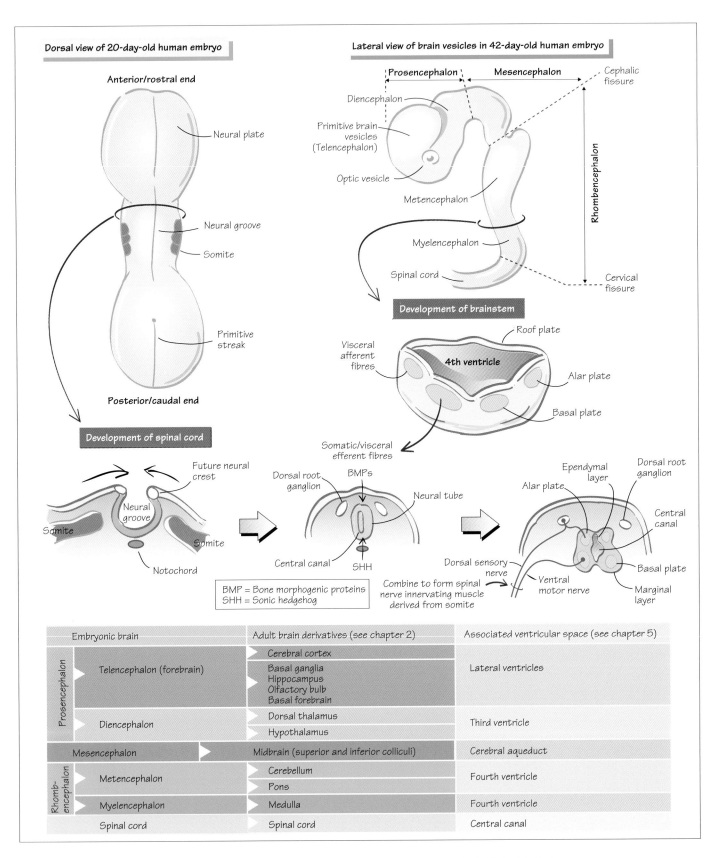

Embryonic brain		Adult brain derivatives (see chapter 2)	Associated ventricular space (see chapter 5)
Prosencephalon	Telencephalon (forebrain)	Cerebral cortex	Lateral ventricles
		Basal ganglia Hippocampus Olfactory bulb Basal forebrain	
	Diencephalon	Dorsal thalamus	Third ventricle
		Hypothalamus	
Mesencephalon		Midbrain (superior and inferior colliculi)	Cerebral aqueduct
Rhomb-encephalon	Metencephalon	Cerebellum	Fourth ventricle
		Pons	
	Myelencephalon	Medulla	Fourth ventricle
	Spinal cord	Spinal cord	Central canal

Neuroanatomy and Neuroscience at a Glance, Fourth Edition. Roger A. Barker, Francesca Cicchetti, Michael J. Neal.

The first signs of nervous system development occur in the third week of gestation, under the influence of secreted factors from the **notochord**, with the formation of a **neural plate** along the dorsal aspect of the embryo. This plate broadens, folds (forming the **neural groove**) and fuses to form the **neural tube**, which ultimately gives rise to the brain at its rostral (i.e. towards the head) end and the spinal cord caudally (i.e. towards the feet/tail end). The fusion begins approximately halfway along the neural groove at the level of the fourth somite and continues caudally and rostrally with the closure of the posterior/caudal and anterior/rostral neuropore during the fourth week of gestation.

The development of the spinal cord

The process of neural tube fusion isolates a group of cells termed the **neural crest**.
- The neural crest gives rise to a range of cells including the **dorsal root ganglia** (DRG) and peripheral components of the autonomic nervous system (ANS; see Chapter 3).
- The DRG contain the sensory cell bodies which send their developing axons into the evolving spinal cord and skin.
- These growing neuronal processes or neurites have an advancing **growth cone** that finds its appropriate target in the periphery and central nervous system (CNS), using a number of cues including cell adhesion molecules and diffusible neurotrophic factors (see Chapter 48).

The neural tube surrounds the neural canal, which forms the central canal of the fully developed spinal cord.
- The tube itself contains the neuroblasts (**ependymal layer**), which divide and migrate out to the **mantle layer**, where they differentiate into neurones to form the grey matter of the spinal cord (see Chapter 2).
- The developing processes from the neuroblasts/neurones grow out into the **marginal layer**, which therefore ultimately forms the white matter of the spinal cord.
- The dividing neuroblasts segregate into two discrete populations, the **alar** and **basal plates**, which in turn will create the dorsal and ventral horns of the spinal cord while a small lateral horn of visceral efferent neurones (part of the ANS) develops at their interface in the thoracic and upper lumbar cord (see Chapter 3).
- This dorso-ventral patterning relies, at least in part, on factors secreted dorsally (bone morphogenic proteins (BMPs)) or ventrally from the notochord (sonic hedgehog (SHH)).

The development of the brain
Adult neurogenesis
Until recently it was believed that no new neurones could be born in the adult mammalian brain. However, it is now clear that neural progenitor cells can be found in the adult CNS, including in humans. These cells are predominantly found in the dentate gyrus of the hippocampus (see Chapter 45) and just next to the lateral ventricles in the subventricular zone (SVZ). They may also exist at other sites of the adult CNS but this is contentious. They respond to a number of signals and appear to give rise to functional neurones in the hippocampus and olfactory bulb, with the latter cells migrating from the SVZ to the olfactory bulb via the rostral migratory stream (RMS). They may therefore fulfil a role in certain forms of memory and possibly in mediating the therapeutic effects of some drugs such as antidepressants (see Chapter 57).

Disorders of central nervous system embryogenesis
- *Anencephaly* occurs when there is failure of fusion of the anterior rostral neuropore. The cerebral vesicles fail to develop and thus there is no brain formation. The vast majority of fetuses with this abnormality are spontaneously aborted.
- *Spina bifida* refers to any defect at the lower end of the vertebral column and/or spinal cord. The most common form of spina bifida refers to a failure of fusion of the dorsal parts of the lower vertebrae (*spina bifida occulta*). This can be associated with defects in the meninges and neural tissue which may herniate through the defect to form a *meningocoele* and *meningomyelocoele*, respectively. The most serious form of spina bifida is when nervous tissue is directly exposed as a result of a failure in the proper fusion of the posterior/caudal neuropore. Spina bifida is often associated with hydrocephalus (see Chapter 5). Occasionally, bony defects are found at the base of the skull with the formation of a *meningocoele*. However, unlike the situation at the lower spinal cord, these can often be repaired without any neurological deficit being accrued.
- *Cortical dysplasia* refers to a spectrum of defects that are the result of the abnormal migration of developing cortical neurones. These defects are becoming increasingly recognized with improved imaging of the human CNS, and are now known to be an important cause of *epilepsy* (see Chapter 61).
- Many intrauterine infections (such as rubella), as well as some environmental agents (e.g. radiation), cause major problems in the development of the nervous system. In addition, a large number of rare genetic conditions are associated with defects of CNS development, but these lie beyond the scope of this book.

Did you know?

The adult human brain continues to make new nerve cells throughout life and that this can be promoted by a whole range of activities including exercising, learning new skills and, for example, socializing.

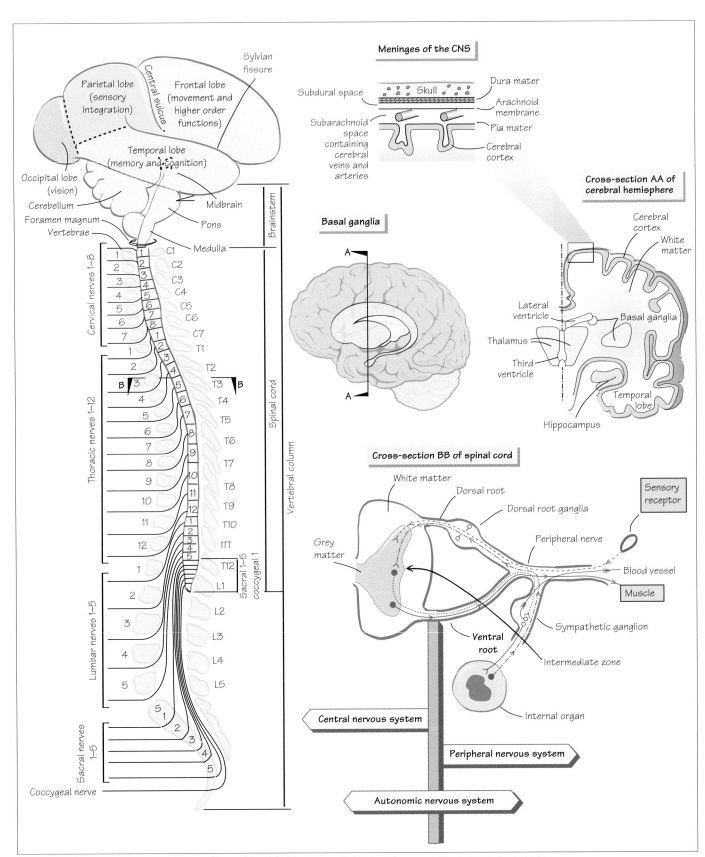

Neuroanatomy and Neuroscience at a Glance, Fourth Edition. Roger A. Barker, Francesca Cicchetti, Michael J. Neal.

12 © 2012 John Wiley & Sons, Ltd. Published 2012 by John Wiley & Sons, Ltd.

The nervous system can be divided into three major parts: the **autonomic** (ANS), **peripheral** (PNS) and **central** (CNS) **nervous systems**. The PNS is defined as those nerves that lie outside the brain, brainstem or spinal cord, while the CNS embraces those cells that lie within these structures.

Autonomic nervous system

• The **ANS** has both a central and peripheral component and is involved with the innervation of internal and glandular organs (see Chapter 3): it has an important role in the control of the endocrine and homoeostatic systems of the body (see Chapter 3, 11). The peripheral component of the ANS is defined in terms of the **enteric** (see Chapter 4), **sympathetic and parasympathetic systems** (see Chapter 3).

• The efferent fibres of the ANS originate either from the **intermediate zone** (or **lateral column**) of the spinal cord or specific cranial nerve and sacral nuclei, and synapse in a **ganglion**, the site of which is different for the sympathetic and parasympathetic systems. The afferent fibres from the organs innervated by the ANS pass via the dorsal root to the spinal cord.

Peripheral nervous system

• The PNS consists of nerve trunks made up of both afferent fibres or axons conducting sensory information to the spinal cord and brainstem, and efferent fibres transmitting impulses primarily to the muscles.

• Damage to an individual nerve leads to weakness of the muscles it innervates and sensory loss in the area from which it conveys sensory information.

• The peripheral nerves occasionally form a dense network or plexus adjacent to the spinal cord (e.g. brachial plexus in the upper limb).

• The peripheral nerves connect with the spinal cord through foramina between the bones (or **vertebrae**) of the spine (or **vertebral column**), or with the brain through foramina in the skull.

Spinal cord

• The **spinal cord** begins at the **foramen magnum**, which is the site at the base of the skull where the lower part of the brainstem (medulla) ends. The spinal cord terminates in the adult at the first lumbar vertebra, and gives rise to 30 pairs (or 31 if the coccygeal nerves are included) of spinal nerves, which exit the spinal cord between the vertebral bones of the spine.

• The first eight spinal nerves originate from the **cervical spinal cord** with the first pair exiting above the first cervical vertebra and the next 12 spinal nerves originate from the **thoracic or dorsal spinal cord**. The remaining 10 pairs of spinal nerves originate from the lower cord, five from the **lumbar** and five from the **sacral** regions.

• The spinal nerves consist of an **anterior or ventral root** that innervates the skeletal muscles, while the **posterior or dorsal root** carries sensation to the spinal cord from the skin that shared a common embryological origin with that part of the spinal cord (see Chapter 1). The dorsal root fibres have their cell bodies in the **dorsal root ganglia** which lie just outside the spinal canal.

• The spinal cord itself consists of **white matter**, which contains the nerve fibres that form the **ascending and descending pathways of the spinal cord**, while the **grey matter** is located in the centre of the spinal cord and contains the cell bodies of the neurones (see Chapter 9).

Brainstem, cranial nerves and cerebellum

• The spinal cord gives way to the **brainstem**, which lies at the base of the brain and is composed of the **medulla**, **pons** and **midbrain** (or mesencephalon as it is sometimes called, although this is strictly a term that should be reserved for this region of the brain in embryonic development) and contains discrete collections of neurones or nuclei for 10 of the 12 cranial nerves, the exceptions being the first (olfactory) and second (optic) nerves (see Chapter 7).

• The brainstem and the **cerebellum** constitute the structures of the posterior fossa.

• The cerebellum is connected to the brainstem via three pairs of cerebellar peduncles, and is involved in the coordination of movement (see Chapter 40).

Cerebral hemispheres

• The **cerebral hemispheres** are composed of **four major lobes**: **occipital**, **parietal**, **temporal** and **frontal**. On the medial part of the temporal lobe are a series of structures that form part of the limbic system (see Chapter 45).

• The outer layer of the cerebral hemisphere is termed the **cerebral cortex**, and contains neurones that are organized in both horizontal layers and vertical columns (see Chapter 10).

• The cerebral cortex is interconnected over long distances via pathways that run subcortically. These pathways, together with those that connect the cerebral cortex to the spinal cord, brainstem and nuclei deep within the cerebral hemisphere, constitute the **white matter of the cerebral hemisphere**. These deep nuclei include structures such as **basal ganglia** (see Chapters 41 and 42) and **thalamus** (Chapter 10).

Meninges

• The CNS is enclosed within the skull and vertebral column Separating these structures are a series of membranes referred to as the **meninges**.

• The **pia mater** is separated from the delicate **arachnoid membrane** by the subarachnoid space (containing the cerebrospinal fluid), which in turn is separated from the **dura mater** by the subdural space (see Chapter 5).

Did you know?

Each hemisphere has a series of dominant functions, which one dominates in you?

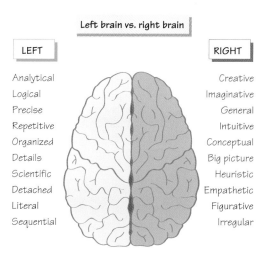

Left brain vs. right brain

LEFT	RIGHT
Analytical	Creative
Logical	Imaginative
Precise	General
Repetitive	Intuitive
Organized	Conceptual
Details	Big picture
Scientific	Heuristic
Detached	Empathetic
Literal	Figurative
Sequential	Irregular

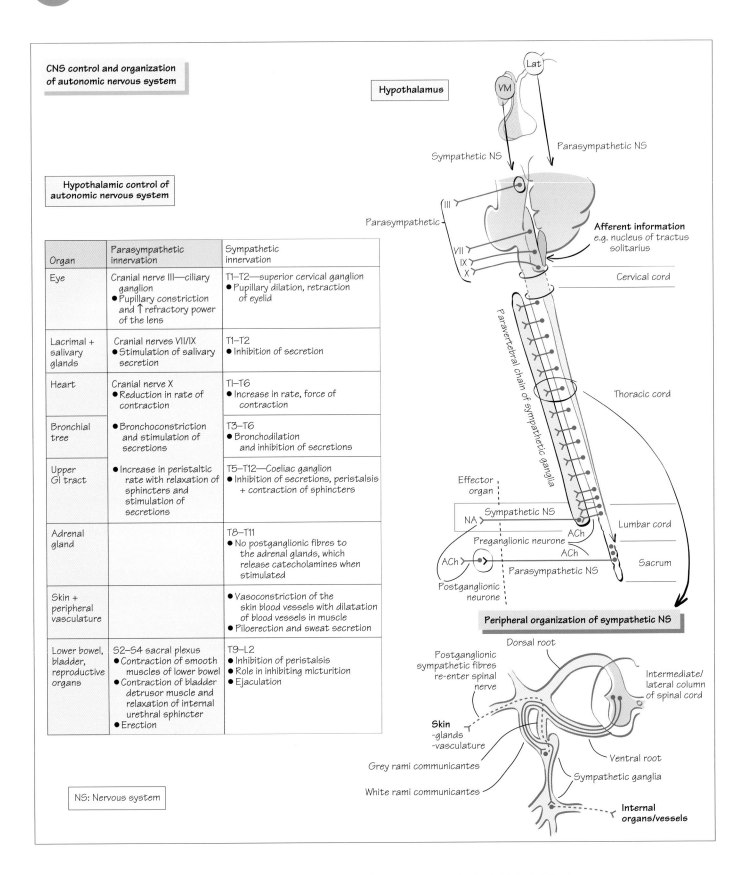

CNS control and organization of autonomic nervous system

Hypothalamus

Hypothalamic control of autonomic nervous system

Organ	Parasympathetic innervation	Sympathetic innervation
Eye	Cranial nerve III—ciliary ganglion • Pupillary constriction and ↑ refractory power of the lens	T1–T2—superior cervical ganglion • Pupillary dilation, retraction of eyelid
Lacrimal + salivary glands	Cranial nerves VII/IX • Stimulation of salivary secretion	T1–T2 • Inhibition of secretion
Heart	Cranial nerve X • Reduction in rate of contraction	TI–T6 • Increase in rate, force of contraction
Bronchial tree	• Bronchoconstriction and stimulation of secretions	T3–T6 • Bronchodilation and inhibition of secretions
Upper GI tract	• Increase in peristaltic rate with relaxation of sphincters and stimulation of secretions	T5–T12—Coeliac ganglion • Inhibition of secretions, peristalsis + contraction of sphincters
Adrenal gland		T8–T11 • No postganglionic fibres to the adrenal glands, which release catecholamines when stimulated
Skin + peripheral vasculature		• Vasoconstriction of the skin blood vessels with dilatation of blood vessels in muscle • Piloerection and sweat secretion
Lower bowel, bladder, reproductive organs	S2–S4 sacral plexus • Contraction of smooth muscles of lower bowel • Contraction of bladder detrusor muscle and relaxation of internal urethral sphincter • Erection	T9–L2 • Inhibition of peristalsis • Role in inhibiting micturition • Ejaculation

NS: Nervous system

Lat

VM

Sympathetic NS

Parasympathetic NS

Parasympathetic

III

VII
IX
X

Afferent information
e.g. nucleus of tractus solitarius

Cervical cord

Paravertebral chain of sympathetic ganglia

Thoracic cord

Effector organ

NA — Sympathetic NS

Lumbar cord

Preganglionic neurone

ACh

ACh

Sacrum

ACh

Postganglionic neurone

Parasympathetic NS

Peripheral organization of sympathetic NS

Dorsal root

Postganglionic sympathetic fibres re-enter spinal nerve

Intermediate/ lateral column of spinal cord

Skin
-glands
-vasculature

Ventral root

Grey rami communicantes

Sympathetic ganglia

White rami communicantes

Internal organs/vessels

Neuroanatomy and Neuroscience at a Glance, Fourth Edition. Roger A. Barker, Francesca Cicchetti, Michael J. Neal.

Anatomy of the autonomic nervous system

The **autonomic nervous system** (ANS) includes those nerve cells and fibres that innervate internal and glandular organs. They subserve the regulation of processes that usually are not under voluntary influence.

• The **efferent conducting pathway** from the central nervous system (CNS) to the innervated organ always consists of two succeeding neurones: a **preganglionic** and a **postganglionic**, with the former having its cell body in the CNS (see Chapter 2).

• The ANS is subdivided into the **enteric**, **sympathetic** and **parasympathetic nervous systems** – the latter two commonly exert opposing influences on the structure they are innervating.

• The sympathetic nervous system preganglionic neurones are found in the **intermediate part** (lateral horn) of the spinal cord from the upper thoracic to mid-lumbar cord (T1–L3).

• The preganglionic parasympathetic neurones have their cell bodies in the brainstem and sacrum.

• The postganglionic cell bodies are found in the vertebral and prevertebral ganglia in the sympathetic nervous system but in the parasympathetic system they are situated either adjacent to or in the walls of the organ they supply.

• In addition to anatomical differences the sympathetic nervous system uses **noradrenaline** (norepinephrine; NA) as its postganglionic transmitter while the parasympathetic nervous system uses **acetylcholine** (ACh). Both systems use ACh at the level of the ganglia.

Central nervous system control of the autonomic nervous system

The **CNS control of the ANS** is complex, involving a number of brainstem structures as well as the **hypothalamus** (see Chapter 11). The main hypothalamic areas involved in the control of the ANS are the **ventromedial hypothalamic** area in the case of the sympathetic nervous system and the **lateral hypothalamic area** in the case of the parasympathetic nervous system. Controlling pathways are direct or indirect via a number of brainstem structures such as the periaqueductal grey matter and parts of the reticular formation (see Chapter 8).

Clinical features of damage to the autonomic nervous system

Damage to the ANS can either be local to a given anatomical structure, or generalized when there is loss of the whole system caused by either a central or peripheral disease process.

• **Focal** peripheral lesions: These are not uncommon and the deficiencies resulting from these lesions can be easily predicted. For example, loss of the sympathetic innervation to the eye results in pupillary constriction (miosis), drooping of the upper eyelid (ptosis) and loss of sweating around the eye (anhydrosis) – a triad of signs known as *Horner's syndrome*. Other examples include the *reflex sympathetic dystrophies* where there is severe pain and autonomic changes confined to a single limb, often in response to some trivial injury. The exact role of the sympathetic nervous system in the genesis of these conditions is not known, as local sympathectomies are not always effective treatments. However, in some instances these treatments can help which may relate to the fact that the nociceptors can start expressing receptors for NA (see Chapters 32 and 33).

• More **global** damage to the ANS: This can occur because of degeneration of the central neurones either in isolation (e.g. *pure autonomic failure*) or as part of a more widespread degenerative process as is seen, for example, in *multiple-system atrophy*, where there may be additional cell loss in the basal ganglia and cerebellum. Alternatively, the autonomic failure may result from a loss of the peripheral neurones, e.g. in diabetes mellitus, certain forms of amyloidosis, alcoholism and *Guillain–Barré syndrome*. Finally, abnormalities in the ANS can be seen with certain toxins (e.g. botulism; see Chapter 16) as well as in *Lambert–Eaton myasthenic syndrome* (see Chapters 16 and 62).

In all these cases the patient presents with orthostatic and postprandial hypotension (syncopal or presyncopal symptoms on standing, exercising or eating a big meal) with a loss of variation in heart rate, bowel and bladder disturbances (urinary urgency, frequency and incontinence), impotence, loss of sweating and pupillary responses. The symptoms are often difficult to treat and a number of agents are used to try to improve the postural hypotension and sphincter abnormalities. Agents for postural hypotension include fludrocortisone, ephedrine, domperidone, midodrine and vasopressin analogues (all of which cause fluid retention).

Did you know?

Lie detectors reflect ANS responses.

4 Enteric nervous system

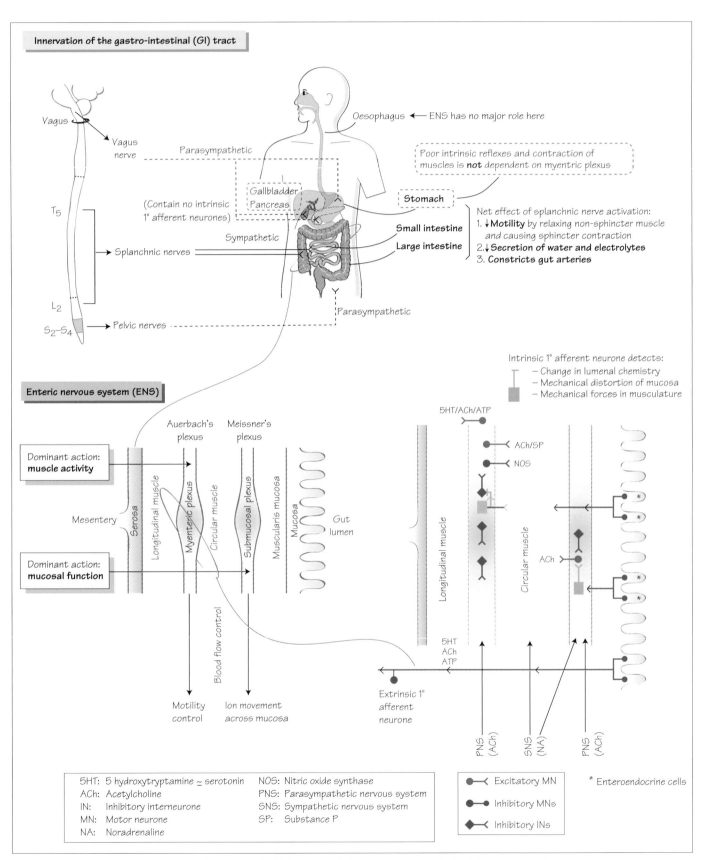

Innervation of the gastro-intestinal (GI) tract

Vagus

Vagus nerve

Parasympathetic

Oesophagus ← ENS has no major role here

Poor intrinsic reflexes and contraction of muscles is **not** dependent on myentric plexus

Gallbladder
Pancreas

(Contain no intrinsic 1° afferent neurones)

T_5

Sympathetic

Splanchnic nerves

Stomach

Small intestine
Large intestine

Net effect of splanchnic nerve activation:
1. ↓**Motility** by relaxing non-sphincter muscle and causing sphincter contraction
2. ↓**Secretion of water and electrolytes**
3. **Constricts gut arteries**

L_2

S_2–S_4 → Pelvic nerves

Parasympathetic

Intrinsic 1° afferent neurone detects:
– Change in lumenal chemistry
– Mechanical distortion of mucosa
– Mechanical forces in musculature

Enteric nervous system (ENS)

5HT/ACh/ATP

Auerbach's plexus

Meissner's plexus

ACh/SP

NOS

Dominant action: **muscle activity**

Serosa
Longitudinal muscle
Myenteric plexus
Circular muscle
Submucosal plexus
Muscularis mucosa
Mucosa

Gut lumen

Mesentery

Longitudinal muscle

Circular muscle

ACh

Dominant action: **mucosal function**

Blood flow control

Motility control

Ion movement across mucosa

5HT
ACh
ATP

Extrinsic 1° afferent neurone

PNS (ACh)

SNS (NA)

PNS (ACh)

* Enteroendocrine cells

5HT: 5 hydroxytryptamine ≈ serotonin
ACh: Acetylcholine
IN: Inhibitory interneurone
MN: Motor neurone
NA: Noradrenaline

NOS: Nitric oxide synthase
PNS: Parasympathetic nervous system
SNS: Sympathetic nervous system
SP: Substance P

○─< Excitatory MN
●─< Inhibitory MNs
◆─< Inhibitory INs

Neuroanatomy and Neuroscience at a Glance, Fourth Edition. Roger A. Barker, Francesca Cicchetti, Michael J. Neal.

Structure of the enteric nervous system

The enteric nervous system is found in the wall of the gut, primarily the small and large intestine, and is involved with normal gastrointestinal motility and secretory function. It contains about 100 million nerve cell bodies. It is heavily innervated/regulated by the autonomic nervous system but is a separate entity with its own intrinsic circuitry and function. It has no major role in the oesophagus and it is less clear what role it fulfils in the stomach.

The enteric nervous system consists of two plexuses:
• **myenteric plexus** or **Auerbach's plexus**, which lies between the longitudinal and circular muscle layers;
• **submucosal plexus** or **Meissner's plexus**, which lies between the circular muscle and muscularis mucosa.

The plexuses consist of:
• excitatory and some inhibitory motor neurones regulate muscle contraction;
• inhibitory interneurones integrate responses;
• intrinsic primary (1°) afferent neurones (IPAN) detect the chemical and mechanical state of the gut.

Multiple neurotransmitters and receptors are found in the different neuronal populations, the activities of which can therefore be modulated by a large number of drugs as well as by the ANS. Many of the neurones of the enteric nervous system contain more than one neurotransmitter.

Functions of the enteric nervous system

• The enteric nervous system can function in isolation to coordinate contraction of the gut musculature.
• It also regulates local food flow and the mucosal movement of ions/electrolytes.
• It allows for changes in local gut behaviour in response to local stimuli – both mechanical and chemical – and this may also rely on the release of substances from non-neuronal cells, e.g. 5-hydroxytryptamine (5HT)/adenosine triphosphate (ATP) from entero-endocrine cells.
• In addition there are ascending and descending neuronal networks that enable the sequential activation of muscles in the gut wall, which allows for the transport of luminal contents down the gut (peristalsis).

Disorders of the enteric nervous system

• *Congenital* or *developmental* abnormalities such as *Hirschsprung's disease* – in which there is a localized absence of enteric nervous system in the colon, causing constipation at birth, and which can only be cured by surgery to remove the atonic bit of bowel.
• *Sporadic* or *acquired* abnormalities, such as *irritable bowel syndrome* or chronic constipation as is seen in *Parkinson's disease*, (see Chapter 42) where it is due to local degeneration of intrinsic neurones.
• *Secondary* to a neuropathy from diabetes mellitus/*Guillain–Barré syndrome*.
• *Iatrogenic*, e.g. laxative abuse/opioid medication.

Did you know?

Many neuroscientists refer to the network of neurones lining the gut as the 'second brain', as these neurones are capable of generating "feelings" such as butterflies in your stomach when you are anxious.

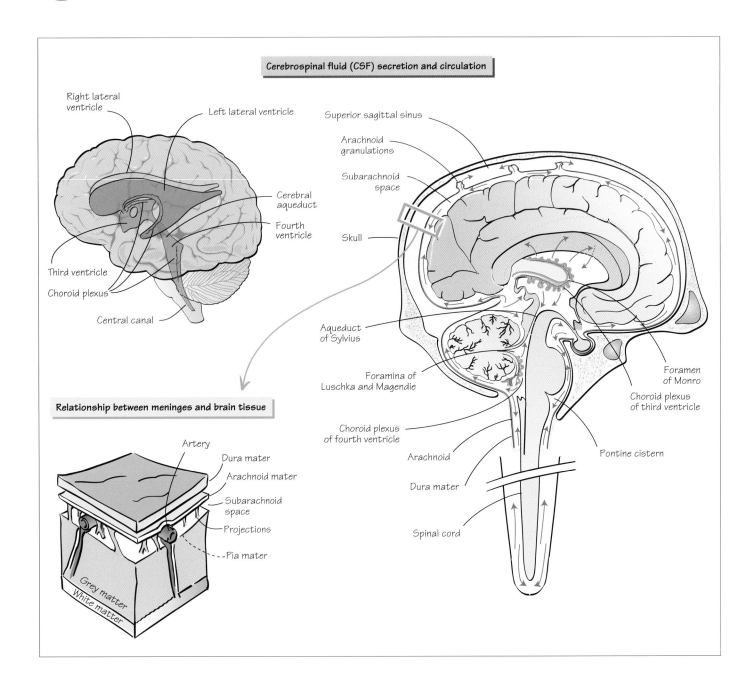

Cerebrospinal fluid (CSF) secretion and circulation

Right lateral ventricle
Left lateral ventricle
Cerebral aqueduct
Fourth ventricle
Third ventricle
Choroid plexus
Central canal

Superior sagittal sinus
Arachnoid granulations
Subarachnoid space
Skull
Aqueduct of Sylvius
Foramina of Luschka and Magendie
Choroid plexus of fourth ventricle
Arachnoid
Dura mater
Spinal cord
Foramen of Monro
Choroid plexus of third ventricle
Pontine cistern

Relationship between meninges and brain tissue

Artery
Dura mater
Arachnoid mater
Subarachnoid space
Projections
Pia mater
Grey matter
White matter

The brain is enclosed by three protective layers, which also extend down the spinal cord.
• The **dura mater** is a thick tough membrane lying close to the skull and vertebrae and innervated by afferent fibres of the trigeminal and upper cervical nerves.
• Adjacent to the dura mater is the **arachnoid mater**, a thin membrane with thread-like processes that project into the subarachnoid space and making contact with the delicate pia mater.
• The **pia mater** envelops the spinal cord and contours of the brain surface and dips into the sulci.

The **subarachnoid space** is filled with cerebrospinal fluid (CSF) and also accommodates major arteries, branches of which project down through the pia into the central nervous system (CNS). At specific sites the size of the subarachnoid space increases to form **cisterns**. These are particularly prevalent in the region of the brainstem and the largest is the **cisterna magna** found between the cerebellum and medulla.

The meninges extend caudally enclosing the spinal cord. Here the dura is attached to the foramen magnum at its upper limit and projects down to the second sacral vertebrae.

Neuroanatomy and Neuroscience at a Glance, Fourth Edition. Roger A. Barker, Francesca Cicchetti, Michael J. Neal.

Cerebrospinal fluid (CSF) production and circulation

• CSF is secreted by the **choroid plexuses**, which are found primarily in the ventricles.
• The rate of production varies between 300 and 500 mL/24 h and the ventricular volume is approximately 75 mL.
• CSF is similar to blood plasma although it contains less albumin and glucose.
• After production, CSF flows from the **lateral ventricles** into the **third ventricle** via the **intraventricular foramina of Monro** and then passes into the **fourth ventricle** through the **central aqueduct of Sylvius** and into the subarachnoid space via the **foramina of Luschka and Magendie**. From the subarachnoid space at the base of the brain, CSF flows rostrally over the cerebral hemispheres or down into the spinal cord.

CSF reabsorption occurs within the superior sagittal and related venous sinuses. Arachnoid **granulations** are minute pouches of the arachnoid membrane projecting through the dura into the venous sinuses. The exact mechanism by which CSF is reabsorbed is not clear but it does involve the movement of all CSF constituents into the venous blood. As well as playing an important part in maintaining a constant intracerebral chemical environment (see below), the CSF also helps protect the brain from mechanical damage by buffering the effects of impact.

Blood–brain barrier

The blood–brain barrier (BBB) used to be thought of as a single physical barrier preventing the passage of molecules and cells into the brain. More recently, however, it has been shown to be made up of a series of different transport systems for facilitating or restricting the movement of molecules across the blood–CSF interface. A characteristic of cerebral capillary endothelial cells is the presence of tight junctions between such cells, which are induced and maintained by astrocytic foot processes (see Chapter 13). These unusually tight junctions reduce opportunities for the movement of large molecules and cells, and thus require the existence of specific transport systems for the passage of certain critical molecules into the brain.

• Small molecules such as glucose pass readily into the CSF despite not being lipid soluble.
• Larger protein molecules do not enter the brain, but there are a number of carrier mechanisms that enable the transport of other sugars and some amino acids.

The rôle of the barrier is to maintain a constant intracerebral chemical environment and protect against osmotic challenges, while granting the CNS relative immunological privilege by preventing cells from entering it (see Chapter 62). However, from a therapeutic point of view the barrier reduces or prevents the delivery of many large-molecular-weight drugs (e.g. antibiotics) into the brain and represents a major problem in the treatment of many CNS disorders.

Clinical disorders
Hydrocephalus

Hydrocephalus is defined as dilatation of the ventricular system and so can be seen in cases of cerebral atrophy, e.g. dementia (compensatory hydrocephalus). However, hydrocephalus can also occur as a result of increased pressure within the ventricular system, secondary to an obstruction in the flow of CSF (obstructive hydrocephalus). This typically occurs at the outlets from the fourth ventricle into the subarachnoid space, where the obstruction may be linked to the presence of a tumour, congenital malformation or the sequelae of a previous infection (see below). Alternatively, the flow of CSF from the third to the fourth ventricle may be impaired as a result of the development of *central aqueduct stenosis*.

Hydrocephalus is also seen in rare conditions of oversecretion of CSF (e.g. tumours of the choroid plexus) as well as in the common situation of reduced absorption as is characteristically seen in *spina bifida*.

The *symptomatology* of hydrocephalus is varied but classically the patient presents with features of raised intracranial pressure (early morning headache, nausea, vomiting) and, in acute rises of pressure, altered levels of consciousness with brief periods of visual loss. Overall, probably the most common cause of raised intracranial pressure is a *glioma tumour* (see Chapter 13) producing these effects by virtue of its mass. Such tumours in the posterior fossa can also directly cause hydrocephalus, which may contribute to the raised intracranial pressure.

In *obstructive hydrocephalus* the treatment focuses on draining excess CSF using a variety of shunts linking the ventricles to either the heart (atrium) or the peritoneal cavity.

Meningitis

Meningitis or inflammation within the meningeal membrane can be caused by a number of different organisms. In acute infection there is the rapid spread of inflammation throughout the entire subarachnoid space of the brain and spinal cord, which produces the symptoms of headache, pyrexia, vomiting, neck stiffness (meningism) and, in severe forms of the disease, reduced levels of consciousness. The early administration of antibiotics is essential although the type of antibiotic employed will depend on the nature of the organism responsible for the inflammation.

In other cases the infection or inflammation may follow a more subacute course, such as *tuberculous meningitis* or *sarcoidosis*. In such cases, secondary hydrocephalus may ensue as a result of meningeal thickening at the base of the brain obstructing CSF flow.

Rarely, tumours can spread up the meninges giving a *malignant meningitis*. This characteristically presents as an evolving cranial nerve or nerve root syndrome with pain. This is to be distinguished from primary tumours of the meninges – *meningiomas* – which are slow growing and benign, and typically present with epileptic seizures or deficits secondary to compression of neighbouring CNS structures.

Did you know?

The CSF contains many important substances that can be measured and that could potentially be used as biomarkers for chronic neurodegenerative disorders of the brain, eg. A β and tau protein in Alzheimer's disease (Chapter 60).

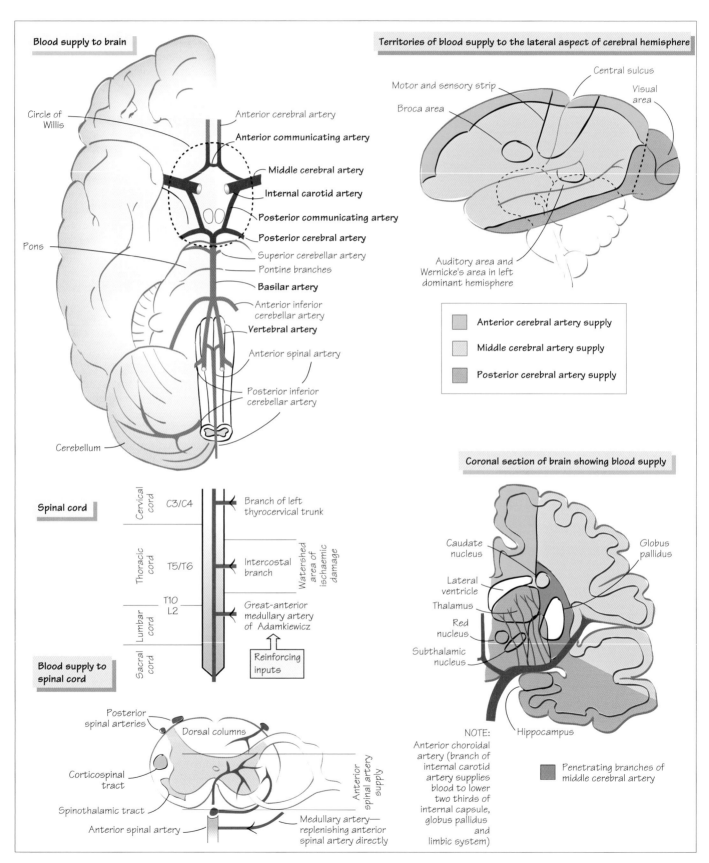

Blood supply to brain

Circle of Willis
Anterior cerebral artery
Anterior communicating artery
Middle cerebral artery
Internal carotid artery
Posterior communicating artery
Posterior cerebral artery
Superior cerebellar artery
Pontine branches
Basilar artery
Anterior inferior cerebellar artery
Vertebral artery
Anterior spinal artery
Posterior inferior cerebellar artery
Pons
Cerebellum

Territories of blood supply to the lateral aspect of cerebral hemisphere

Central sulcus
Motor and sensory strip
Visual area
Broca area
Auditory area and Wernicke's area in left dominant hemisphere

Anterior cerebral artery supply
Middle cerebral artery supply
Posterior cerebral artery supply

Spinal cord

Cervical cord — C3/C4 — Branch of left thyrocervical trunk
Thoracic cord — T5/T6 — Intercostal branch — Watershed area of ischaemic damage
Lumbar cord — T10 L2 — Great-anterior medullary artery of Adamkiewicz
Sacral cord

Reinforcing inputs

Blood supply to spinal cord

Posterior spinal arteries
Dorsal columns
Corticospinal tract
Anterior spinal artery supply
Spinothalamic tract
Anterior spinal artery
Medullary artery—replenishing anterior spinal artery directly

Coronal section of brain showing blood supply

Caudate nucleus
Globus pallidus
Lateral ventricle
Thalamus
Red nucleus
Subthalamic nucleus
Hippocampus

NOTE:
Anterior choroidal artery (branch of internal carotid artery supplies blood to lower two thirds of internal capsule, globus pallidus and limbic system)

Penetrating branches of middle cerebral artery

Neuroanatomy and Neuroscience at a Glance, Fourth Edition. Roger A. Barker, Francesca Cicchetti, Michael J. Neal.

20 © 2012 John Wiley & Sons, Ltd. Published 2012 by John Wiley & Sons, Ltd.

Blood supply to the brain

The arterial blood supply to the brain comes from four vessels: both the right and left internal carotid as well as the vertebral arteries.

• The **vertebral arteries** enter the skull through the foramen magnum and unite to supply blood to the brainstem (**basilar artery**) and posterior parts of the cerebral hemisphere (**posterior cerebral arteries**) – the whole network constituting the posterior circulation.

• The **internal carotid arteries (ICAs)** traverse the skull in the carotid canal and the cavernous sinus before piercing the dura and entering the middle cranial fossa just lateral to the optic chiasm. They then divide and supply blood to the anterior and middle parts of the cerebral hemispheres (**anterior [ACA] and middle [MCA] cerebral arteries**). In addition, the posterior and anterior cerebral circulations anastomose at the base of the brain in the **circle of Willis**, with the **anterior** and **posterior communicating arteries** offering the potential to maintain cerebral circulation in the event of a major arterial occlusion. The ICA prior to their terminal bifurcation supply branches to the pituitary (hypophysial arteries), the eye (ophthalmic artery), parts of the basal ganglia (globus pallidus) and limbic system (anterior choroidal artery) as well as providing the posterior communicating artery.

• The **MCA** forms one of the two terminal branches of the ICA and supplies the sensorimotor strip surrounding the central sulcus (with the exception of its medial extension which is supplied by the ACA) as well as the auditory and language cortical areas in the dominant (usually left) hemisphere. Therefore, *occlusion of the MCA* causes a contralateral paralysis that affects the lower part of the face and arm especially, with contralateral sensory loss or inattention and a loss of language if the dominant hemisphere is involved (see Chapters 28, 31, 34, 35, 38, and 39). In addition, there are a number of small penetrating branches of the MCA that supply subcortical structures such as the basal ganglia and internal capsule (see below).

• The two **ACAs**, which form the other major terminal vessels of the ICAs, are connected via the anterior communicating artery and supply blood to the medial portions of the frontal and parietal lobes as well as the corpus callosum. Occlusion of an ACA characteristically gives paresis of the contralateral leg with sensory loss, and on occasions deficits in gait and micturition accompanied with mental impairment and *dyspraxia* (see Chapter 34).

• The **vertebral arteries**, which arise from the subclavian artery, ascend to the brainstem via foramina in the transverse processes of the upper cervical vertebrae. At the level of the lower part of the pons the vertebral arteries unite to form the **basilar artery**, which then ascends before dividing into the two **posterior cerebral arteries (PCAs)** at the superior border of the pons. Each vertebral artery en route to forming the basilar artery gives off a number of branches including the posterior spinal artery, **the posterior inferior cerebellar artery (PICA)** and the **anterior spinal artery**. These spinal arteries supply the upper cervical cord (see below), whereas the PICA supplies the lateral part of the medulla and cerebellum.

Occlusion of this vessel gives rise to the *lateral medullary syndrome of Wallenberg*.

• The **PCAs** supply blood to the posterior parietal cortex, the occipital lobe and inferior parts of the temporal lobe. Occlusion of these vessels causes a visual field defect (usually a *homonymous hemianopia with macular sparing*, as this cortical area receives some supply from the MCA; see Chapter 25), amnesic syndromes (see Chapters 45 and 46), disorders of language (see Chapter 26) and, occasionally, complex visual perceptual abnormalities (see Chapter 28). The PCA has a number of central perforating or penetrating branches that supply the midbrain, thalamus, subthalamus, posterior internal capsule, optic radiation and cerebral peduncle, and these are commonly affected in hypertension, when occlusion of the PCA produces small **lacunar infarcts**.

Apart from occlusion, **haemorrhage** from cerebral vessels may involve the brain substance (intracerebral), the subarachnoid space or both. Such haemorrhages usually occur in the context of either trauma, hypertension or rupture of congenital aneurysms in the circle of Willis (*berry aneurysms*) (see Chapter 64).

Venous drainage of the brain

The brainstem and cerebellum directly drains into the dural venous sinuses adjacent to the posterior cranial fossa. The cerebral hemispheres, in contrast, have internal and external veins – the external cerebral veins drain the cortex and empty into the superior sagittal sinus (see Chapter 5). This sinus drains into the transverse sinus, then the lateral sinus, before emptying into the internal jugular vein. The internal cerebral veins drain the deep structures of the cerebral hemisphere to the great vein of Galen and thence into the straight sinus. Occlusion of either of these venous systems can occur, causing raised intracranial pressure with or without focal deficits.

Blood supply to the spinal cord

The blood supply to the spinal cord comes in the form of a **single anterior spinal artery** and paired **posterior spinal arteries**. The anterior spinal artery arises from the **vertebral arteries** and extends from the level of the lower brainstem to the tip of the conus medullaris. The posterior spinal arteries take their origin from the vertebral arteries. At certain sites along the spinal cord there are a number of reinforcing inputs from other arteries (see figure).

Vascular insults to the spinal cord occur most commonly at the watershed areas in the cord, namely the lower cervical and lower thoracic cord. Occlusion of the anterior spinal artery produces a loss of power and spinothalamic sensory deficit with preservation of the dorsal column sensory modalities (joint position sense and vibration perception; see Chapters 9 and 54).

Did you know?

There are over 100000 miles of blood vessels in your brain.

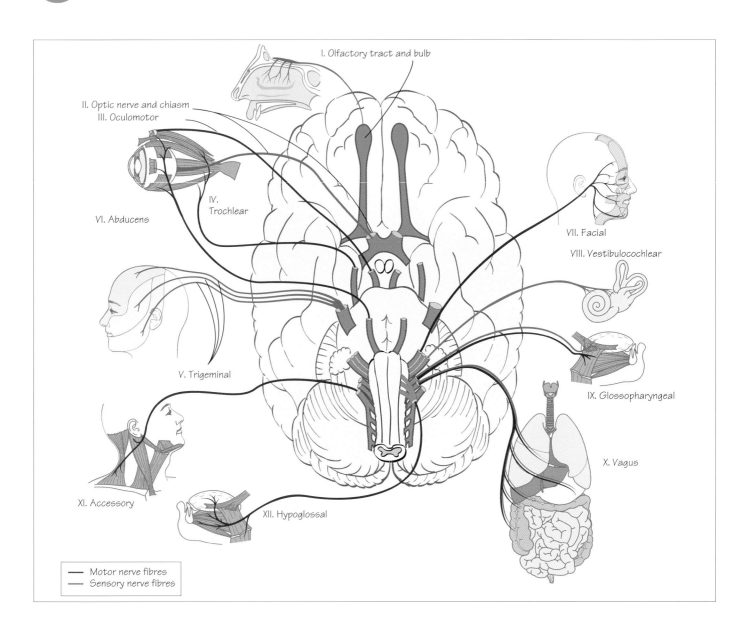

I. Olfactory tract and bulb

II. Optic nerve and chiasm
III. Oculomotor

IV. Trochlear

VI. Abducens

VII. Facial

VIII. Vestibulocochlear

V. Trigeminal

IX. Glossopharyngeal

XI. Accessory

XII. Hypoglossal

X. Vagus

— Motor nerve fibres
— Sensory nerve fibres

Olfactory nerve

The receptors for olfaction are found within the nasal mucosa, and their axons project through the cribriform plate to the olfactory bulb on the undersurface of the frontal lobe (see Chapter 30). This cranial nerve therefore does not originate or pass through the brainstem and conveys information on smell.

• Damage to this nerve occurs most commonly with head trauma and shearing of the olfactory axons as they pass through the cribriform plate causing *anosmia*.

Optic nerve

The photoreceptors in the eye project onto bipolar cells to ganglion cells and then to the CNS via the optic nerve. The nerve passes through the optic canal at the back of the orbit into the brain and unites with the optic nerve from the other eye to form the optic chiasm. The fibres from here pass ultimately to the visual cortex as well as to a number of subcortical sites (see Chapters 24–26).

• Damage to this nerve will affect vision, although the extent and type of this visual loss depends on the site of injury (see Chapter 25).

Oculomotor nerve

This originates in the midbrain at the level of the superior colliculus and supplies all the extraocular muscles apart from the lateral rectus, and superior oblique. It also carries the parasympathetic innervation to the eye and provides the major innervation of levator palpebrae superioris.

• A complete third nerve palsy causes the eye to lie 'down and out' with a fixed dilated unresponsive pupil and *ptosis* (droopy eyelid).

Neuroanatomy and Neuroscience at a Glance, Fourth Edition. Roger A. Barker, Francesca Cicchetti, Michael J. Neal.

Common causes of this are a ***posterior communicating artery aneurysm*** or a microvascular insult to the nerve itself as occurs in diabetes mellitus, for example.

Trochlear nerve

This nerve originates in the midbrain at the level of the inferior colliculus, and exits out of the brainstem dorsally. It supplies the superior oblique muscle.

• Damage to this nerve causes double vision (***diplopia***) when looking down. A common cause of fourth cranial nerve palsy is head trauma.

Fifth cranial or trigeminal nerve

The trigeminal nerve has both a motor and sensory function. The motor nucleus is situated at the mid-pontine level, medial to the main sensory nucleus of the trigeminal nerve, and receives an input from the motor cortex (see Chapter 38 and 39). It supplies the muscles of mastication. Sensation from the whole face (including the cornea) passes to the brainstem in the trigeminal nerve, and synapses in three major nuclear complexes: the nucleus of the spinal tract and the main sensory nucleus of the trigeminal nerve; and the mesencephalic nucleus. Sensation from the face is relayed via three branches: the ophthalmic division that supplies the forehead; the maxillary division that innervates the cheek; and the mandibular branch from the jaw – with the more rostral fibres (ophthalmic branch fibres) passing to the lowest part of the nucleus of the spinal tract in the upper cervical cord. These brainstem trigeminal nuclei in turn project to the thalamus as part of the somatosensory and pain systems (see Chapters 31 and 32).

• Damage to the trigeminal nerve results in weak jaw opening and chewing, coupled to facial sensory loss and an absent corneal reflex.

Sixth cranial or abducens nerve

This originates from the dorsal lower portion of the pons and supplies the lateral rectus muscle.

• Damage to this nerve results in horizontal ***diplopia*** when looking to the lesioned side and can be caused by local brainstem pathology or can be a false localizing sign in raised intracranial pressure.

Seventh cranial or facial nerve

This is predominantly a motor nerve, although it does carry parasympathetic fibres to the lacrimal and salivary glands (the greater superficial petrosal nerve and chorda tympani) as well as sensation from the anterior two-thirds of the tongue (the chorda tympani). The motor nucleus for the facial nerve originates in the pons, and supplies all the muscles of the face except for those involved in mastication.

• A lesion of this nerve produces a lower facial nerve palsy with weakness of all the facial muscles ipsilateral to the side of the lesion. In addition, there is a loss of taste on the anterior two-thirds of the tongue if the lesion occurs proximal to the origin of the chorda tympani. This is most commonly seen in ***Bell's palsy***. In contrast, damage to the descending motor input to the facial nucleus from the cortex (an upper motor neurone facial palsy) causes weakness of the lower part of the contralateral face only, as the musculature of the upper part of the face has upper motor neurone innervation from the motor cortex of both hemispheres.

Eighth cranial or vestibulocochlear nerve

This conveys information from the cochlea (the auditory or cochlear nerve; see Chapters 27 and 28) as well as the semicircular canals and otolith organs (the vestibular nerve; see Chapter 29).

• Damage to this nerve (e.g. in ***acoustic neuromas***) causes disturbances in balance with deafness and tinnitus (a ringing noise).

Ninth cranial or glossopharyngeal nerve

The glossopharyngeal nerve contains motor, sensory and parasympathetic fibres. The motor fibres originate from the rostral nucleus ambiguus and supply the stylopharyngeus muscle, while the sensory fibres synapse in the tractus solitarius (or nucleus of the solitary tract) and provide taste and sensation from the posterior tongue and pharynx. The parasympathetic fibres originate in the inferior salivatory nucleus and provide an input to the parotid gland.

• Damage to this nerve usually occurs in conjunction with the vagus nerve (see below).

Tenth cranial or vagus nerve

This nerve provides a motor input to the soft palate, pharynx and larynx, which originates in the dorsal motor nucleus of the vagus and nucleus ambiguus. It also has a minor sensory role, conveying taste from the epiglottis and sensation from the pinna, but has a significant parasympathetic role (see Chapter 3).

• Damage to the vagus nerve causes ***dysphagia*** and articulation disturbances and, as with glossopharyngeal nerve lesions, there may be a loss of the gag reflex.

Eleventh cranial or spinal accessory nerve

This is purely motor in nature and originates from the nucleus ambiguus in the medulla and the accessory nucleus in the upper cervical spinal cord. It supplies the sternocleidomastoid and trapezius muscles.

• Damage to the eleventh nerve causes weakness in these muscles.

Twelfth cranial or hypoglossal nerve

The hypoglossal nerve provides the motor innervation of the tongue. Its fibres originate from the hypoglossal nucleus in the posterior part of the medulla.

• Damage to this nerve causes wasting and weakness in the tongue, which leads to problems of swallowing and speech, and is most commonly seen in ***motor neurone disease*** (see Chapter 60). Isolated damage of this nerve is rare and it is more commonly affected with other lower cranial nerves (e.g. the ninth, tenth and eleventh cranial nerves) and in such cases the patient may present with a ***bulbar palsy***. A ***pseudobulbar palsy***, in contrast, refers to a loss of the descending cortical input to these cranial nerve nuclei.

Did you know?

Some people with damage to their facial nerve cry when they eat – these are called crocodile tears.

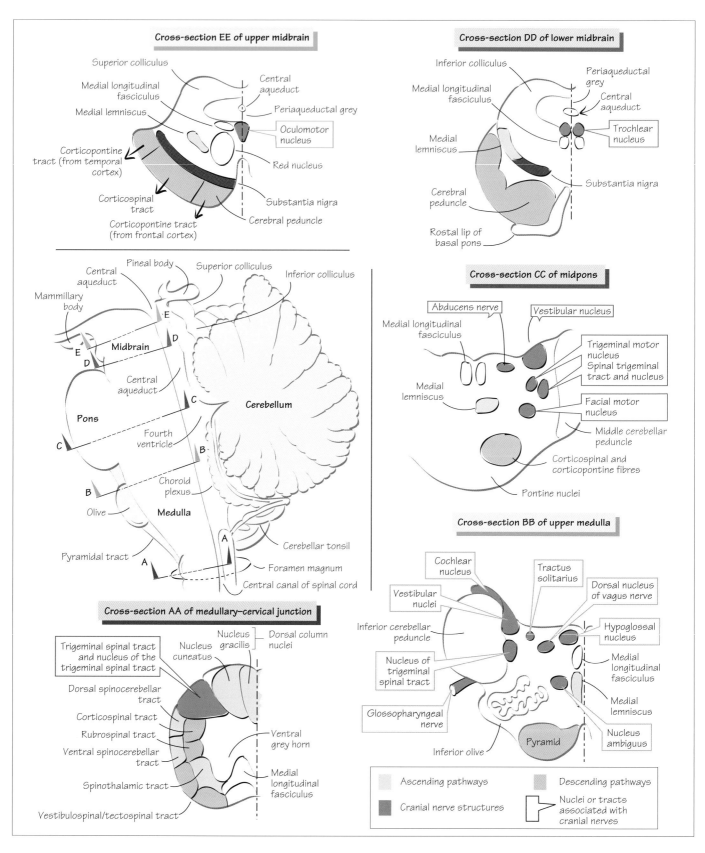

Neuroanatomy and Neuroscience at a Glance, Fourth Edition. Roger A. Barker, Francesca Cicchetti, Michael J. Neal.

The brainstem begins at the **foramen magnum** and extends to the cerebral peduncles and thalamus. It consists of the **medulla, pons** and **midbrain** and is located anterior to the cerebellum to which it is connected by three cerebellar peduncles. It contains the following:

• nuclei for 10 of the 12 pairs of **cranial nerves** (see Chapter 7), the exceptions being the olfactory and optic nerves;
• networks of neurones for controlling eye movements, which includes the third, fourth and sixth cranial nerves (see Chapter 56);
• monoaminergic nuclei that project widely throughout the central nervous system (see Chapter 18);
• areas that are vital in the control of respiration and the cardiovascular system, as well as the autonomic nervous system (see Chapter 3);
• areas important in the control of consciousness including sleep and associated monoaminergic nuclei (see Chapter 43);
• ascending and descending pathways linking the spinal cord to supraspinal structures, such as the cerebral cortex and cerebellum, some of which take their origin from the brainstem (see Chapters 9, 31, 32 and 35–39).

Important structures in the brainstem

• The **dorsal column nuclei** represent the primary site of termination of the fibres conveyed in the dorsal columns (DCs), responsible for light touch, vibration perception and joint position sense. The relay neurones in this structure send axons that decussate in the lower medulla to form the **medial lemniscus**, which synapses within the thalamus (see Chapter 31).
• The **pyramid** which represents the descending corticospinal tract (CoST) in the medulla, a pathway that decussates at the lower border of this structure.
• The **tractus solitarius** and **nucleus ambiguus** are associated with taste and the motor innervation of the pharynx by the glossopharyngeal and vagus nerves (see Chapter 7).
• The **inferior olive** in the medulla receives inputs from a number of sources and provides the climbing fibre input to the cerebellum (see Chapters 40 and 49).
• The **cerebellar peduncles** convey information to and from the cerebellum (see Chapter 40).
• The **medial longitudinal fasciculus** originates in the vestibular nucleus and projects rostrally connecting some of the oculomotor nuclei (third and sixth cranial nerves) as well as caudally to form part of the vestibulospinal tract.
• The **vestibular nucleus** has important connections from the balance organs within the inner ear and projects to the spinal cord

and cerebellum as well as other brainstem structures (see Chapters 20, 40 and 49).
• The **substantia nigra** in the midbrain contains both dopamine and γ-aminobutyric acid (GABA) neurones, forms part of the basal ganglia and is involved in the control of movement (see Chapters 41 and 42). The loss of its dopaminergic neurones is the major pathological event in Parkinson's disease (see Chapter 42).
• The **red nucleus** in the midbrain is intimately associated with the cerebellum, and is the site of origin for the rubrospinal tract which, with the CoST, forms the lateral descending pathway of motor control (see Chapter 37).
• The **periaqueductal grey matter** of the mesencephalon is an area rich in endogenous opioids and thus is important in the supraspinal modulation of nociception (see Chapter 32).
• The **central aqueduct of Sylvius** running through the midbrain connects the third to the fourth ventricle, and narrowing of it (stenosis) can cause hydrocephalus (see Chapter 5).
• The **cerebral peduncles** contain the descending motor pathways from the cerebral cortex to the spinal cord and brainstem, especially the pons (see Chapter 35).
• The **inferior colliculi** in the midbrain are part of the auditory system (see Chapter 28) while the **superior colliculi** are more involved with visual processing and eye movement control (see Chapters 25 and 56).

Thus, damage to the brainstem can have devastating consequences, although small lesions can often be localized with great accuracy because of the number of structures located within this small area of the brain. The most common causes of lesions in this part of the brain are either inflammatory (e.g. *multiple sclerosis*; see Chapter 62) or vascular in nature (see Chapter 64). However, disorders of the brainstem can also be seen with tumours (see Chapter 13) and a host of other conditions, and if damage is severe and extensive then it can be fatal.

Testing specifically for brainstem functions is undertaken to assess if an individual with extensive brain injury (e.g. massive stroke or head injury) is brain dead, which has implications for further interventional therapy and organ donation. This assessment involves looking at reflex eye movements to head movement, eye movement responses to stimulation of the vestibular system and spontaneous respiration.

Did you know?

It has been reported that brainstem damage can cause colourful, vivid hallucinations of small little people and animals.

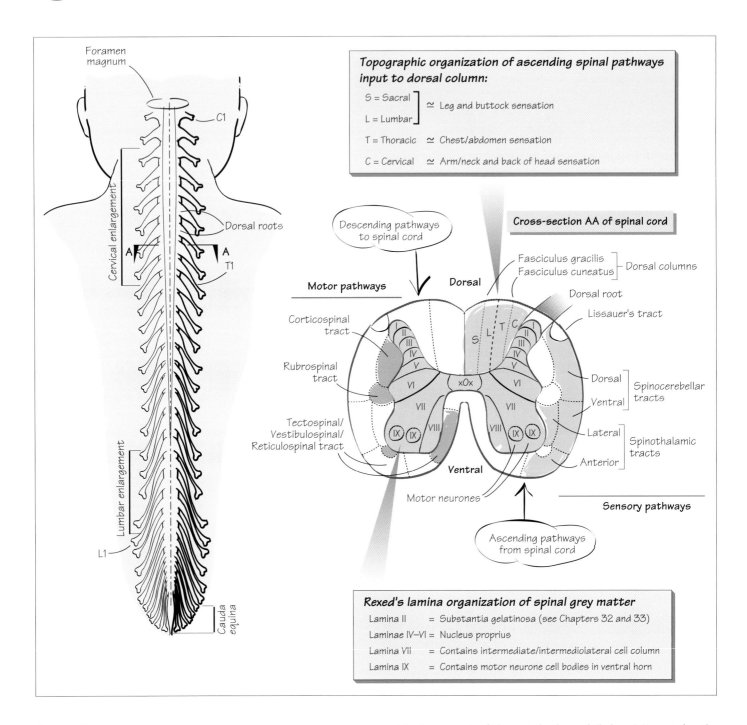

Topographic organization of ascending spinal pathways input to dorsal column:

S = Sacral ⎤
L = Lumbar ⎦ ≃ Leg and buttock sensation

T = Thoracic ≃ Chest/abdomen sensation

C = Cervical ≃ Arm/neck and back of head sensation

Cross-section AA of spinal cord

Rexed's lamina organization of spinal grey matter

Lamina II = Substantia gelatinosa (see Chapters 32 and 33)
Laminae IV–VI = Nucleus proprius
Lamina VII = Contains intermediate/intermediolateral cell column
Lamina IX = Contains motor neurone cell bodies in ventral horn

Overall structure

The spinal cord lies within the vertebral canal and extends from the foramen magnum to the lower border of the first lumbar vertebra.

• It is enlarged at two sites (cervical and lumbar regions) corresponding to the innervations of the upper and lower limbs (see Chapter 2).

• The lower part of the vertebral canal (below L1) contains the lower lumbar and sacral nerves and is known as the **cauda equina**.

Sensory nerve fibres enter the spinal cord via the **dorsal (posterior) roots** and their accompanying cell bodies are located in the dorsal root ganglia, while the motor and preganglionic autonomic fibres exit via the **ventral (or anterior) root**, together with some mostly unmyelinated afferent fibres.

Neuroanatomy and Neuroscience at a Glance, Fourth Edition. Roger A. Barker, Francesca Cicchetti, Michael J. Neal.

The **motor cell bodies (or motor neurones [MNs])** are found in the ventral horn of the spinal cord, while the preganglionic cell bodies of the sympathetic nervous system are found in the **intermediolateral column** of the spinal cord (see Chapter 3).

The neuronal cell bodies that make up the central grey matter of the cord are organized into a series of **laminae (of Rexed)**. The white matter surrounding this is composed of myelinated and unmyelinated axons constituting the ascending and descending spinal tracts.

Organization of sensory afferent fibres entering the spinal cord

Sensory information from the peripheral receptors is relayed by primary afferent nerve fibres which terminate in layers I–V of the **dorsal horn**, the site for termination being different for different receptors. However, in reality, many afferent fibres divide (into an ascending and a descending branch) as they enter the spinal cord so that synaptic contact can be made both with many interneurones in the dorsal horn, and up and down the cord through **Lissauer's tract**.

Sensory processing in the dorsal horn

• Typically, a number of primary afferents make synaptic contact with a single dorsal horn neurone.
• This **convergence** of input has the effect of reducing the acuity (accuracy) of stimulus location, but the process of **lateral inhibition** helps minimize this loss of acuity by promoting the inhibition of submaximally activated fibre inputs and thus increasing spatial contrast in the sensory input (see Chapter 22).
• The dorsal horn receives a number of descending inputs from supraspinal structures that are important in modulating the processing of sensory information through the spinal cord (see, for example, Chapter 32).

Ascending sensory pathways in spinal cord

The major ascending pathways of the spinal cord are (see also Chapter 22):
• spinothalamic tract (STT), also known as the anterolateral system;
• spinocerebellar tracts;
• dorsal columns (DCs; sometimes called the dorsal column-medial lemniscus system).

Each tract relays specific information in a topographical fashion, i.e. the sensory information from different parts of the body is conserved in the organization of the ascending pathways. Inputs from the more rostral parts of the body (arm as opposed to leg) supply fibres that lie more laterally in the ascending pathway.

Both the DC and STT **decussate** (fibres cross the midline) and therefore the sensory information they relay is ultimately processed in the **contralateral** cerebral hemisphere. However, the site at which this decussation occurs is different for the two pathways, with the anterolateral system crossing the midline in the spinal cord while the DCs decussate in the lower medulla after synapsing in the DC nuclei and forming the medial lemniscus (see Chapters 31 and 32).

Spinal motor neurones

• α- and γ-MNs are both found in the ventral (anterior) horn.
• The α-MNs are some the largest neurones found in the nervous system and innervate skeletal muscle fibres, while the γ-MNs innervate the intrafusal muscle fibres of the muscle spindle (see Chapter 36).
• The cervical cord MNs innervate the arm muscles while the lumbar and sacral MNs innervate the leg musculature.
• The MNs are arranged **somatotopically** across the ventral horn such that the more medially placed MNs innervate proximal muscles, while those located more laterally innervate distal muscles (see Chapter 35–37).

Descending motor tracts

There are a number of descending motor pathways that are defined by their site of origin within the brain (see Chapter 37):
• corticospinal (CoST) or pyramidal tract originates in the cerebral cortex;
• rubrospinal tract originates from the red nucleus in the midbrain and along with the CoST innervates the laterally placed MNs that supply the distal musculature;
• The vestibulospinal, reticulospinal and tectospinal tracts – known as the extrapyramidal tracts – innervate the more ventromedially placed MNs that control the axial musculature (see Chapters 35–37).

Clinical features of spinal cord damage (see Chapter 55)

A knowledge of the organizational anatomy of the spinal cord allows one to predict the pattern of deficits with damage, which is of great value in clinical neurology. Examples of specific spinal cord lesions and syndromes illustrating this point are discussed in Chapters 54 and 55.

Did you know?

Two million people worldwide live with a spinal cord injury.

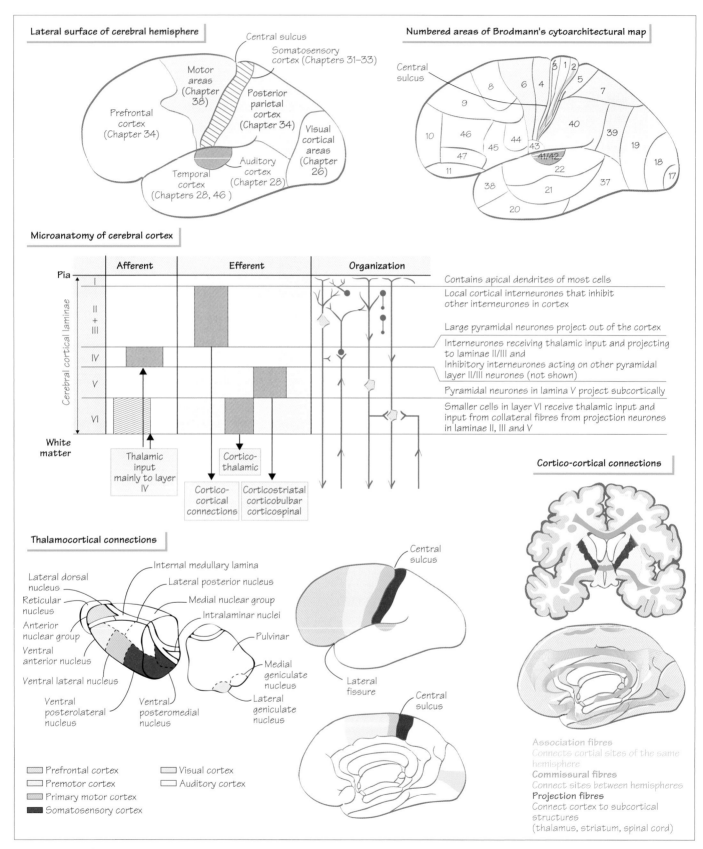

Lateral surface of cerebral hemisphere

Central sulcus

Somatosensory cortex (Chapters 31–33)

Motor areas (Chapter 38)

Posterior parietal cortex (Chapter 34)

Prefrontal cortex (Chapter 34)

Visual cortical areas (Chapter 26)

Temporal cortex (Chapters 28, 46)

Auditory cortex (Chapter 28)

Numbered areas of Brodmann's cytoarchitectural map

Central sulcus

Microanatomy of cerebral cortex

Pia

Cerebral cortical laminae

I, II + III, IV, V, VI

White matter

	Afferent	Efferent	Organization

Contains apical dendrites of most cells

Local cortical interneurones that inhibit other interneurones in cortex

Large pyramidal neurones project out of the cortex

Interneurones receiving thalamic input and projecting to laminae II/III and
Inhibitory interneurones acting on other pyramidal layer II/III neurones (not shown)

Pyramidal neurones in lamina V project subcortically

Smaller cells in layer VI receive thalamic input and input from collateral fibres from projection neurones in laminae II, III and V

Thalamic input mainly to layer IV

Cortico-thalamic

Cortico-cortical connections

Corticostriatal corticobulbar corticospinal

Cortico-cortical connections

Thalamocortical connections

Lateral dorsal nucleus
Reticular nucleus
Anterior nuclear group
Ventral anterior nucleus
Ventral lateral nucleus
Ventral posterolateral nucleus
Internal medullary lamina
Lateral posterior nucleus
Medial nuclear group
Intralaminar nuclei
Pulvinar
Medial geniculate nucleus
Ventral posteromedial nucleus
Lateral geniculate nucleus

Central sulcus
Lateral fissure
Central sulcus

Prefrontal cortex
Premotor cortex
Primary motor cortex
Somatosensory cortex
Visual cortex
Auditory cortex

Association fibres
Connects cortial sites of the same hemisphere
Commissural fibres
Connect sites between hemispheres
Projection fibres
Connect cortex to subcortical structures (thalamus, striatum, spinal cord)

Neuroanatomy and Neuroscience at a Glance, Fourth Edition. Roger A. Barker, Francesca Cicchetti, Michael J. Neal.

The organization of the outer layer of the **cerebral cortex** (neocortex) can be considered in various ways. One way uses cyto-architectural maps such as **Brodmann's areas** – which equates to some extent with the functional organization of this structure into motor, sensory and associative areas, as evidenced by the **laminar organization** of the cortex. An area of cortex that is predominantly *sensory* in character has a prominent layer IV, while cortical *motor* areas have a prominent layer V.

An alternative approach is to view the cortex as being organized vertically. This vertical organization has become known as the **columnar hypothesis** and proposes that the 'column' of cortex is the basic unit of cortical processing.

Anatomical organization of the cerebral cortex

The neocortex is classically described as consisting of six layers, although in certain areas of the cerebral cortex further subdivisions are used, e.g. the primary visual cortex (see Chapter 26).
• The thalamic afferent fibres, relaying sensory information, project to layer IV often with a smaller input to layer VI. They terminate in discrete patches.
• This input then synapses onto interneurones within the cortex which in turn project vertically to neurones in layers II, III and V, and from there project to other cortical and subcortical sites, respectively.

Thus, the weight of synaptic relations within the cerebral cortex is in the vertical direction. This arrangement of synaptic connections is well seen in the somatosensory and visual cortices (see Chapters 26 and 31). In many cortical areas with a motor function, the motor output from that cortical area is such that it is directed back at the motor neurones controlling the muscles that move the sensory receptors which ultimately project to that same area of cortex – so-called input–output coupling (see Chapter 39).

Developmental organization of the cerebral cortex

In the mammalian CNS the entire population of cortical neurones is produced by a process of migration from the proliferative zones that are situated around the cavities of the cerebral ventricles. The **radial glial fibres**, which guide and may even give rise to the migrating neurones, span the fetal cerebral wall and direct the neurones to their correct cortical location in the developing **cortical plate** from the **ventricular and subventricular zones** (see Chapter 1). Thus, developmentally, the cortex forms in a vertical fashion.

Neurophysiological organization of the cerebral cortex

Neurophysiologically, if a recording electrode is passed at right angles through the cortex, it encounters cells with similar properties. However, if the electrode is passed tangentially then cells shift their response characteristics. This has been shown in many cortical areas (eg. Chapter 26).

This columnar organization of the cortex ensures that topography can be maintained and that the reorganization of the cortex in the event of a change in the peripheral input is relatively straightforward (see Chapter 49).

Functional organization of the cerebral cortex
Serial processing models
The original models proposed that information processing was performed in a serial fashion, such that the cortical cells form a series of **hierarchal levels**. Thus, one set of cells performs a relatively straightforward analysis, which then converges on another population of neurones that perform a more complex analysis (see, for example, Chapter 26). The ultimate prediction of these hierarchical models is that one neurone at the top of the hierarchy will register the percept – the '**grandmother' cell**.
Parallel processing models
The discovery of the X, Y and W classes of ganglion cells in the retina (see Chapter 24) led to the development of a competing theory that proposed that information is analysed by a series of **parallel pathways**, with each pathway analysing one specific aspect of the sensory stimulus (e.g. colour or motion with visual stimuli; see Chapter 26). This theory does not exclude hierarchical processing but relegates it to the mode of analysis within separate parallel pathways. In practice, the cortex employs both modes of analysis.
Distributed processing models
It should be stressed that cortical columns are not to be viewed as a static mosaic structure, as one column may be a member of a number of different pathways of analysis. This organization has been termed the **distributed system theory** and describes the brain as a complex of widely and reciprocally interconnected systems, with the dynamic interplay of neural activity within and between these systems as the very essence of brain function. Consequently, one column may be a member of many distributed systems, because each distributed system is specific for one feature of a stimulus and one column may code for several features of the stimulus.

Anatomical and functional organization of the thalamus

The thalamus is made up of a number of discrete nuclei and is more than a simple relay station as it receives extensive connections from the cortex and brainstem structures and is also critically involved in levels of arousal. The main nuclei of the thalamus are:
• The anterior nucleus – which is associated with the limbic system and prefrontal cortex (Chapters 34 and 45).
• The ventroanterior and ventrolateral nuclei – which are associated with motor systems (see Chapters 38–41).
• The ventroposterior nuclei – which are associated with somatosensory systems (see Chapters 31 and 32).
• The pulvinar – which is associated with posterior parietal cortex (see Chapter 34).
• The medial geniculate nucleus – which is associated with the auditory pathways (see Chapter 28).
• The lateral geniculate nucleus – which is associated with the visual system (see Chapter 25).
• The intralaminar nuclei – which is associated with pain pathways and basal ganglia (see Chapters 33 and 41).
• The reticular nucleus – which is associated with levels of arousal and some forms of epilepsy (see Chapters 43 and 44).

Did you know?

Korbinian Brodmann was the first to define the distinct cortical areas back in 1909. He proposed 50 distinct areas with the last one called Area 52!

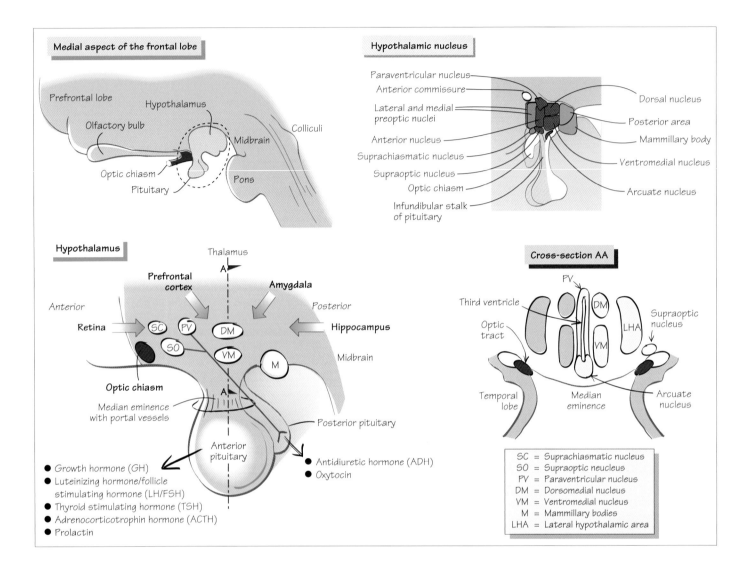

Medial aspect of the frontal lobe

Prefrontal lobe
Hypothalamus
Olfactory bulb
Colliculi
Midbrain
Optic chiasm
Pons
Pituitary

Hypothalamic nucleus

Paraventricular nucleus
Anterior commissure
Lateral and medial preoptic nuclei
Anterior nucleus
Suprachiasmatic nucleus
Supraoptic nucleus
Optic chiasm
Infundibular stalk of pituitary
Dorsal nucleus
Posterior area
Mammillary body
Ventromedial nucleus
Arcuate nucleus

Hypothalamus

Thalamus
Prefrontal cortex
Amygdala
Anterior
Posterior
Retina
Hippocampus
SC PV DM
SO VM
M
Midbrain
Optic chiasm
Median eminence with portal vessels
Anterior pituitary
Posterior pituitary

- Growth hormone (GH)
- Luteinizing hormone/follicle stimulating hormone (LH/FSH)
- Thyroid stimulating hormone (TSH)
- Adrenocorticotrophin hormone (ACTH)
- Prolactin

- Antidiuretic hormone (ADH)
- Oxytocin

Cross-section AA

PV
DM
Third ventricle
Optic tract
LHA
Supraoptic nucleus
VM
Temporal lobe
Median eminence
Arcuate nucleus

SC = Suprachiasmatic nucleus
SO = Supraoptic neuclus
PV = Paraventricular nucleus
DM = Dorsomedial nucleus
VM = Ventromedial nucleus
M = Mammillary bodies
LHA = Lateral hypothalamic area

The hypothalamus lies on either side of the third ventricle, below the thalamus and between the optic chiasm and the midbrain. It receives a significant input from limbic system structures (see Chapter 45) as well as from the retina. It contains a large number of neurones that are sensitive to changes in hormone levels, electrolytes and temperature.

It has an efferent output to the autonomic nervous system (ANS), as well as a critical role in the control of pituitary endocrine function (a detailed discussion on the endocrinology of the hypothalamic–pituitary system is beyond the scope of this book). Thus, the hypothalamus, while being important in the control of the ANS, has a much greater role in the homoeostasis of many physiological systems (e.g. thirst, hunger, sodium and water balance, temperature regulation), the control of circadian and endocrine functions, the ability to form anterograde memories (in conjunction with the limbic system; see Chapters 45 and 46) and the translation of the response to emotional stimuli into endocrinological and autonomic responses.

The hypothalamus performs a number of other functions, all of which can be lost or deranged in the disease state. The most common cause is as a side-effect of surgical removal of *pituitary tumours*.

Functions of the hypothalamus

- The hypothalamus controls the ANS and damage to it can cause autonomic instability. The **ventromedial part** of the hypothalamus has a major role in controlling the sympathetic nervous system while the **lateral hypothalamic area** controls the parasympathetic nervous system (see Chapter 3).

Neuroanatomy and Neuroscience at a Glance, Fourth Edition. Roger A. Barker, Francesca Cicchetti, Michael J. Neal.

• It controls the endocrine functions of the pituitary by the production of releasing and inhibiting hormones as well as producing antidiuretic hormone (ADH, also known as vasopressin) and oxytocin. Hypothalamic damage can have profound systemic effects because of the endocrinological disturbances associated with it, of which perhaps the most common example is neurogenic *diabetes insipidus*, in which there is a loss of the production of ADH from the hypothalamus. In this condition the patient passes many litres of urine each day, which needs to be compensated for by increased fluid intake. This is to be distinguished from nephrogenic diabetes insipidus, where the problem lies within the ADH receptor in the kidney.

• It has a major role in coordinating autonomic and endocrinological responses, both under physiological conditions, and in the expression of emotional states as coded for by the limbic system. In cases of hypovolaemia or extreme anxiety, for example, the hypothalamus mediates not only increased sympathetic activity, but also enhanced cortisol production via the stimulated release of adrenocorticotrophic hormone (ACTH) from the anterior pituitary. This is termed the stress response, which is defined by the rise in cortisol.

• It has an important role in thermoregulation. Lesions to the **anterior hypothalamic area** cause hyperthermia, while stimulation of this same area lowers body temperature via the ANS, in contrast to the **posterior hypothalamic area**, which behaves in an opposite fashion. It may also mediate some of the more long-term responses seen with prolonged changes in ambient temperature, such as increased thyrotrophin-releasing hormone (TRH) production in patients exposed to a chronically cold environment. Damage to the hypothalamus can lead to profound changes in the central control of temperature. In septic states, the production of some cytokines (e.g. interleukin-1) may reset the thermostat in the hypothalamus to a higher than normal temperature, accounting for the paradoxical situation of a fever with physiological evidence of mechanisms designed to conserve or generate heat (e.g. shivering).

• It has a role in the control of feeding. In simple terms, the ventromedial hypothalamus is often called the satiety centre, in that damage to it causes excessive eating (hyperphagia) and weight gain, while damage to the lateral hypothalamic (or hunger) area produces aphagia (no eating at all). The control of these centres involves a number of hormones, including insulin and the more recently described leptins.

• It has a role in the control of thirst and water balance by virtue of its osmoreceptors; the afferent input from a host of peripheral sensory receptors (e.g. atrial stretch receptors in the heart, arterial baroreceptors); the activation of hypothalamic hormone receptors (e.g. angiotensin II receptors); and its efferent output via the ANS to the heart and kidney as well as the production of ADH.

• It has a role in the control of circadian rhythms via the retinal input to the **suprachiasmatic nucleus**. This nucleus appears to be critical in setting the circadian rhythm as lesion and transplant experiments have shown. Although the exact mechanism by which these rhythms are mediated is not known, it may involve the production of melatonin by the pineal gland.

• It has a role with the limbic system in memory. Damage to the **mammillary bodies**, which receive a significant input from the hippocampal complex as occurs in chronic alcoholism with thiamine deficiency, produces a profound amnesia (*Korsakoff's syndrome*) of both an anterograde (inability to lay down new memories) and retrograde (inability to recover old memories) nature. The latter feature distinguishes these patients from those who have hippocampal damage (see Chapters 45 and 46) and may explain why patients with Korsakoff's syndrome tend to invent missing information (confabulation).

• The hypothalamus may also have a role in sexual and emotional behaviour independent of its endocrinological influences.

Did you know?

The hypothalamus is not only different in men and women but has been said to differ in homo- and heterosexual individuals.

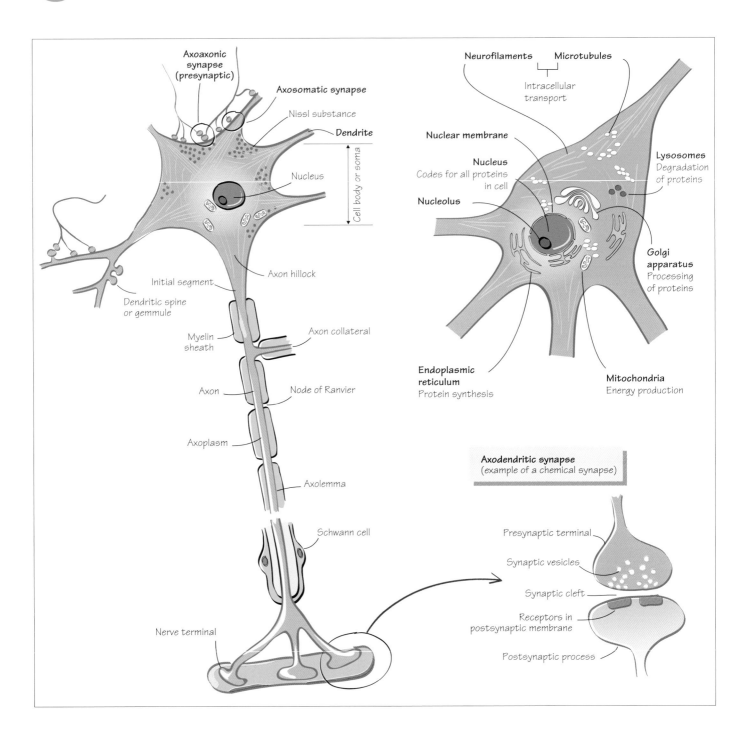

There are two major classes of cells in the nervous system: the neuroglial cells and neurones, with the latter making up only 10–20% of the whole population. The neurones are specialized for excitation and nerve impulse conduction (see Chapters 14, 15 and 17), and communicate with each other by means of the synapse (see Chapter 16) and so act as the structural and functional unit of the nervous system.

Neurones

The **cell body (soma)** is that part of the neurone containing the nucleus and surrounding cytoplasm. It is the focus of cellular metabolism, and houses most of the neurone's intracellular organelles (**mitochondria**, **Golgi apparatus** and peroxisomes). It is typically associated with two types of neuronal processes: the **axon** and **dendrites**. Most neurones also contain basophilic staining,

Neuroanatomy and Neuroscience at a Glance, Fourth Edition. Roger A. Barker, Francesca Cicchetti, Michael J. Neal.

termed **Nissl substance**, which is composed of granular endoplasmic reticulum and ribosomes and is responsible for protein synthesis. This is located within the cell body and dendritic processes but is absent from the **axon hillock** and axon itself, for reasons that are not clear. In addition, throughout the cell body and processes are **neurofilaments** which are important in maintaining the architecture or cytoskeleton of the neurone. Furthermore, two other fibrillary structures within the neurone are important in this respect: microtubules and microfilaments, structures that are also important for axoplasmic flow (see below) and axonal growth.

The **dendrites** are neuronal cell processes that taper from the soma outwards, branch profusely and are responsible for conveying information towards the soma from **synapses** on the dendritic tree (**axodendritic synapses**; see also Chapter 17). Most neurones have many dendrites (**multipolar neurones**) and while some inputs synapse directly onto the dendrite, some do so via small **dendritic spines or gemmules**. Thus, the primary role of dendrites is to increase the surface area for synapse formation allowing integration of a large number of inputs that are relayed to the cell body.

In contrast, the **axon**, of which there is only one per neurone, conducts information away from the soma towards the **nerve terminal** and synapses (see Chapter 15). Although there is only one axon per neurone, it can branch to give several processes. This branching occurs close to the soma in the case of sensory neurones (**pseudo-unipolar** neurones; see Chapter 31), but more typically occurs close to the synaptic target of the axon. The axon originates from the soma at the **axon hillock** where the **initial segment** of the axon emerges. This is the most excitable part of a neurone because of its high density of sodium channels, and so is the site of initiation of the action potential (see Chapter 15). All neurones are bounded by a lipid bilayer (**cell membrane**) within which proteins are located, some of which form ion channels (see Chapter 14); others form receptors to specific chemicals that are released by neurones (see Chapters 18 and 19) and others act as ion pumps moving ions across the membrane against their electrochemical gradient, e.g. Na^+–K^+ exchange pump (see Chapter 15).

The axonal surface membrane is known as the **axolemma** and the cytoplasm contained within it, the **axoplasm**. The ion channels within the axolemma imbue the axon with its ability to conduct action potentials while the axoplasm contains neurofilaments, microtubules and mitochondria. These latter organelles are not only responsible for maintaining the ionic gradients necessary for action potential production, but also allow for the transport and recycling of proteins away from (and to a lesser extent towards) the soma to the nerve terminal. This **axoplasmic flow or axonal transport** is either slow (~1 mm/day) or fast (~100–400 mm/day) and is not only important in permitting normal neuronal/synaptic activity but may also be important for neuronal survival and development and as such may be abnormal in some neurodegenerative disorders

such as motor neurone disease as well as disorders associated with abnormalities of certain proteins such as tau (see Chapter 60).

Many axons are surrounded by a layer of lipid, or **myelin sheath**, which acts as an electrical insulator. This myelin sheath alters the conducting properties of the axon, and allows for rapid action potential propagation without a loss of signal integrity (see Chapter 15). This is achieved by means of gaps, or **nodes (of Ranvier)**, in the myelin sheath where the axolemma contains many ion channels (typically Na^+ channels) which are directly exposed to the tissue fluid. The nodes of Ranvier are also those sites from which axonal branches originate, and these branches are termed **axon collaterals**. The myelin sheath encompasses the axon just beyond the initial segment and finishes just prior to its terminal arborization. The myelin sheath is formed by **Schwann cells** in the PNS and by **oligodendrocytes** in the central nervous system (CNS) (see Chapter 13), with many CNS axons being ensheathed by a single oligodendrocyte while in the PNS, one Schwann cell provides myelin for one internode.

Synapses

The **synapse** is the junction where a neurone meets another cell, which in the case of the CNS is another neurone. In the PNS the target can be muscle, glandular cells or other organs. The typical synapse in the nervous system is a **chemical** one, which is composed of a **presynaptic nerve terminal (bouton or end-bulb)**, and a **synaptic cleft**, which physically separates the nerve terminal from the **postsynaptic membrane** and across which the chemical or neurotransmitter from the presynaptic terminal must diffuse (see Chapter 16). This synapse is typically between an axon of one neurone and the dendrite of another (**axodendritic synapse**) although synapses are found where the point of contact between the axon and the postsynaptic cell is either at the level of the cell body (**axosomatic synapses**) or, less frequently, the presynaptic nerve terminal (**axoaxonic synapse**; see Chapter 17). A few synapses within the CNS do not possess these features but are low-resistance junctions (gap junctions) and are termed **electrical synapses**. These synapses allow for rapid conduction of action potentials without any integration and as such tend to enable populations of cells to fire together or in synchrony (see Chapters 16 and 61). They may also be important in the coupling of activity across cortical areas which may be important in some of the synchronized responses seen in the brain in sleep-wakefulness (see Chapters 43 and 44).

The specific loss of neurones is seen in a number of neurological disorders, and those diseases in which this is the primary event are discussed in Chapter 60.

Did you know?

The adult human brain contains 100 billion nerve cells.

13 Cells of the nervous system II: neuroglial cells

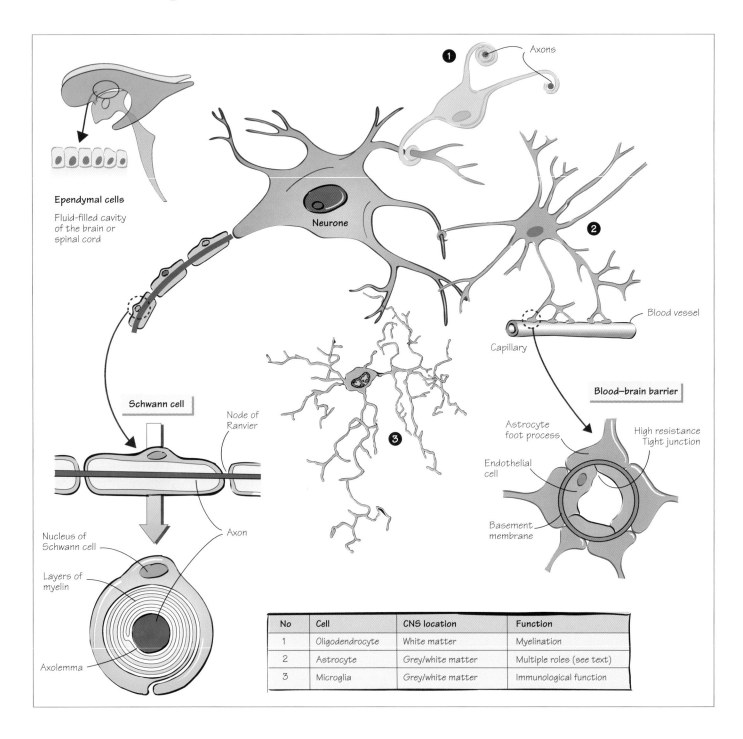

No	Cell	CNS location	Function
1	Oligodendrocyte	White matter	Myelination
2	Astrocyte	Grey/white matter	Multiple roles (see text)
3	Microglia	Grey/white matter	Immunological function

There are four main classes of neuroglial cells within the central nervous system (CNS): oligodendrocytes, astrocytes, microglia and ependymal cells, all of which have different functions. In contrast, in the peripheral nervous system (PNS), Schwann cells are the glial cells involved in myelination and facilitating axonal regeneration.

Astrocytes are small stellate cells that are found throughout the CNS and classified either morphologically or ontogenetically. They have many important functions within the CNS and are not simply passive support elements.
• They form a structural and supporting framework for neuronal cells and capillaries by virtue of their cytoplasmic processes, which

Neuroanatomy and Neuroscience at a Glance, Fourth Edition. Roger A. Barker, Francesca Cicchetti, Michael J. Neal.

end in close apposition not only to neurones but also to capillaries. In this respect they form the glia limitans – where the astrocytic foot processes cover the basal laminae around blood vessels and at the pia mater.

• They maintain the integrity of the **blood–brain barrier** (**BBB**), by promoting the formation of high-resistance junctions between brain capillary endothelial cells (see Chapter 5).

• They are capable of taking up, storing and releasing some neurotransmitters (e.g. glutamate, γ-aminobutyric acid [GABA]) and thus may be an important adjunct in chemical neurotransmission within the CNS.

• They can remove and disperse excessive ion concentration in the extracellular fluid, especially K^+.

• They participate in neuronal guidance during development (see Chapter 1), and may be involved in the response to injury (see Chapter 49), and adult neurogenesis.

• They may have a role in presenting antigen to the immune system in situations where the CNS and BBB are damaged (see Chapter 62).

• The most common clinical disorder involving astrocytes is their abnormal proliferation in tumours called *astrocytomas*. These tumours produce effects by compressing adjacent CNS tissue and this presents as an evolving neurological deficit (with or without epileptic seizures) depending on its site of origin. In adults, the tumours most commonly arise in the white matter of the cerebral hemispheres.

Microglial cells are the macrophages of the brain, and are found throughout the white and grey matter of the CNS. They are phagocytic in nature and are important in mediating immune responses within the CNS (see Chapter 62). They have a role in inflammation seen in some neurodegenerative disorders of the CNS, such as Parkinson's disease (see Chapters 42 and 60), where there is great interest in whether they can be both neurotrophic as well as neurotoxic (see Chapter 62).

Ependymal cells are important in facilitating the movement of cerebrospinal fluid (CSF) as well as interacting with astrocytes to form a barrier separating the ventricles and the CSF from the neuronal environment. They also line the central canal in the spinal cord (see Chapter 5). These ependymal cells are termed ependymocytes to distinguish them from those ependymal cells that are involved in the formation of CSF (the choroid plexus) and those that transport substances from the CSF to the blood (tanycytes).

Tumours of the ependyma (*ependymomas* or *choroid plexus papillomas*) occur either in the ventricles, where they tend to produce *hydrocephalus* (see Chapter 5), or in the spinal cord, where they cause local destruction of the neural structures.

Oligodendrocytes are responsible for the myelination of CNS neurones, and are therefore found in large numbers in the white matter. Each oligodendrocyte forms internodal myelin for 3–50 fibres and also surrounds many other fibres without forming myelin sheaths. In addition, they have a number of molecules associated with them that are inhibitory to axonal growth, and thus contribute to the failure of axonal regeneration in the CNS (see Chapter 49).

Clinical disorders of oligodendrocyte function cause central demyelination which is seen in a number of conditions including *multiple sclerosis* (see Chapter 62), while abnormal proliferation of oligodendrocytes produces a slow-growing tumour (an *oligodendroglioma*) which tends to present with epileptic seizures (see Chapter 61).

Schwann cells are found only in the PNS and are responsible for the myelination of peripheral nerves by a process that involves the wrapping of the cell around the axon. Thus, the final myelin sheath is composed of multiple layers of Schwann cell membrane in which the cytoplasm has been extruded. Unlike oligodendrocytes, one Schwann cell envelops one axon and provides myelin for one internode. In addition, Schwann cells are important in the regeneration of damaged peripheral axons, in contrast to the largely inhibitory functions of the central neuroglial cells (see Chapter 48).

A number of genetic and inflammatory neuropathies are associated with the loss of peripheral myelin (as opposed to the loss of axons), which results in peripheral nerve dysfunction (*demyelinating neuropathies*; see Chapters 17 and 63). In addition, benign tumours of Schwann cells can occur (*schwannomas*), especially in certain genetic conditions such as *neurofibromatosis type I*, where there is the loss of the tumour suppressor gene, neurofibromin.

These tumours are typically asymptomatic but if they arise in areas of limited space they can produce symptoms by compression of the neighbouring neural structures; e.g. at the cerebellopontine angle in the brainstem or spinal root (see Chapters 8, 9, 54 and 55).

Finally, there is a group of rare disorders, typically inherited, that cause a central abnormality of myelination, which together are called leucodystrophies.

Did you know?

Einstein's genius has been attributed to the fact that he had a much larger than normal number of glial cells.

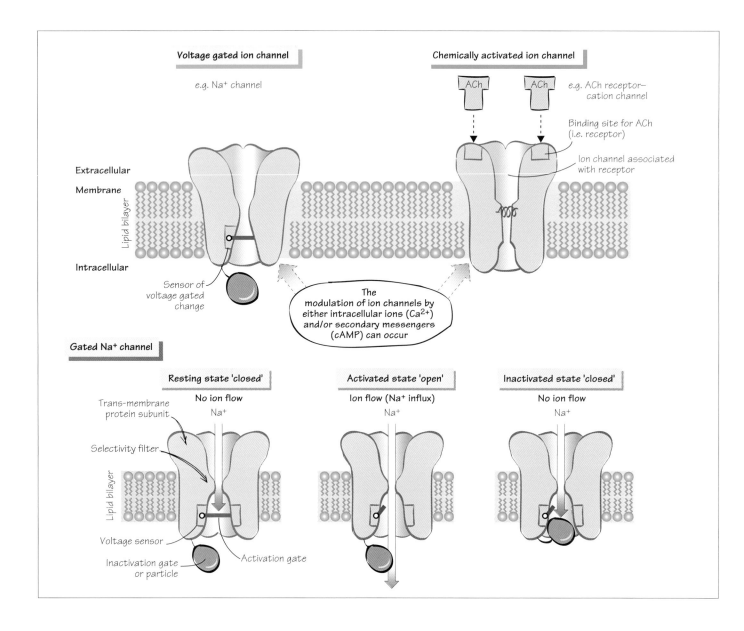

An **ion channel** is a protein macromolecule that spans a biological membrane and allows ions to pass from one side of the membrane to the other. The ions move in a direction determined by the electrochemical gradient across the membrane. In general, ions will tend to flow from an area of high concentration to one of low concentration. However, in the presence of a voltage gradient it is possible for there to be no ion flow even with unequal concentrations. The ion channel itself can be either open or closed. Opening can be achieved either by changing the voltage across the membrane (e.g. a depolarization or the arrival of an action potential) or by the binding of a chemical substance to a receptor in or near the channel.

The two types of channel are called **voltage gated** (or **voltage sensitive**) and **chemically activated** (or **ligand gated**) channels, respectively. However, this distinction is somewhat artificial as a number of voltage sensitive channels can be modulated by neurotransmitters as well as by Ca^{2+}. Furthermore, some ion channels are not opened by voltage changes or chemical messengers but are directly opened by mechanical stretch or pressure (e.g. the somatosensory and auditory receptors; see Chapters 23, 27, 31 and 32).

The most important property of ion channels is that they imbue the neurone with electrical excitability (see Chapter 16) and while they are found in all parts of the neurone, and to a lesser extent in neuroglial cells, they are also seen in a host of non-neural cells.

Neuroanatomy and Neuroscience at a Glance, Fourth Edition. Roger A. Barker, Francesca Cicchetti, Michael J. Neal.

All biological membranes, including the neuronal membrane, are composed of a lipid bilayer that has a high electrical resistance, i.e. ions will not readily flow through it. Therefore, in order for ions to move across a membrane, it is necessary to have either 'pores' (ion channels) in the lipid bilayer or 'carriers' that will collect the ions from one side of the membrane and carry them across to the other side where they are released. In neurones, the rate of ion transfer necessary for signal transmission is too fast for any carrier system and so ion channels (or 'pores') are employed by neurones for the transfer of ions across the membrane.

The **fundamental properties of an ion channel** are as follows:

• It is composed of a number of protein subunits that traverse the membrane and allow ions to cross from one side to the other – a **transmembrane pore**.

• The channel so formed must be able to move from a **closed** to an **open** state and back, although intermediate steps may be required.

• It must be able to open in response to specific stimuli. Most channels possess a sensor of voltage change and so open in response to a depolarizing voltage, i.e. one that moves the resting membrane potential from its resting value of approximately -70 to -80 mV to a less negative value.

In contrast, some channels, especially those found at synapses, are not opened by a voltage change but by a chemical, e.g. acetylcholine (ACh). These channels have a **receptor** for that chemical and binding to this receptor leads to channel opening. However, many channels possess both voltage and chemical sensors and the presence of an intracellular ion or secondary messenger molecule (e.g. cyclic adenosine monophosphate [cAMP]) leads to a **modulation** of the ion flow across the membrane that the voltage-dependent process has produced.

Activation of the voltage sensor or chemical receptor leads to the opening of a 'gate' within the channel which allows ions to flow through the channel. The channel is then closed by either a process of **deactivation** (which is simply the reversal of the opening of the gate) or **inactivation** which involves a **second gate** moving into the channel more slowly than the activation gate moves out, so that there is a time when there is no gate in the channel and ions can flow through it.

The flow of ions through the channel can be either **selective or non-selective**. If the channel is selective then it only allows certain ions through and it achieves this by means of a **filter**. The selectivity filter is based on energetic considerations (thermodynamically) and gives the channel its name, e.g. sodium channel. However, certain channels are non-selective in that they allow many different types of similarly charged ions through, e.g. ACh cation channel.

The overall description of an ion channel is in terms of a number of different physical measures. The net flow of ions through a channel is termed the **current**; while the **conductance** is defined as the reciprocal of resistance (current/voltage) and represents the ease with which the ions can pass through the membrane. **Permeability**, on the other hand, is defined as the rate of transport of a substance or ion through the membrane for a given concentration difference.

There are many different types of ion channel and even within a single family of ion-specific channels there are multiple subtypes, e.g. there are at least five different types of potassium channels.

The number and type of ion channel govern the response characteristics of the cell. In the case of neurones, this is expressed in terms of the rate of action potential generation and its response to synaptic inputs (see Chapters 15, 17, 45 and 61).

Clinical disorders of ion channels

A number of pharmacological agents work at the level of ion channels, including local anaesthetics and some antiepileptic drugs. However, in recent years a number of neurological disorders, primarily involving muscle, have been found to be caused by mutations in the sodium and chloride ion channels. These conditions include various forms of *myotonia* (delayed relaxation of skeletal muscle following voluntary contraction, i.e. an inability to let go of objects easily) and various forms of *periodic paralyses* in which patients develop a transient flaccid weakness which can be either partial or generalized.

Furthermore, certain forms of familial hemiplegic *migraine* (see Chapter 50) and cerebellar dysfunction (see Chapter 40) are associated with abnormalities in the Ca^{2+} channel, and some forms of *epilepsy* (see Chapter 61) may be caused by a disorder of specific ion channels. In other disorders there is a redistribution or exposing of normally non-functioning ion channels. This commonly occurs next to the node of Ranvier as a result of central demyelination in *multiple sclerosis* and peripheral demyelination in the *Guillain–Barré syndrome*, and results in an impairment in action potential propagation (see Chapters 17 and 62). Finally, in some conditions, antibodies are produced in the body (sometimes in response to a tumour) which react with voltage gated ion channels, producing disorders in the central nervous system (e.g. *limbic encephalitis* and anti-voltage gated potassium channels) as well as in the peripheral nervous system (*Lambert–Eaton myasthenic syndrome* and anti-voltage gated calcium channels).

Did you know?

The second-most dangerous vertebrate in the world is the puffer fish, which produces a toxin (colloquially known as zombie powder) that specifically binds to sodium channels (tetrotodoxin) and can kill a person in less than 24 hours.

15 Resting membrane and action potential

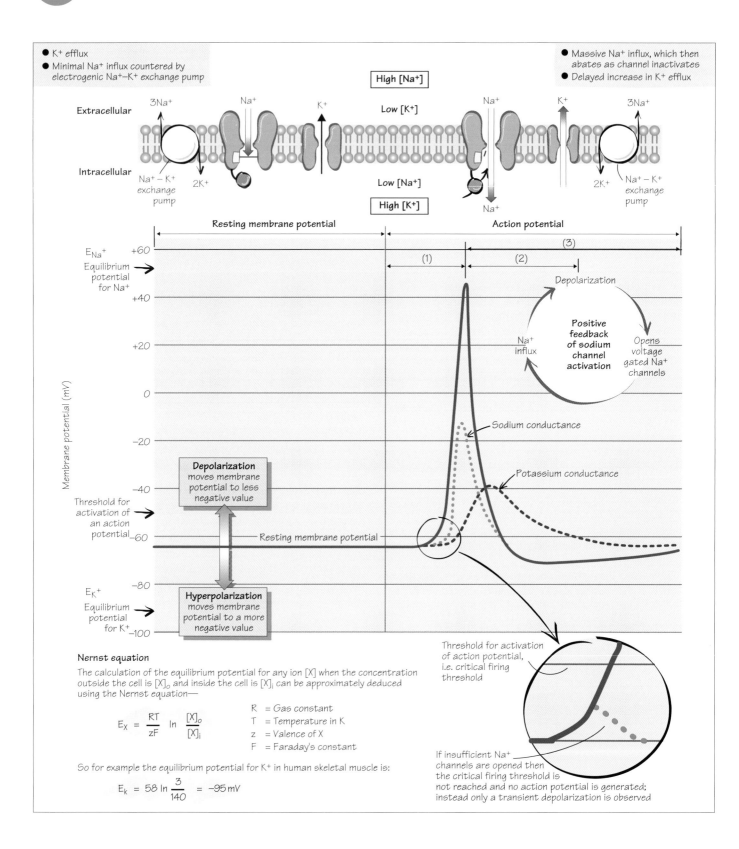

Nernst equation

The calculation of the equilibrium potential for any ion [X] when the concentration outside the cell is $[X]_o$ and inside the cell is $[X]_i$ can be approximately deduced using the Nernst equation—

$$E_X = \frac{RT}{zF} \ln \frac{[X]_o}{[X]_i}$$

R = Gas constant
T = Temperature in K
z = Valence of X
F = Faraday's constant

So for example the equilibrium potential for K+ in human skeletal muscle is:

$$E_k = 58 \ln \frac{3}{140} = -95 \, mV$$

Neuroanatomy and Neuroscience at a Glance, Fourth Edition. Roger A. Barker, Francesca Cicchetti, Michael J. Neal.

Resting membrane potential

In the resting state, the neuronal cell membrane is relatively impermeable to ions. This is important in the generation of the **resting membrane potential**.

The major intracellular ion is potassium, compared to sodium in the extracellular fluid, and so the natural flow of ions according to their concentration gradients is for K^+ to leave the cell (or efflux) and for Na^+ to enter (or influx). The movement of positive ions out of the cell leads to the generation of a negative membrane potential or **hyperpolarization**, while the converse is true for positive ion influx (a process of **depolarization**). However, the resting membrane is relatively impermeable to Na^+ ions while being relatively permeable to K^+ ions. At rest therefore, K^+ will tend to efflux from the cell down its concentration gradient, leaving excess negative charge behind, and this will continue until the chemical concentration gradient driving K^+ out of the cell is exactly offset by the electrical potential difference generated by this efflux (the membrane potential) drawing K^+ back into the cell.

The membrane potential at which this steady state is achieved is the **equilibrium potential** for $K^+(E_{K^+})$ and can be derived using the **Nernst equation** (see figure for details). In fact, the measured resting membrane potential in axons is slightly more positive than expected because there is some small permeability to Na^+ of the membrane in the resting state. The small Na^+ influx is countered by an adenosine triphosphate (ATP) dependent **Na^+–K^+ exchange pump** which is itself slightly electrogenic. This pump is essential in maintaining the ionic gradients, and is electrogenic by virtue of the fact that it pumps out three Na^+ ions for every two K^+ ions brought in. It makes only a small contribution to the level of the resting membrane potential.

Action potential generation

One of the fundamental features of the nervous system is its ability to generate and conduct electrical impulses (see Chapters 17 and 18). These can take the form of generator potentials, synaptic potentials and action potentials – the latter being defined as a single electrical impulse passing down an axon.

This **action potential (nerve impulse or spike)** is an **all-or-nothing phenomenon**, that is to say once the threshold stimulus intensity is reached an action potential will be generated. Therefore information in the nervous system is coded by frequency of firing rather than size of the action potential (see Chapter 22). The threshold stimulus intensity is defined as that value at which the net inward current (which is largely determined by Na^+ ions) is just greater than the net outward current (which is largely carried by K^+ ions), and is typically around −55 mV (**critical firing threshold**). This occurs most readily in the region of the axon hillock where there is the highest density of Na^+ channels, and is thus the site of action potential initiation in the neurone. However, if the threshold is not reached, the graded depolarization will not generate an action potential and the signal will not be propagated along the axon.

Sequence of events in the generation of an action potential

1. The depolarizing voltage activates the voltage sensitive Na^+ channels in the neuronal membrane, which allows some Na^+ ions to flow down their electrochemical gradient (increased Na^+ conductance). This depolarizes the membrane still further, opening more Na^+ channels in a **positive feedback loop**. When sufficient Na^+ channels are opened to produce an inward current greater than that generated by the K^+ efflux, there is rapid opening of all the Na^+ channels producing a large influx of Na^+ which depolarizes the membrane towards the **equilibrium potential for Na^+** (approximately +55 mV). The spike of the action potential is therefore generated, but fails to reach the equilibrium potential for Na^+ because of the persistent and increasing K^+ efflux.

2. The falling phase of the action potential then follows as the voltage sensitive Na^+ channels become inactivated (see Chapter 14). This inactivation is voltage dependent, in that it is in response to the depolarizing stimulus, but has slower kinetics than the activation process and so occurs later (see Chapter 14). During this falling phase, a voltage dependent K^+ current becomes important as its activation by the depolarization of the membrane has even slower kinetics than sodium channel inactivation. This voltage activated K^+ channel leads to a brief period of membrane hyperpolarization before it deactivates and the membrane potential is returned to the resting state.

3. Immediately after the spike of the action potential there is a **refractory period** when the neurone is either inexcitable (**absolute refractory period**) or only activated to submaximal responses by suprathreshold stimuli (**relative refractory period**). The absolute refractory period occurs at the time of maximal Na^+ channel inactivation, while the relative refractory period occurs at a later time when most of the Na^+ channels have returned to their resting state but the voltage activated K^+ current is well developed. The refractory period has two important implications for action potential generation and conduction. First, action potentials can be conducted only in one direction, away from the site of its generation and, secondly, they can be generated only up to certain limiting frequencies (see Chapter 17).

Did you know?

Nerves can conduct action potentials at velocities of up to 402 km (250 miles) per hour.

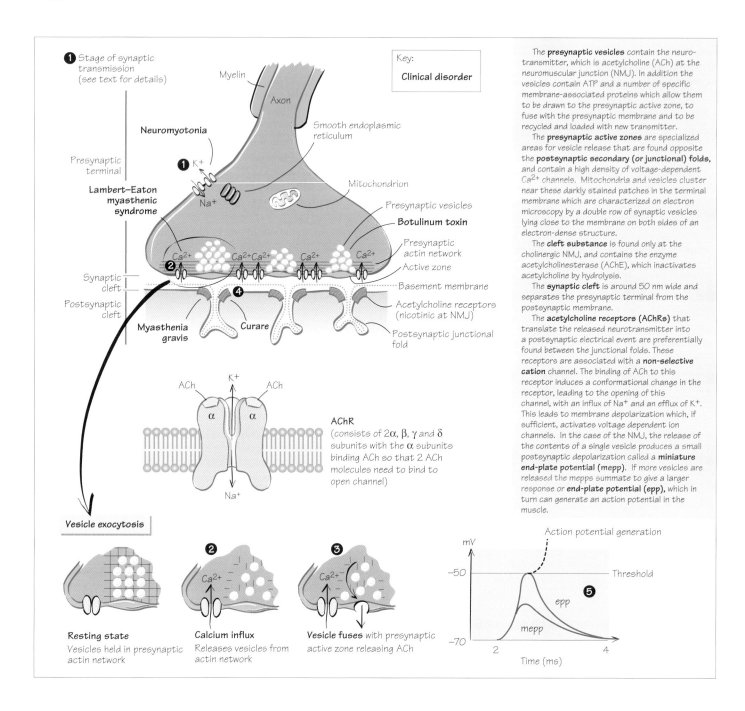

The **presynaptic vesicles** contain the neurotransmitter, which is acetylcholine (ACh) at the neuromuscular junction (NMJ). In addition the vesicles contain ATP and a number of specific membrane-associated proteins which allow them to be drawn to the presynaptic active zone, to fuse with the presynaptic membrane and to be recycled and loaded with new transmitter.

The **presynaptic active zones** are specialized areas for vesicle release that are found opposite the **postsynaptic secondary (or junctional) folds**, and contain a high density of voltage-dependent Ca^{2+} channels. Mitochondria and vesicles cluster near these darkly stained patches in the terminal membrane which are characterized on electron microscopy by a double row of synaptic vesicles lying close to the membrane on both sides of an electron-dense structure.

The **cleft substance** is found only at the cholinergic NMJ, and contains the enzyme acetylcholinesterase (AChE), which inactivates acetylcholine by hydrolysis.

The **synaptic cleft** is around 50 nm wide and separates the presynaptic terminal from the postsynaptic membrane.

The **acetylcholine receptors (AChRs)** that translate the released neurotransmitter into a postsynaptic electrical event are preferentially found between the junctional folds. These receptors are associated with a **non-selective cation** channel. The binding of ACh to this receptor induces a conformational change in the receptor, leading to the opening of this channel, with an influx of Na^+ and an efflux of K^+. This leads to membrane depolarization which, if sufficient, activates voltage dependent ion channels. In the case of the NMJ, the release of the contents of a single vesicle produces a small postsynaptic depolarization called a **miniature end-plate potential (mepp)**. If more vesicles are released the mepps summate to give a larger response or **end-plate potential (epp)**, which in turn can generate an action potential in the muscle.

In 1897 Sherrington coined the term **synapse** to mean the junction of two neurones. Much of the early work on the synapse was carried out on the cholinergic **neuromuscular junction (NMJ)**, although it appears that this chemical synapse is similar in its mode of action to those found in the central nervous system (CNS). The chemical synapse is the predominant synapse type found in the nervous system, but electrical synapses are found in certain sites, e.g. glial cells (see Chapter 13).

Neuromuscular transmission (a model for synaptic transmission)

The sequence of events at a chemical synapse is as follows:
1. The arrival of the action potential leads to the depolarization of the presynaptic terminal (labelled (**1**) on figure) with the opening of **voltage-dependent Ca^{2+} channels** in the **active zones** of the presynaptic terminal and subsequent Ca^{2+} influx (**2**) (this is the stage that represents the major delay in synaptic transmission).

Neuroanatomy and Neuroscience at a Glance, Fourth Edition. Roger A. Barker, Francesca Cicchetti, Michael J. Neal.

2. The influx of Ca^{2+} leads to the phosphorylation and alteration of a number of presynaptic calcium-binding proteins (some of which are found in the vesicle membrane) which liberates the **vesicle** from its **presynaptic actin network** allowing it to bind to the **presynaptic membrane (3)**. These proteins include various different soluble NSF attachment proteins (SNAPs) and SNAP receptors (SNAREs).

3. The fusion of the two hemichannels (presynaptic vesicle and presynaptic membrane) leads to the formation of a small pore that rapidly expands with the release of vesicular contents into the **synaptic cleft**. The vesicle membrane can then be recycled by **endocytosis** into the presynaptic terminal, either by a non-selective or more selective clathrin- and dynamin-mediated process.

More recently an alternative form of vesicle release has been described called 'kiss and run' exocytosis or flicker-fusion and this describes the formation of a transient fusion pore between the vesicle and the presynaptic membrane.

4. Most of the released neurotransmitter then diffuses across the synaptic cleft and binds to the **postsynaptic receptor (4)**. Some transmitter molecules diffuse out of the synaptic cleft and are lost, while others are inactivated before they have time to bind to the postsynaptic membrane receptor. This **inactivation** is essential for the synapse to function normally and, although enzymatic degradation of acetylcholine (ACh) is employed at the NMJ, other synapses use uptake mechanisms with the recycling of the transmitter into the presynaptic neurone (see Chapter 18).

5. The activation of the postsynaptic receptor leads to a change in the postsynaptic membrane potential. Each vesicle contains a certain amount or quantum of neurotransmitter, whose release generates a small postsynaptic potential change of a fixed size – the **miniature end-plate potential (mepp)**. The release of transmitter from several vesicles leads to mepp summation and the generation of a larger depolarization or **end-plate potential (epp)** which, if sufficiently large, will reach threshold for action potential generation in the postsynaptic muscle fibre (**5**).

This **vesicle hypothesis** has been criticized, because not all CNS synapses contain neurotransmitters in vesicles and because electrical synapses are found in some neural networks. However, it is clear that electrical and chemical synapses can coexist in the same neurones and also it is increasingly recognized that neurones may communicate with each other through a range of non-synaptic mechanisms.

Disorders of neuromuscular transmission

A number of naturally occurring toxins can affect the NMJ.

• **Curare** binds to the acetylcholine receptor (AChR) and prevents ACh from acting on it and so induces paralysis. This is exploited clinically in the use of curare derivatives for muscle paralysis in certain forms of surgery.

• **Botulinum toxin** prevents the release of ACh presynaptically. In this case an exotoxin from the bacterium *Clostridium botulinum* binds to the presynaptic membrane of the ACh synapse and prevents the quantal release of ACh. The accidental ingestion of this toxin in cases of food poisoning produces paralysis and autonomic failure (see Chapter 3). However, the toxin can be used therapeutically in small quantities by injecting it into muscles that are abnormally overactive in certain forms of focal *dystonia* – a condition in which a part of the body is held in a fixed abnormal posture by overactive muscular activity (see Chapter 42). It is also used in cosmetic surgery to get rid of wrinkles.

A number of neurological conditions affect the NMJ selectively. These include *myasthenia gravis*, *Lambert–Eaton myasthenic syndrome* (*LEMS*) and *neuromyotonia or Isaac's syndrome*.

• In *neuromyotonia* the patient complains of muscle cramps and stiffness as a result of continuous motor activity in the muscle. This is often caused by an antibody directed against the presynaptic voltage gated K^+ channel, so the nerve terminal is always in a state of depolarization with transmitter release.

• In *LEMS* there is an antibody directed against the presynaptic Ca^{2+} channel, so that on repeated activation of the synapse there is a steady increase in Ca^{2+} influx as the blocking antibody is competitively overcome by exogenous Ca^{2+}. The patient complains of weakness, especially of the proximal muscles, which transiently improves on exercise.

• *Myasthenia gravis*, on the other hand, is caused by an antibody against the AChR, and patients complain of weakness that increases with exercise (fatigability) involving the eyes, throat and limbs. This weakness is due to the number of AChRs being reduced and the ACh released presynaptically competes for the few available receptors. More recently, a second antibody has been recognized in myasthenia gravis in patients without antibodies to the AChR. This antibody is directed to a muscle specific kinase (MUSK), although exactly how this causes the syndrome is not fully known.

Electrical synapses

Electrical transmission occurs at a small number of sites in the brain. The presence of fast conducting gap junctions promotes the rapid and widespread propagation of electrical activity and thus may be important in synchronizing some aspects of cortical function (see Chapter 43). However unlike chemical synapses, electrical synapses:

• are not unidirectional in terms of transmission of electrical information;

• do not contain a synaptic cleft;

• do not allow for synaptic integration.

The abnormal absence of gap junctions in Schwann cells leads to one form of peripheral hereditary motor sensory neuropathy.

Did you know?

Eating the meat of curare poisoned animals is not dangerous, because the toxin is only poisonous when it gets into the bloodstream.

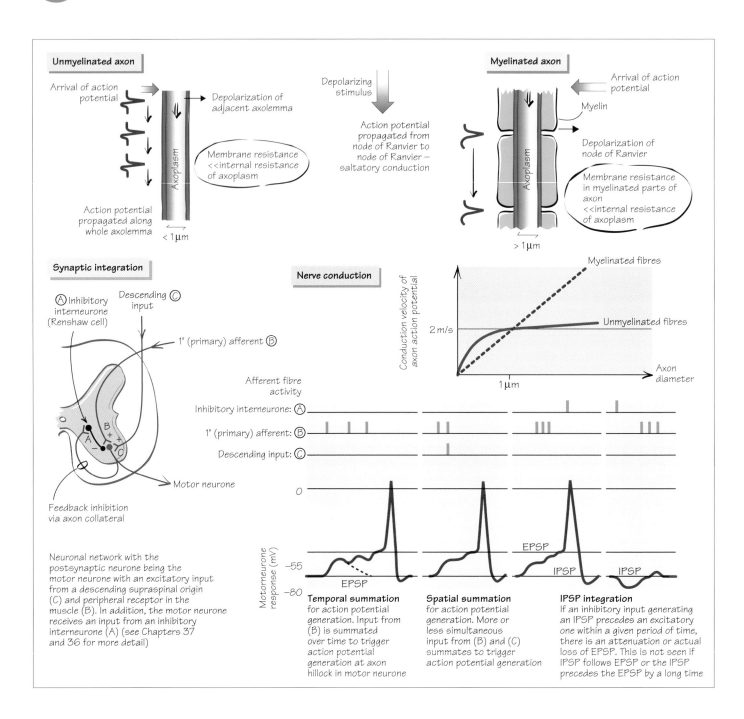

Nerve conduction

Action potential propagation is achieved by local current spread and is made possible by the large safety factor in the generation of an action potential as a consequence of the positive feedback of Na$^+$ channel activation in the rising phase of the nerve impulse (see Chapter 15). However, the use of local current spread does set constraints, not only on the velocity of nerve conduction; it also influences the fidelity of the signal being conducted. The nervous system overcomes these difficulties by insulating nerve fibres above a given diameter with myelin, which is periodically interrupted by the nodes of Ranvier.

• In **unmyelinated axons** an action potential at one site leads to depolarization of the membrane immediately in front and theoretically behind it, although the membrane at this site is in its refractory state and so the action potential is only conducted in one direction (see Chapter 15). The current preferentially passes across

Neuroanatomy and Neuroscience at a Glance, Fourth Edition. Roger A. Barker, Francesca Cicchetti, Michael J. Neal.

the membrane (because of the high internal resistance of the axoplasm) and is greatest at the site closest to the action potential. However, while nerve impulse conduction is feasible and accurate in unmyelinated axons, especially in the very small diameter fibres where the internal axoplasmic resistance is very high, it is nevertheless slow. Conduction velocity can therefore be increased by either increasing the axon diameter (of which the best example is the squid giant axon with a diameter of ~1 mm) or insulating the axon using a high-resistance substance such as the lipid-rich myelin.

• Conduction in **myelinated fibres** follows exactly the same sequence of events as in unmyelinated fibres, but with a crucial difference: the advancing action potential encounters a high-resistance low-capacitance structure in the form of a nerve fibre wrapped in myelin. The depolarizing current therefore passes along the axoplasm until it reaches a low-resistance **node of Ranvier** with its high density of Na^+ channels and an action potential is generated at this site. The action potential therefore appears to be conducted down the fibre, from node to node – a process termed **saltatory conduction**. The advantage of myelination is that it allows for rapid conduction while minimizing the metabolic demands on the cell. It also increases the packing capacity of the nervous system, so that many fast-conducting fibres can be accommodated in smaller nerves. As a result most axons over a certain diameter (~1 μm) are myelinated.

Disturbances in nerve conduction are clinically seen when there is a disruption of the myelin sheath, e.g. in the peripheral nervous system (PNS) in inflammatory demyelinating neuropathies such as the *Guillain–Barré syndrome* and in the central nervous system (CNS) with *multiple sclerosis* (see Chapter 62). In both conditions there is a loss of the myelin sheath, especially in the area adjacent to the node of Ranvier, which exposes other ion channels, as well as reducing the length of insulation along the axon. The result is that the propagated action potential has to depolarize a greater area of axolemma, part of which is not as excitable as the normal node of Ranvier because it contains fewer Na^+ channels. This leads to slowing of the action potential propagation and, if the demyelination is severe enough, actually leads to an attenuation of the propagated action potential to the point that it can no longer be conducted – so-called conduction block.

Synaptic integration

Each central neurone receives many hundreds of synapses and each input is integrated into a response by that neurone, a process that involves the summation of inputs from many different sites at any one time (**spatial summation**) as well as the summation of one or several inputs over time (**temporal summation**).

Presynaptic

The presynaptic nerve terminal usually contains one neurotransmitter, although the release of two or more transmitters at a single presynaptic terminal has been described – a process termed **cotransmission** (see Chapter 18). The amount of neurotransmitter released is dependent not only on the degree to which the presynaptic terminal is depolarized, but also the rate of neurotransmitter synthesis, the presence of inhibitory presynaptic autoreceptors and presynaptic inputs from other neurones in the form of axoaxonic synapses (see Chapter 18). These synapses are usually inhibitory (presynaptic inhibition) and are more common in sensory pathways (see, for example, Chapter 32).

Postsynaptic

The released neurotransmitter acts on a specific protein or **receptor** in the postsynaptic membrane and in certain synapses on **presynaptic autoreceptors** (see Chapter 18). When this binding leads to an opening of ion channels with a cation influx in the postsynaptic process with depolarization, the synapse is said to be **excitatory**, while those ion channels that allow postsynaptic anion influx or cation efflux with hyperpolarization are termed **inhibitory**.

• **Excitatory postsynaptic potentials (EPSPs)** are the depolarizations recorded in the postsynaptic cell to a given excitatory synaptic input. The depolarizations associated with the EPSPs can go on to induce action potentials if they are summated in either time or space. **Spatial summation** involves the integration by the postsynaptic cell of several EPSPs at different synapses with the summed depolarization being sufficient to induce an action potential. **Temporal summation**, in contrast, involves the summation of inputs in time such that each successive EPSP depolarizes the membrane still further until the threshold for action potential generation is reached.

• **Inhibitory postsynaptic potentials (IPSPs)** are hyperpolarizations of the postsynaptic membrane, usually as a result of an influx of Cl^- and an efflux of K^+ through their respective ion channels. IPSPs are very important in modulating the neurone's response to excitatory synaptic inputs (see figure). Therefore inhibitory synapses tend to be found in strategically important sites on the neurone – the proximal dendrite and soma – so that they can have profound effects on the input from large parts of the dendritic tree. In addition, some neurones can inhibit their own output by the use of axon collaterals and a local inhibitory interneurone (**feedback inhibition**), e.g. motor neurones and Renshaw cells of the spinal cord (see Chapter 37).

More **long-term modulations of synaptic transmission** are discussed in Chapters 40, 45 and 49, and in some disorders of the nervous system (e.g. *epilepsy, multiple sclerosis*) abnormal transmission of information may occur via non-synaptic mechanisms.

Did you know?

A single Purkinje cell in the cerebellum receives in excess of 200 000 synapses.

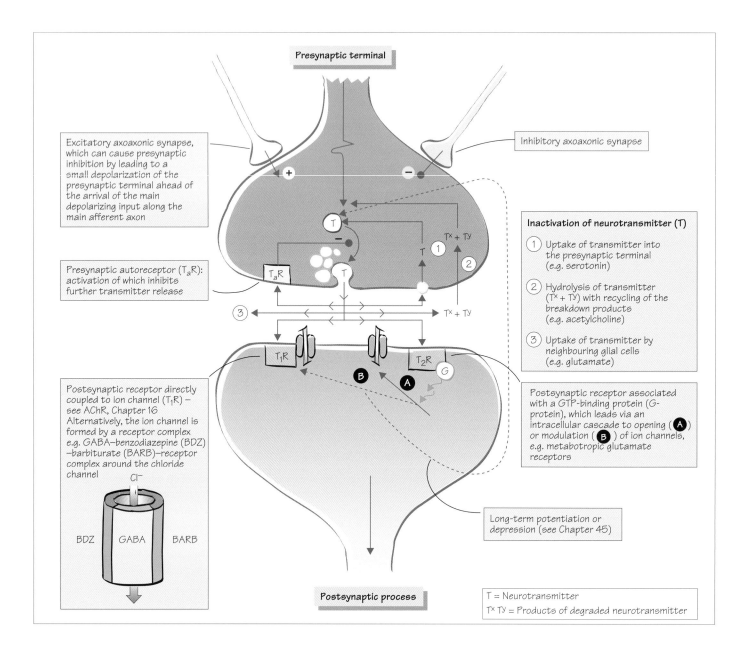

Neurotransmitters and synaptic function

The neurotransmitter released at a synapse interacts with a specific protein in the postsynaptic membrane, known as a **receptor**. At some synapses the neurotransmitter also binds to a **presynaptic autoreceptor** that regulates the amount of transmitter that is released.

Receptors are usually specific for a given neurotransmitter, although several different types of that receptor may exist. In some cases co-released neurotransmitters can either modulate the binding of another neurotransmitter to its receptor or act synergistically on a common single ion channel (e.g. the **γ-aminobutyric acid [GABA]–benzodiazepine–barbiturate receptor**).

Receptors for specific neurotransmitters are either **coupled directly to ion channels** (T_1R on figure, e.g. acetylcholine receptors (AChR); see Chapter 16) or **to a membrane enzyme (T_2R)**. In these latter instances the binding of the neurotransmitter to the receptor either opens an ion channel via an intracellular enzyme cascade (e.g. cyclic adenosine monophosphate [cAMP] and G-proteins) or indirectly modulates the probability of other ion channels opening in response to voltage changes (**neuromodulation**). These receptors therefore mediate slower synaptic events, unlike those receptors directly coupled to ion channels that relay fast synaptic information.

The activated receptor can only return to its resting state once the neurotransmitter has been removed either by a process of

Neuroanatomy and Neuroscience at a Glance, Fourth Edition. Roger A. Barker, Francesca Cicchetti, Michael J. Neal.

enzymatic **hydrolysis** or **uptake** into the presynaptic nerve terminal or neighbouring glial cells. Even then there are often intermediate steps in the process of returning the receptor and its associated ion channel to the resting state. At some synapses the affinity and, ultimately, the number of receptors is dependent on the previous activity of the synapse. For example, at catecholaminergic synapses the receptors become less sensitive to the released transmitter when the synapse is very active – a process of **desensitization and down-regulation**. This process involves a decrease in the affinity of the receptor for the transmitter in the short term, which goes on in the long term to an actual decrease in the number of receptors. The converse is true with synapses that are rarely activated (**super-sensitivity and up-regulation**), and in this way synaptic activity is modulated by its ongoing activity.

In addition, at some synapses the activation of the postsynaptic receptor–ion channel complex can modulate the long-term activity of the synapse, either by affecting the presynaptic release of neurotransmitter or the postsynaptic receptor response – a process known as either **long-term potentiation (LTP) or long-term depression (LTD)** depending on the actual change in synaptic efficacy over time (see Chapters 45 and 49). Therefore the state, number and types of receptor for a specific neurotransmitter as well as the presence of receptors to other neurotransmitters are all important in determining the extent of synaptic activity at any given synapse.

Diversity and anatomy of neurotransmitter pathways

The nervous system employs a large number of neurotransmitters, which can be divided into groups (see also Chapter 19).

Excitatory amino acids

These represent the main excitatory neurotransmitters in the central nervous system (CNS) and are important at most synapses in maintaining ongoing synaptic activity. The main excitatory amino acid is **glutamate**, which acts at a number of receptors (which are defined by the agonists that activate them). The **inotropic** receptors consist of the *N*-methyl-D-aspartate (**NMDA**) and **non-NMDA receptors**, and the former receptor with its associated calcium channel may be important in the generation of LTP (see Chapter 45), excitotoxic cell death (see Chapter 60) and possibly *epilepsy* (see Chapter 61).

A separate group of G-protein associated glutamate receptors, the **metabotropic receptors**, respond on activation by initiating a number of intracellular biochemical events that modulate synaptic transmission and neuronal activity. These receptors may underlie long-term depression in the hippocampus.

Inhibitory amino acids

The major CNS inhibitory neurotransmitters are **GABA**, which is present throughout the CNS, and **glycine** which is predominantly found in the spinal cord. Abnormalities of GABA neurones may underlie some forms of movement disorders as well as anxiety states and epilepsy (see Chapters 59 and 61). While mutations in the glycine receptor have now been linked to some forms of *hyperexplexia* – a condition in which there is an excessive startle response, such that any stimulus induces a stiffening of the body with collapse to the ground without any impairment of consciousness.

Monoamines

The monoaminergic systems of the CNS originate from small groups of neurones in the brainstem, which then project widely to all areas of the CNS. They are found at many other sites within the body, including the autonomic nervous system (ANS; see Chapter 3). In all locations they bind to a host of different receptors and thus can have complex actions including a role in depression, schizophrenia, cognition and movement control (see Chapters 41, 42, 47, 57 and 58).

Acetylcholine

This neurotransmitter is widely distributed throughout the nervous system, including the neuromuscular junction (see Chapter 16) and ANS (see Chapter 3). Therefore, many agents have been developed that target the different cholinergic synapses in the periphery and which are used routinely in surgical anaesthesia. Several disease processes can affect the peripherally located cholinergic synapses (see Chapter 16), while secondary abnormalities in the central cholinergic pathways may be important in *dementia of the Alzheimer type* and *Parkinson's disease* (see Chapters 42 and 60).

Neuropeptides

These neurotransmitters, of which there are many different types, are found in all areas of the nervous system and are often co-released with other neurotransmitters. They can act as conventional neurotransmitters as well as having a role in neuromodulation (e.g. pain pathways; see Chapters 32 and 38).

Did you know?

John Eccles won the Nobel prize in 1963 for his work demonstrating that synapses could be inhibitory as well as excitatory.

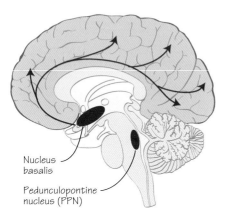

Basal forebrain cholinergic projections

Nucleus basalis

Pedunculopontine nucleus (PPN)

Nucleus basalis projects to the neocortex

PPN projects to the thalamus and spinal cord

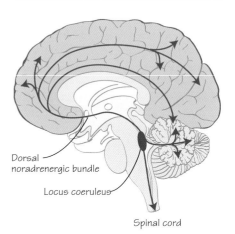

Locus coeruleus noradrenergic projections

Dorsal noradrenergic bundle

Locus coeruleus

Spinal cord

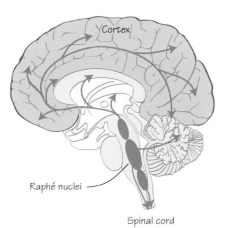

Raphé serotoninergic projections

Cortex

Raphé nuclei

Spinal cord

Raphé projects throughout the CNS

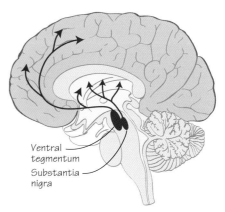

Midbrain dopaminergic projections

Ventral tegmentum

Substantia nigra

Mesocortical pathway projects to the frontal cortex
Mesolimbic pathway projects to the nucleus accumbens
Nigrostriatal pathway projects to the striatum

Neuroanatomy and Neuroscience at a Glance, Fourth Edition. Roger A. Barker, Francesca Cicchetti, Michael J. Neal.

Neurotransmitter	Distribution	Receptor types	Associated neurological disorders
Amino acids *Excitatory*			
Glutamate	Widespread throughout CNS	1. Inotropic: *N*-methyl-D-aspartate (NMDA); and non-NMDA receptors including α-amino-5-hydroxy-3-methyl-4-isoxazole propionic acid (AMPA); kainate and quisqualate receptors	Epilepsy (Ch. 61)
		2. Metabotropic	Excitotoxic cell death (Ch. 60)
Inhibitory γ-aminobutyric acid (GABA)	Widespread throughout CNS	GABA-A	Spinal cord motor disorders (Ch. 37)
		GABA-B	Epilepsy (Ch. 61) Anxiety (Ch. 59)
Glycine	Spinal cord	Glycine	Startle syndromes (Ch. 35)
Monoamines*			
Noradrenaline (norepinephrine)	Locus coeruleus to whole CNS (Ch. 57)	α1; α2	Depression (Ch. 57)
	Postganglionic sympathetic nervous system (Ch. 3)	β1; β2	Autonomic failure (Ch. 3)
Serotonin (5-hydroxytryptamine; 5-HT)	Raphé nucleus in brainstem to whole CNS (Ch. 57)	5-HT1 (A–F) 5-HT2 (A–C) 5-HT3–5-HT7	Depression (Ch. 57) Anxiety (Ch. 59) Migraine
Dopamine	Nigrostriatal pathway in basal ganglia (Ch. 41)	D1–D5 receptors cause an increase in intracellular	Parkinson's disease (Ch. 42)
	Mesolimbic and mesocortical pathways (Chs 47)	cAMP on activation	Schizophrenia (Ch. 58)
	Retina (Ch. 24)	D2 receptors cause a decrease in intracellular cAMP on activation	Control of pituitary hormone secretion (Ch. 11)
	Hypothalamic–pituitary projection (Ch. 11)	D3–D4 are independent of cAMP signalling system	Control of vomiting Drug addiction (Ch. 47)
Acetylcholine	Neuromuscular junction (Ch. 16)	Nicotinic	Disorders of the neuromuscular junction (Ch. 16)
	Autonomic nervous system (Ch. 3)	Muscarinic (M1–M3 subtypes)	Autonomic failure (Ch. 3)
	Basal forebrain to cerebral cortex and limbic system (Ch. 45 and 60)		Dementia of the Alzheimer type (Ch. 60)
	Interneurones in many CNS structures including striatum (Ch. 41)		Parkinson's disease (Ch. 42) Epilepsy (Ch. 61) Sleep–wake cycle (Ch. 43)
Neuropeptides	Widespread distribution in CNS but especially found in: • dorsal horn of spinal cord (Ch. 32 and 33) • basal ganglia (Ch. 41) • autonomic nervous system (Ch. 3)	Various	See: • Pain systems (Ch. 33 and 37) • Basal ganglia (Ch. 41) • Autonomic nervous system (Ch. 3) • Neural plasticity (Ch. 48) • Anxiety (Ch. 60) • Sleep (Ch. 43)
Others Purinergic Adenosine triphosphate (ATP) Endozapines			

*Histamine and adrenaline (noradrenaline) are monoamines that are found primarily in the hypothalamus and adrenal medulla, respectively.

Did you know?

Eating chocolate releases natural endorphins which dulls pain and may also explain why many believe that chocolate is addictive in the same way as people can become dependent on opioid drugs. If the opioid receptors are blocked, the craving and euphoric feelings for chocolate diminish.

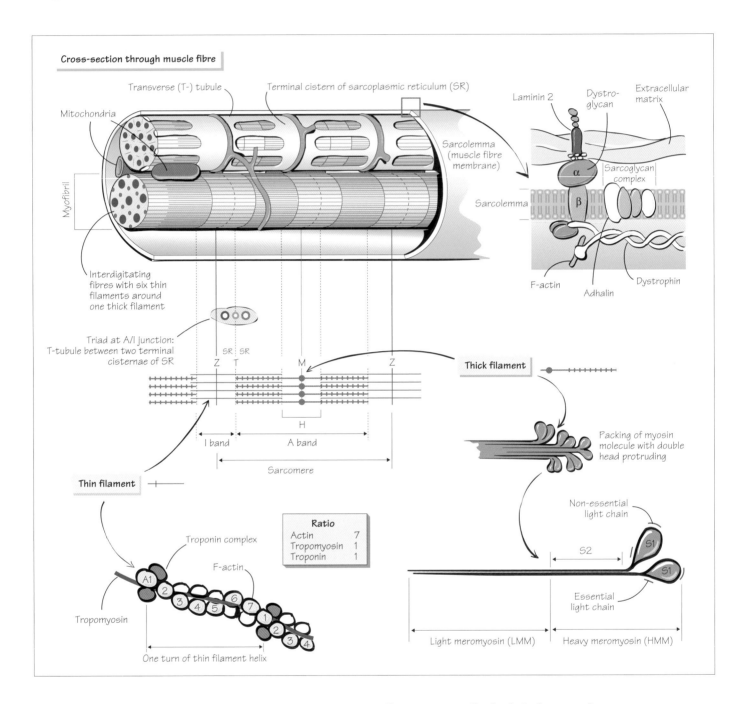

Skeletal muscle is responsible for converting the electrical impulse from a lower motor neurone that arrives at the neuromuscular junction (NMJ) into a mechanical force by means of contraction. The arrival of the action potential leads to the release of acetylcholine (ACh) which activates the nicotinic ACh receptor (AChR) in the postsynaptic muscle, which in turn leads to the depolarization of the muscle fibre (see Chapter 16). This produces a calcium influx into the muscle fibre which leads to muscle contraction (see Chapter 21).

Structure of skeletal muscle

Skeletal muscle is composed of groups of muscle fibres which are long, multinucleated cells. These fibres contain **myofibrils**, which in turn are made up of thick and thin filaments that overlap to some extent giving this type of muscle its striated appearance. The myofibrils are bounded by the **sarcolemma**, which invaginates between the myofibrils in the form of **transverse** or **T-tubules**. This structure is separate from the **sarcoplasmic reticulum** (**SR**), which envelops the myofibrils and is important as an intracellular store

Neuroanatomy and Neuroscience at a Glance, Fourth Edition. Roger A. Barker, Francesca Cicchetti, Michael J. Neal.

of Ca^{2+}. The sarcolemma is a complex structure and abnormalities in its membrane components have recently been found to underlie some forms of inherited muscular dystrophies.

The **thick filament** is composed of myosin and lies at the centre of the **sarcomere**.

• Myosin is composed of two heavy chains that are form by the **light and heavy meromyosin proteins** (LMM and HMM, respectively).

• The HMM portion contains **S1 and S2 subfragments**.

• The S1 fragment consists of two heads and associated with each of these heads are two light chains.

• The light chain found at the tip of the S1 head is termed **non-essential** and is responsible for breaking down adenosine triphosphate (ATP) at the end of the power stroke of crossbridge formation.

• The remaining **essential** light chain is attached at the point where the S1 head swings out towards the actin and is important in the process of myosin head movement.

• By virtue of the properties of LMM, myosin filaments spontaneously pack together so that the S1 heads are on the outside towards the actin filaments. The S1 heads therefore form the major part of the crossbridge with the actin.

Thin filaments are composed of F-actin, tropomyosin and troponin. Troponin is itself composed of three subunits (troponin-I, -C and -T).

• These three components of the troponin complex all subserve different functions but as a whole they regulate muscle contraction by holding the tropomyosin in position so that it physically blocks the S1 head of the myosin from binding to the actin.

• The depolarization of the muscle leads to a calcium influx which then binds to troponin, producing a conformational change in the thin filament such that the tropomyosin shifts off the binding site for myosin on actin.

• Thus, tropomyosin and troponin regulate muscle contraction by a process of **stearic block**. In some muscles in other animals, the regulation of the interaction between actin and myosin lies with the myosin associated light chains.

At the point of overlap of these two sets of filaments is found the **triad** structure of a T-tubule, linked to two terminal cisternae of SR by foot processes.

Disorders of structural proteins in skeletal muscle – the muscular dystrophies

There are many disorders, including:

• Disorders of excitability through mutations in the ion channels (see Chapter 14).

• Inflammation within the muscle (see Chapter 62).

• Abnormalities in the structural proteins.

These latter conditions underlie many of the inherited muscular dystrophies, of which the best characterized are Duchenne's and the limb girdle muscular dystrophies.

Duchenne's muscular dystrophy (DMD) is an X-linked disorder in which there is a deletion of the gene coding for the structural protein dystrophin, with the milder form of the disease (*Becker's muscular dystrophy*) having a reduced amount of this same protein. Patients with DMD typically present early in life with clumsiness and difficulty in walking, with an associated wasting of the proximal limb muscles and pseudohypertrophy of the calf muscles. As the disease progresses the patient becomes increasingly disabled, with the development of cardiac and other abnormalities which lead to death, typically in the third decade. Characteristically, these patients have a raised creatine kinase (a marker of muscle damage) as the muscles in these patients are prone to necrosis as a result of the absence of dystrophin. This protein lies beneath the sarcolemma of skeletal (as well as smooth and cardiac) muscle and provides stability and flexibility to the muscle membrane, such that when absent the membrane can be easily disrupted. This allows entry of large quantities of Ca^{2+}, which precipitates necrosis by excessive activation of proteases.

The *limb girdle muscular dystrophies (LGMD)*, in contrast, can present at any age with progressive weakness of the proximal limb muscles and a raised creatine kinase. The condition can be inherited in a number of different ways, and recently the autosomal recessive forms of this condition have been found to contain abnormalities in the **dystrophin** associated glycoproteins, adhalin and the **sarcoglycan complex**. These proteins link the intracellular dystrophin with components of the extracellular matrix and so are important in maintaining the integrity of the sarcolemma.

There is also some evidence that in myasthenia gravis (see Chapter 16) antibodies can also be found against some of these structural proteins such as the ryanodine receptor and titin.

Disorders with inflammation of skeletal muscle – the myositides

In a number of disorders there is selective inflammation in skeletal muscle, including:

• inflammation for unknown reasons with a predominant T-cell infiltrate (polymyositis);

• inflammation with a predominant B-cell mediated process (dermatomyositis) that can be paraneoplastic in nature;

• a degenerative disorder that has a significant secondary inflammatory response (inclusion body myositis).

The former two conditions tend to respond to immunotherapy, while inclusion body myositis does not. In all cases the inflammation damages the muscle, causing weakness often with pain, and a raised serum creatine kinase.

Did you know?

The biggest single muscle in the human body is gluteus maximus (in the buttocks), while the smallest is the stapedius muscle, which is found in the ear, and the strongest are the masseters, which help you chew.

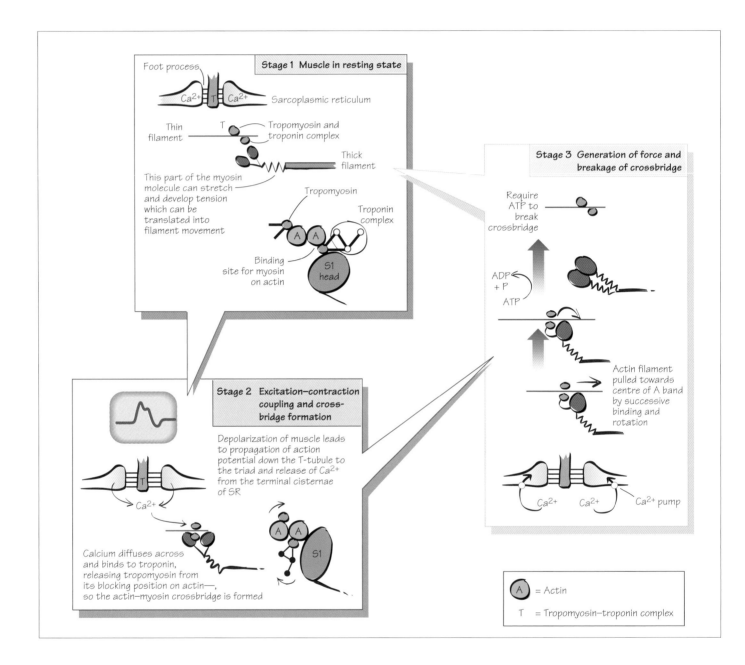

Summary of sequence of events in the contraction of muscle

1. The arrival of the action potential at the neuromuscular junction (NMJ) leads to an influx of Ca^{2+} and the release of vesicles containing acetylcholine (ACh).

2. ACh then binds to the nicotinic ACh receptor (AChR) on the muscle fibre leading to its depolarization.

3. Ca^{2+} is then released from the sarcoplasmic reticulum (SR) of the muscle.

4. Ca^{2+} release leads to the removal of the blocking calcium-binding protein complex of **tropomyosin** and **troponin** from **actin**, the main component of the **thin filament**.

5. Removal of this stearic block allows **myosin**, the major component of the **thick filaments**, to bind to actin via a **cross-bridge**.

Neuroanatomy and Neuroscience at a Glance, Fourth Edition. Roger A. Barker, Francesca Cicchetti, Michael J. Neal.

6. The fibres are then pulled past each other; the cross-bridge between the two fibres is broken at the end of this power stroke by the **hydrolysis of adenosine triphosphate (ATP)**.

The cycle of cross-bridge formation and breakage can then be repeated and the muscle contracts in a ratchet-like fashion.

Sequence of events in the contraction of muscle

- *Stage 1*

In the resting state the troponin complex holds the tropomyosin in such a position that it blocks myosin from binding to actin (stearic block).

- *Stage 2*

The arrival of an action potential at the NMJ causes a postsynaptic action potential to be initiated, which is propagated down the specialized invagination of the muscle membrane known as the **transverse tubule (T-tubule)**. This T-tubule conducts the action potential down into the muscle, so that all the muscle fibres can be activated. It lies adjacent to the terminal cisternae of the SR in a structure known as a **triad**, i.e. a T-tubule lies between two terminal cisternae of the SR (muscle equivalent of smooth endoplasmic reticulum) which contain high concentrations of Ca^{2+}.

The T-tubules are linked to the SR by foot processes, which are part of a calcium ion channel. The arrival of the action potential at the triad leads to the release of Ca^{2+} from the terminal cisternae, by a process of mechanical coupling. The action potential opens a common Ca^{2+} ion channel between the T-tubule and SR, which then allows Ca^{2+} to influx down its electrochemical gradient towards the myofibrils. The Ca^{2+} then binds to the troponin complex and this leads to a rearrangement of the tropomyosin so that the myosin head can now bind to the actin, forming a cross-link or cross-bridge.

- *Stage 3*

Once the myosin has bound to the actin there is a delay before tension develops in the cross-bridge. The tension pulls and rotates the actin past the myosin and this causes the muscle to contract. The cross-bridge at the end of this power stroke detaches the myosin from actin with hydrolysis of ATP, a process that is also calcium dependent.

The whole cycle can then be repeated. The process of cross-bridge formation with filament movement is called the **sliding filament hypothesis** of muscle contraction, as the two filaments slide past each other in a ratchet-like fashion as the cycle repeats. The Ca^{2+} released by the terminal cisternae of the SR, allowing the process of cross-bridge formation and breakage, is actively taken back up into this structure by a specific Ca^{2+} pump.

Disorders of muscle contraction

Diseases of the muscles, which disrupt their anatomy, will lead to weakness as a consequence of a disorganization of contractile proteins. However, there are some disorders in which there is a disruption of the contractile process itself and examples of this are the rare *periodic paralyses* and *malignant hyperthermia/hyperpyrexia*. In this latter condition there is an abnormality in the ryanodine receptor which is part of the protein complex linking the T-tubule to the SR. This leads, under certain circumstances such as general anaesthesia, to sustained depolarization, contraction and necrosis of muscles resulting in an increase in body temperature and multiorgan dysfunction. In contrast, the *periodic paralyses* involve abnormalities in the ion channels that can lead to prolonged inexcitability of muscles, which thus become weak and paralysed. These are rare disorders and respiratory muscles are not involved; the paralysis can be provoked by a number of insults such as exercise or high carbohydrate meals.

It is also important to remember that disorders of muscle contraction occur as a consequence of abnormalities at the NMJ (see Chapter 16), as well as with some inborn errors of metabolism. These latter *metabolic myopathies* involve inherited defects in either carbohydrate or lipid metabolism, which lead to either episodic exercise-induced symptoms or chronic progressive weakness.

Did you know?

Rigor mortis is the stiffening of muscles after death and is caused by calcium leaking through the walls of the dead muscle fibres.

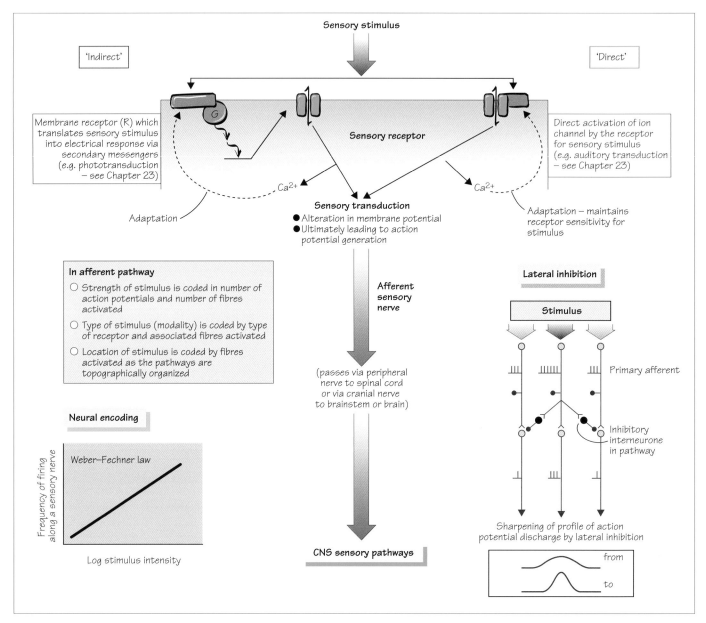

A sensory system is one in which information is conveyed to the spinal cord and brain from peripheral sensory receptors, which in themselves are either specialized neurones or nerve endings.

• The specialized **sensory receptor**, **afferent axon** and **cell body** together with the synaptic contacts in the spinal cord are known as the **primary afferent**. The process by which stimuli from the external environment are converted into electrical signals for transmission through the nervous system is known as **sensory transduction** (see Chapter 23).

• The signal produced by the sensory receptor is relayed to the central nervous system (CNS) via peripheral or cranial nerves and through a series of synapses eventually projects to a given area of cortex that is then capable of detailed analysis of that sensory input.

There are five main sensory systems in the mammalian nervous system:

1. touch/pressure, proprioception, temperature and pain or the somatosensory system (see Chapters 31–33);
2. vision (see Chapters 24–26);
3. hearing and balance (see Chapters 27–29);
4. taste (see Chapter 30);
5. smell or olfaction (see Chapter 30).

All but the somatosensory pathways are regarded as 'special' senses.

Sensory receptors

Sensory receptors transduce the sensory stimulus either by a process of **direct ion channel activation** (e.g. the auditory system)

Neuroanatomy and Neuroscience at a Glance, Fourth Edition. Roger A. Barker, Francesca Cicchetti, Michael J. Neal.

or **indirectly via a secondary intracellular messenger network** (e.g. the visual system). In both cases the sensory stimulus is converted into an electrical signal that can then be relayed to the CNS in the form of either graded depolarizations/hyperpolarizations leading on to action potentials (e.g. visual system) or the direct generation of action potentials at the level of the receptor.

The **specificity** or **modality** of a sensory system relies on the activation of specialized nerve cells or fibres which are highly specific for different forms of afferent stimuli.

The receptor will only respond to stimuli when they are applied within a given region around it (its **receptive field**). This area or receptive field from which the receptor can be activated is recognized by the CNS as corresponding to a specific site or position in the body or outside world. The receptor will only transmit electrical information to the CNS when it receives a stimulus of sufficient intensity to reach the firing **threshold**.

The incremental response to a change in stimulus intensity by the receptor gives the receptor its **sensitivity**. Many receptors have high sensitivity both to the absolute level of stimulus detection and to changes in stimulus intensity. This is because they are capable of both amplifying the original signal by the use of secondary messenger systems and **adapting** to the presence of a continuous unchanging stimulus (see below and Chapter 23).

Ascending sensory pathways in the spinal cord

With very sensitive receptors the intrinsic instability of the transduction process is termed the **noise** and the challenge for the nervous system is to detect a sensory stimulus response or signal over this background noise (termed the **signal to noise ratio**).

The strength of a sensory stimulus can be coded for at the level of the receptor and its first synapse, either in the form of action potentials or graded membrane potentials within the receptor. The **afferent sensory nerve** can code (among other things) for the strength of the stimulus, first by increasing the number of afferent fibres activated (**recruitment** or **spatial coding**) and, second, by increasing the number of action potentials generated in each axon per unit time (**temporal** or **frequency coding**). There is a complex relationship between the stimulus intensity and action potential firing frequency in the afferent nerve – this is defined by the **Weber–Fechner law**.

Tract	Spinothalamic tract (STT)	Dorsal column–medial lemniscal pathway	Spinocerebellar tract (SCT)
Relevant chapter	32, 33	31	40
Site of origin	Dorsal horn (laminae I, III, IV and V) Crosses midline in spinal cord	Primary afferents from mechanoreceptors, muscle and joint receptors	Spinal cord interneurones and proprioceptive information from muscles and joint
Termination	• Somatotopic organization with more caudal fibres added laterally • Projects to brainstem and contralateral thalamus	• Somatotopic organization with fibres terminating in dorsal column nuclei of medulla • Decussate at this level to form medial lemniscus that synapses in the ventroposterior nucleus of the thalamus	Two tracts: (1) dorsal SCT relays information from muscle and joint receptors to cerebellum via inferior cerebellar peduncle (2) ventral SCT relays information from spinal cord interneurones to cerebellum via superior cerebellar peduncle
Function	Conveys pain and temperature	Conveys proprioception, light touch and vibration	Conveys proprioceptive information as well as information of ongoing activity in spinal cord interneurones

Sensory pathways

Each sensory pathway has its own unique input to the CNS, although ultimately most sensory pathways provide an input to the thalamus – the site of that projection being different for each sensory system. This in turn projects to the cortex, although the olfactory pathway primarily projects to limbic structures (see Chapter 30) and the muscle spindle to the cerebellum (see Chapter 40).

Each sensory system has its own area of cortex that is primarily concerned with analysing the sensory information and this area of cortex – the **primary sensory area** – is connected to adjacent cortical areas that perform more complex sensory processing (**secondary sensory areas**). This in turn projects into the **association areas** (posterior parietal, prefrontal and temporal cortices; see Chapter 34) which then project to the motor and limbic systems (see Chapter 35). These latter areas are more involved in the processing of sensory information as a cue for moving and generating complex behavioural responses.

The primary sensory cortical areas project also subcortically to their thalamic (and/or brainstem) projecting nuclei. This may be important in augmenting the detection of significant ascending sensory signals. This augmentation probably involves at least two major processes: **lateral inhibition** and **feature detection**. Lateral inhibition is a process by which those cells and axons with the greatest activity are highlighted by the inhibition of adjacent less active ones, which produces greater contrast in the afferent information. Feature detection, on the other hand, corresponds to the selective detection of given features of a sensory stimulus, which can occur at any level from the receptor to the cortex.

Did you know?

The first sense to develop while *in utero* is the sense of touch and it begins in the face at around 8 weeks of age.

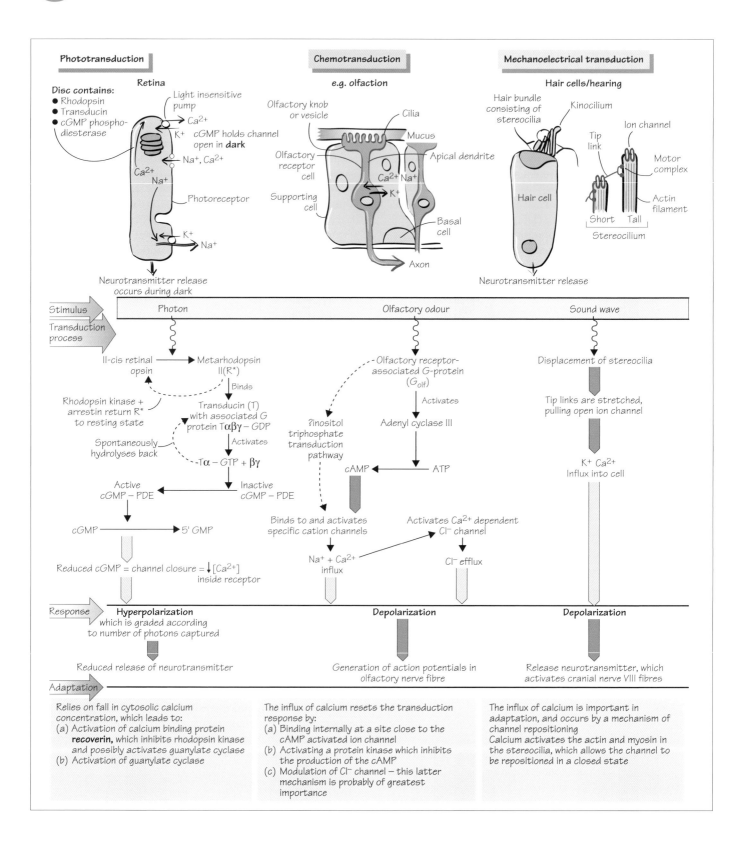

Neuroanatomy and Neuroscience at a Glance, Fourth Edition. Roger A. Barker, Francesca Cicchetti, Michael J. Neal.

54 © 2012 John Wiley & Sons, Ltd. Published 2012 by John Wiley & Sons, Ltd.

Sensory transduction involves the conversion of a stimulus from the external or internal environment into an electrical signal for transmission through the nervous system. This process is performed by all sensory systems and in general involves either:

• a **chemical process** in the retina, tongue or olfactory epithelium; or

• a **mechanical process** in the cochlea and somatosensory systems.

These contrasting modes of transduction are best characterized in some of the special senses.

Phototransduction

Phototransduction is the process by which light energy in the form of photons is translated into electrical energy in the form of potential changes in the photoreceptors (rods and cones) in the retina. The following sequence of events defines it:

1. Photons are captured in pigments in the photoreceptor outer segment.

2. This results in an amplification process using the G-protein, transducin and cyclic guanosine monophosphate (cGMP) as the secondary messenger.

3. This causes a reduction in cGMP concentrations which leads to channel closure.

4. The closure of these channels, which allows Na^+ and Ca^{2+} to enter the photoreceptor in the dark, leads to a hyperpolarization response, the degree of which is graded according to the number of photons captured by the photoreceptor pigment.

The hyperpolarization response leads to reduced glutamate release by the photoreceptor on to bipolar and horizontal cells (see Chapter 24). The termination of the photoreceptor response to a continuous unvarying light stimulus is multifactorial, but changes in intracellular Ca^{2+} concentration are important. The light insensitive Ca^{2+} pump in the outer segment coupled to the closure of the cation channel leads to a significant reduction in intracellular Ca^{2+} concentrations which is important in terminating the photoreceptor response as well as mediating light (or background) adaptation.

A number of rare congenital forms of **night blindness** have now been associated with specific deficits within the phototransduction pathway.

Olfactory transduction

Olfactory transduction is similarly a chemically mediated process. The olfactory receptor cells are bipolar neurones consisting of a dendrite with a knob on which are found the cilia, and an axonal part that projects as the olfactory nerve to the olfactory bulb on the underside of the frontal lobe. The presence of cilia, which contain the olfactory receptors, greatly increases the surface area of the olfactory neuroepithelium and so increases the probability of trapping odorant molecules. The following sequence of events defines it:

1. The binding of the odorant molecule to the receptor leads to the activation of G_{olf}.

2. This activates adenylate cyclase type III which hydrolyses adenosine triphosphate (ATP) to cyclic adenosine monophosphate (cAMP).

3. cAMP then binds to and activates specific cation channels, thus allowing Na^+ and Ca^{2+} to influx down their concentration gradients.

4. This not only partly depolarizes the receptor, but also leads to the activation of a Ca^{2+}-dependent Cl^- channel and the subsequent Cl^- efflux then further depolarizes the olfactory receptor.

5. There are probably additional transduction processes present in the olfactory receptor using inositol triphosphate as the secondary messenger.

6. This can lead to the generation of action potentials at the cell body, which are then conducted down the olfactory nerve axons to the olfactory bulb.

The Ca^{2+} influx is also important in adaptation by resetting the transduction response.

Auditory transduction

In contrast to both phototransduction and olfactory transduction, the process of **auditory transduction** in the inner ear involves the mechanical displacement of **stereocilia** on the hair cells of the cochlea (see Chapter 27). The following sequence of events defines it:

1. The sensory stimulus, a sound wave, causes displacement of the stapedial foot process in the oval window which generates waves in the perilymphatic filled scala vestibuli and tympani of the cochlea.

2. This leads to displacement of the basilar membrane on which the hair cells are to be found in the organ of Corti. These cells transduce the sound waves into an electrical response by a process of mechanotransduction. The stereocilia at the apical end of the hair cell are linked by tip links, which are attached to ion channels.

3. The sound causes the stereocilia to be displaced in the direction of the largest stereocilia (or kinocilium) which creates tension within the tip links which then pull open an ion channel.

4. This ion channel then allows K^+ (not Na^+, as the endolymph within the scala media is rich in K^+ and low in Na^+) and Ca^{2+} to flow into the hair cell and by so doing depolarizes it.

5. This depolarization leads to the release of neurotransmitter at the base of the hair cell which activates the afferent fibres of the cochlear nerve.

The continued displacement of the stereocilia in response to a sound is countered by a process of adaptation with a repositioning of the ion channel such that it is now shut in response to that degree of tip link tension. This is achieved by the influx of Ca^{2+} through the ion transduction channels which leads via actin–myosin in the stereocilia to a new repositioning of the ion channel.

A number of syndromes with congenital deafness have now been identified as being caused by abnormalities in the myosin found in hair cells.

Other transduction processes

Transduction in the somatosensory receptors, nociceptors, thermoreceptors, taste receptors and muscle spindle are discussed in Chapters 30, 31, 32 and 36 respectively.

Did you know?

In an experiment performed in 1942, it was established that on average, an individual rod was sensitive to a single photon!

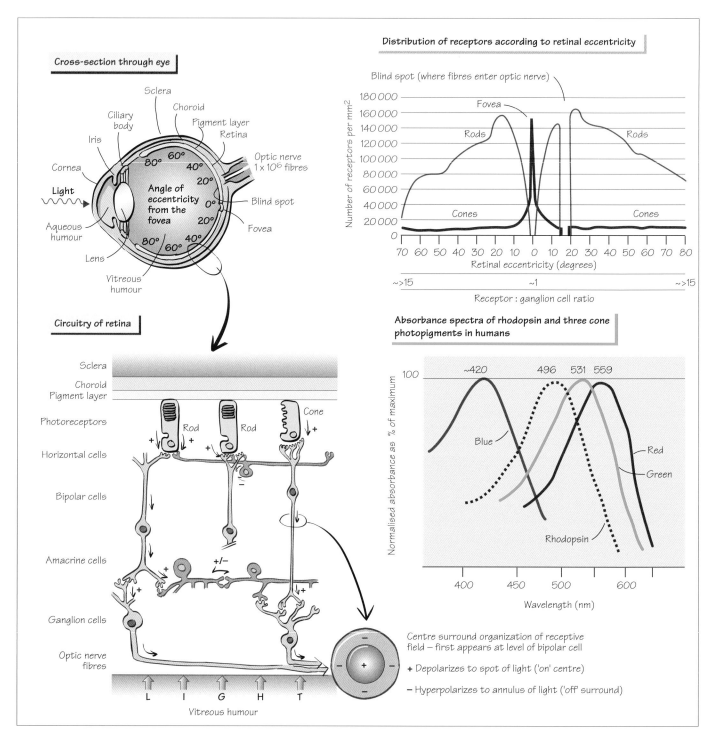

The visual system is responsible for converting all incident light energy into a visual image of the world. This information is coded for in the retina which lies at the back of the eye, and transmits that information to the visual cortical areas, the hypothalamus and upper brainstem (see Chapters 25 and 26). The process of visual transduction is detailed in Chapter 23.

Optical properties of the eye

On reaching the eye, light has to be precisely focused on to the retina, and this process of **refraction** is dependent on the curvature of the cornea and the axial length of the eye. Failure to do this accurately leads to an inability either to see clearly when reading (*long-sightedness or hypermetropia*), or to see distant objects clearly

Neuroanatomy and Neuroscience at a Glance, Fourth Edition. Roger A. Barker, Francesca Cicchetti, Michael J. Neal.

(*short-sightedness or myopia*), or both. In the latter case there is often an additional problem of *astigmatism*, in which the refraction of the eye varies in different meridians.

In addition to the need to be refracted precisely on to the retina, light must also be transmitted without any loss of quality and this relies on the cornea, anterior and posterior chambers and lens all being clear. Injuries or disease of any of these components can lead to a reduced **visual acuity** (the ability to discriminate detail). The most common conditions affecting these parts of the eye are infections and damage to the cornea (*keratitis*) or opacification of the lens (*cataracts*).

Retinal anatomy and function

Photoreceptors

The light on striking the **retina** is transduced into electrical signals by the **photoreceptors** that lie on the innermost layer of the retina, furthest from the vitreous humour. There are two main types of photoreceptors: **rods and cones**.
• *Rods*: The rods are found in all areas of the retina, except the **fovea**; they are sensitive to low levels of light and are thus responsible for our vision at night (**scotopic vision**). Many rods relay their information to a single ganglion cell, and so this system is sensitive to absolute levels of illumination while not being capable of discriminating fine visual detail and colour. Thus, at night we can detect objects but not in any detail or colour.
• *Cones*: The cones are found at highest density in the **fovea** and contain one of three different **photopigments**. They are responsible for our daytime or **photopic vision**. This, coupled to the high density of these receptors at the **fovea**, where they have an almost one-to-one relationship with ganglion cells, means that they are the receptors responsible for visual acuity and colour vision. Alterations in the photopigments contained within these receptors leads to *colour blindness*. Diseases of the receptors leading to their death, such as *retinitis pigmentosa*, lead to a progressive loss of vision that typically affects the peripheral retina and rods in the early stages, resulting in night blindness and constricted visual fields, although with time the disease process can spread to affect the cones.

Horizontal cells

The photoreceptors make synapses with both horizontal and bipolar cells. The **horizontal cells** have two major roles: (i) they create the centre surround organization of the receptive field of the bipolar cell; and (ii) they are responsible for shifting the spectral sensitivity of the bipolar cell to match the level of background illumination (part of the light adaptation response; see Chapter 23).

The **centre surround receptive field** means that a bipolar cell will respond to a small spot of light in the middle of its receptive field in one way (depolarization or hyperpolarization), while an annulus or ring of light around that central spot of light will produce an opposite response. The horizontal cells, by receiving inputs from many receptors and synapsing onto the photoreceptor bipolar cell, can provide the necessary information for this receptive field to be generated. The mechanism by which they fulfil their other role in light adaptation is not fully understood.

Bipolar cells

The **bipolar cells** relay information from the photoreceptors to the ganglion cells and receive synapses from photoreceptors, horizontal and amacrine cells. They can be classified according to the receptor they receive from (cone only, rod only, or both) or their response to light. Bipolar cells that are hyperpolarized by a small spot of light in the centre of their receptive fields are termed **off-centre (on-surround)** while the converse is true for those bipolar cells that are depolarized by a small spot of light in the centre of their receptive field.

Ganglion cells

The **ganglion cells** are found closest to the vitreous humour; they receive information from both bipolar and amacrine cells and send their axons to the brain via the optic nerve. These nerve fibres course over the inner surface of the retina before leaving at a site which forms the **optic disc** and which is responsible for the **blind spot** as no receptors are located at this site. This blind spot is not usually apparent in normal vision. The ganglion cells can be classified in a number of different ways: according to their morphology; their response to light as for bipolar cells ('on' or 'off' centre); or a combination of these properties (the **XYW system in cats** or the **M and P channels in primates**). The X ganglion cells, which make up 80% of the retinal ganglion cell population, are involved in the analysis of detail and colour while the Y ganglion cells are more involved in motion detection. The W ganglion cells, which make up the remaining 10% of the population, project to the brainstem, but as yet have no clearly defined function. The X and Y ganglion cell system defined initially in cats is equivalent to the P and M channel in primates, which is broadly responsible for 'form' and 'movement' coding, respectively. In addition, there is a small population of ganglion cells that contain a protein called melanopsin, which allows them to detect light independently of photoreceptors. These ganglion cells project to multiple sites within the central nervous system, especially the suprachiasmatic nucleus of the hypothalamus (see Chapters 11 and 25).

Amacrine cells

The **amacrine cells** of the retina, which make up the final class of retinal cells, receive and relay signals from and to bipolar, other amacrine and ganglion cells. There are many different types of amacrine cells, some of which are exclusively related to rods and others to cones, and they contain a number of different transmitters. They tend to have complex responses to light stimuli and are important in generating many of the response properties of ganglion cells, including the detection and coding of moving objects and the onset and offset of illumination.

Did you know?

The octopus has no blind spot as its retina is everted such that the photoreceptors lie directly behind the lens.

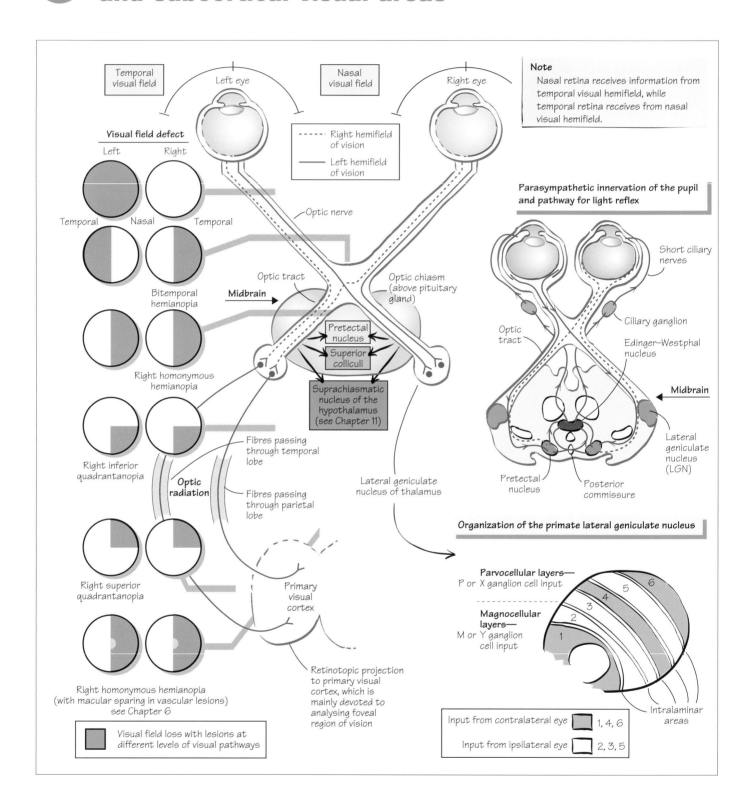

Neuroanatomy and Neuroscience at a Glance, Fourth Edition. Roger A. Barker, Francesca Cicchetti, Michael J. Neal.

58 © 2012 John Wiley & Sons, Ltd. Published 2012 by John Wiley & Sons, Ltd.

The **retina** conveys its information from the ganglion cells to a number of different sites, including:
- several cortical areas, via the lateral geniculate nucleus (LGN) of the thalamus to the primary visual cortex (V1 or Brodmann's area 17). Other cortical areas (known collectively as the extrastriate areas) receive information from the LGN as well as the pulvinar region of the thalamus (see Chapter 26);
- the hypothalamus;
- the midbrain.

The projection from the retina to V1 maintains its retinotopic organization, such that a lesion along the course of the pathway produces a predictable visual field defect. Lesions in front of the optic chiasm typically produce uniocular field defects, while lesions of the chiasm (e.g. from pituitary tumours) cause a bitemporal hemianopia. Lesions behind the chiasm typically produce similar field defects in both eyes, e.g. a homonymous hemianopia or quadrantanopia.

Lateral geniculate nucleus
- The LGN consists of six layers in primates, with each layer receiving an input from either the ipsilateral or contralateral eye.
- The inner two with their large neurones form the magnocellular laminae while the remaining four layers constitute the parvocellular laminae. The morphological distinction between the neurones in these two laminae is also evident electrophysiologically.
- The parvocellular neurones display chromatic or colour sensitivity and sensitivity to high spatial frequency (detail) with sustained responses to visual stimuli. In contrast, the magnocellular neurones show no colour selectivity, respond best to low spatial frequencies and often have a transient response on being stimulated.
- Thus, the magnocellular layer neurones have similar properties to the Y ganglion cells and the parvocellular neurones to the X ganglion cells, a similarity that is reflected in the retinogeniculate projection of these two classes of ganglion cells. The X ganglion cells and the parvocellular laminae neurones are responsible for the detection of colour and form (or *Pattern*) and constitute the **P channel**, while the **M channel** of the Y ganglion cells and the magnocellular laminae of the LGN are responsible primarily for motion detection (or *Movement*).
- The LGN mainly projects to **V1**, where the afferent fibres synapse in layer IV, and to a lesser extent layer VI, with the M and P channels having different synaptic targets within these laminae. In addition, there is a projection from cells that lie between the laminae of the LGN (intralaminar part of the LGN) directly to layers II and III of V1 (see Chapter 26).

Superior colliculi
The superior colliculus in the midbrain is a multilayered structure, wherein the superficial layers are involved in mapping the visual field and the deep layers with complex sensory integration involving visual, auditory and somatosensory stimuli. The intermediate layers are involved in saccadic eye movements and receive connections from the occipitoparietal cortex, the frontal eye fields and the substantia nigra (see Chapter 56). The saccadic eye movements are mapped in the superior colliculus to the visual field representation. So stimulation in this structure will cause a saccadic eye movement that brings the point of fixation to that point in the visual field that is represented in the more superficial layers of this structure. In the superior colliculus all the different sensorimotor representations lie in register. In other words, a vertical descent through this structure encounters, in the following order:
1. neurones that respond to visual stimuli in a given part of the visual field;
2. neurones that cause saccadic eye movements that bring the fovea to bear onto that same part of the visual scene;
3. auditory and somatosensory neurones that are maximally activated by sounds that originate from that part of the visual environment and by areas of skin that would most likely be activated by a physical contact with an object located in that part of the extrapersonal space. This latter feature accounts for the fact that in the superior colliculus the somatosensory representation is primarily skewed towards the nose and face.

Thus, the superior colliculus not only codes for saccades, but tends to code specifically for those saccades that are triggered by stimuli of immediate behavioural significance as well as having a more widespread function in orienting responses. This role for the superior colliculus is reflected in its efferent connections to a number of brainstem structures as well as the spinal cord (tectospinal tract). Clinically, damage is rarely confined to this structure, but when it is, there is a profound loss of saccadic eye movements with neglect.

Pretectal structures and the pupillary response to light
There is a projection from the optic tract to the **pretectal nuclei** of the midbrain which in turn projects bilaterally to the **Edinger–Westphal nucleus**, which provides the parasympathetic input to the pupil allowing it to constrict.
- Light shone in one eye will cause constriction of both pupils (direct and consensual response).
- Damage to one of the optic nerves will cause a reduced direct and consensual response but that same eye will constrict normally to light shone in the unaffected eye, producing a *relative afferent pupillary defect*.

Suprachiasmatic nucleus of the hypothalamus
This nucleus receives a direct retinal input and is important in the generation and coordination of circadian rhythms (see Chapter 11).

Did you know?

Palinopsia is a rare condition which refers to the delayed persistence of a visual image in the absence of its original stimulus and is usually associated with a lesion in the visual cortical association areas.

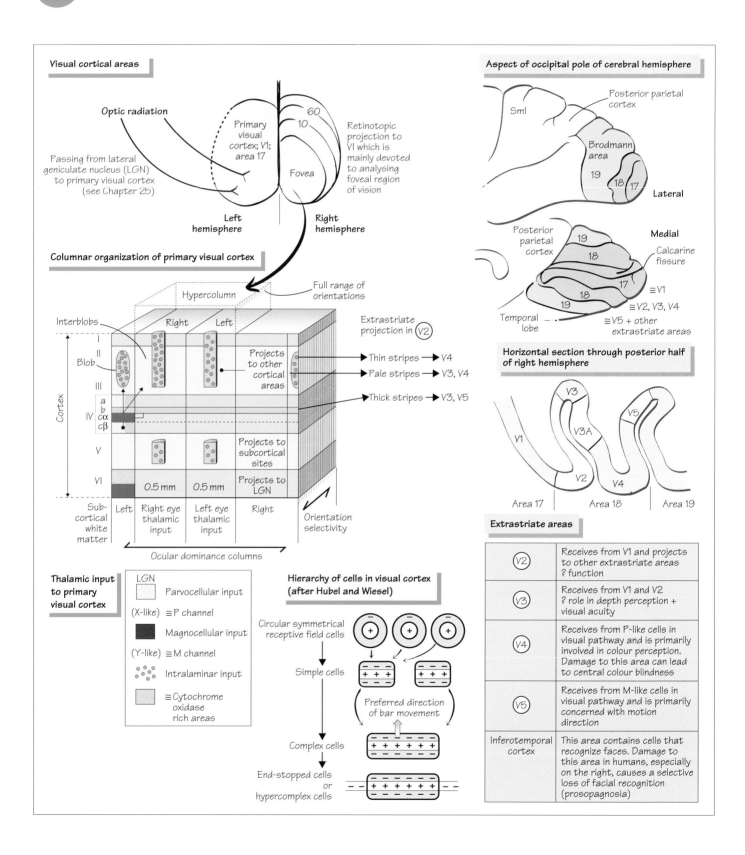

Visual cortical areas

Optic radiation

Passing from lateral geniculate nucleus (LGN) to primary visual cortex (see Chapter 25)

Primary visual cortex; V1; area 17

Fovea

Retinotopic projection to V1 which is mainly devoted to analysing foveal region of vision

60

10

Left hemisphere

Right hemisphere

Columnar organization of primary visual cortex

Hypercolumn

Full range of orientations

Interblobs

Blob

Right Left

Projects to other cortical areas

Extrastriate projection in V2

Thin stripes → V4

Pale stripes → V3, V4

Thick stripes → V3, V5

Cortex

I
II
III
IV a b cα cβ
V
VI

0.5 mm   0.5 mm

Projects to subcortical sites

Projects to LGN

Orientation selectivity

Sub-cortical white matter

Left | Right eye thalamic input | Left eye thalamic input | Right

Ocular dominance columns

Thalamic input to primary visual cortex

LGN
- Parvocellular input (X-like) ≅ P channel
- Magnocellular input (Y-like) ≅ M channel
- Intralaminar input
- ≅ Cytochrome oxidase rich areas

Hierarchy of cells in visual cortex (after Hubel and Wiesel)

Circular symmetrical receptive field cells

Simple cells

Preferred direction of bar movement

Complex cells

End-stopped cells or hypercomplex cells

Aspect of occipital pole of cerebral hemisphere

Sml

Posterior parietal cortex

Brodmann area

19

18 17

Lateral

Posterior parietal cortex

19
18
17
18
19

Medial

Calcarine fissure

≅V1
≅V2, V3, V4
≅V5 + other extrastriate areas

Temporal lobe

Horizontal section through posterior half of right hemisphere

V3

V1

V3A

V5

V2

V4

Area 17 | Area 18 | Area 19

Extrastriate areas

V2	Receives from V1 and projects to other extrastriate areas ? function
V3	Receives from V1 and V2 ? role in depth perception + visual acuity
V4	Receives from P-like cells in visual pathway and is primarily involved in colour perception. Damage to this area can lead to central colour blindness
V5	Receives from M-like cells in visual pathway and is primarily concerned with motion direction
Inferotemporal cortex	This area contains cells that recognize faces. Damage to this area in humans, especially on the right, causes a selective loss of facial recognition (prosopagnosia)

Neuroanatomy and Neuroscience at a Glance, Fourth Edition. Roger A. Barker, Francesca Cicchetti, Michael J. Neal.

60 © 2012 John Wiley & Sons, Ltd. Published 2012 by John Wiley & Sons, Ltd.

Primary visual cortex (V1 or Brodmann's area 17)

The primary visual cortex (V1) lies along the calcarine fissure of the occipital lobe and receives its major input from the lateral geniculate nucleus (LGN).

• These connections are organized **retinotopically** so that adjacent areas of the retina project up the visual pathway via neighbouring axons. However, this retinal projection is not a simple map, as the critical factor is the relationship of the photoreceptors to the projecting ganglion cell of the retina. This means that the centre of vision (especially the fovea) dominates the retinal projection to V1 because of the near one-to-one relationship of photoreceptor to ganglion cell at the fovea in contrast to the peripheral retina (see Chapter 24).

• The LGN projection to V1 is mainly to layer IV and is different for the M and P channels, while the projection from the intralaminar part of the LGN is to layers II and III of V1 (see below).

• The LGN input to layer IV of V1 is so large that this cortical layer is further subdivided into IVa, IVb, IVcα and IVcβ, with each subdivision having slightly different connections. In general, however, the cortical neurones in layer IVc of V1 have **centre surround or circular symmetrical receptive field organization** (see Chapter 24). These layer IVc neurones then project to other adjacent neurones within the cortex, in such a way that several neurones of this type converge onto a single neurone, whose receptive field is now more complex in terms of the optimal activating stimulus.

• These cells respond most effectively to a line or bar of illumination of a given orientation and are termed **simple cells**. These cells in turn project in a convergent fashion onto other neurones (**complex cells**), which are predominantly found in layers II and III, and which are maximally activated by stimuli of a given orientation moving in a particular direction. This direction is often orthogonal to the line orientation.

• The complex cells project to the **hypercomplex** or **end-stopped cells**, which respond to a line of a given orientation and length. This series of cells originally described by Hubel and Wiesel is thus organized in a hierarchical fashion, with each cell deriving its receptive field from the cells immediately beneath it in the hierarchy.

The Hubel and Wiesel model

Hubel and Wiesel further discovered that these neurones were organized into columns of cells with similar properties; the two properties that they originally studied being the eye that provides the dominant input to that neurone (giving **ocular dominance columns**) and the orientation of the line needed to activate neurones maximally (giving **orientation selective columns**).

They represented these two sets of columns as running orthogonally to each other, with the area of cortex containing an ocular dominance column from each eye with a complete set of orientation selective columns being termed the **hypercolumn**.

This hypercolumn, which is 1 mm² in size, is capable of analysing a given section of the visual field that is defined by the corresponding retinal inputs from both eyes. In the case of the fovea, where there is near unity of photoreceptors to ganglion cells, this visual field is very small, while the converse is true for more peripheral retinal inputs. Therefore a shift of 1 mm in the cortex from one hypercolumn to another leads to a shift in the location of the visual field being analysed, with most of these being concerned with foveal vision (see below).

However, there are two main complicating factors with this model:
• the accommodation of the M and P channels;
• the discovery of cytochrome oxidase (a marker of metabolic activity) – rich areas in layers II, III and IVb (and, to a lesser extent, layers V and VI), which show no orientation selectivity but colour and high spatial frequency sensitivity.

These cytochrome oxidase-rich areas in layers II and III are grouped together to form **blobs**, at least one of which is associated with each ocular dominance column, with the areas between them being termed **interblobs**. Both the blobs and interblobs, together with the cytochrome-rich layer IVb, have distinct projections to V2 and other extrastriate areas – projections that correlate well with the M and P channels. This arrangement of channels and connections suggests that visual information is processed not so much in a hierarchical fashion, but by a series of parallel pathways (see Chapter 10).

Functions of V1

The major function of V1, apart from being the first site of binocular interactions, is to deconstruct the visual field into small line segments of various orientation as well as segregating and integrating components of the visual image, which can then be relayed to more specialised visual areas. These areas perform more complex visual analysis but rely on their interaction with V1 for the conscious perception of the whole visual image. This occasionally presents itself clinically in patients with bilateral damage to V1, in which they deny being able to see any visual stimulus even though on formal testing they are capable of localizing visual targets accurately (a phenomenon known as *blindsight*).

Visual association or extrastriate areas

The **extrastriate areas** are those cortical areas outside V1 that are primarily involved in visual processing. The number of such areas varies from species to species, with the greatest number being found in humans. These areas are found within Brodmann's areas 18 and 19 and the inferotemporal cortex. They are involved in more complex visual processing than V1, with one aspect of the visual scene tending to be dominant in terms of the analysis undertaken by that cortical area (e.g. colour or motion detection). In general, damage to these areas tends to produce complex visual deficits, such as the ability to recognize objects visually (visual agnosia) or selective attributes of the image such as colour (central achromatopsia) or motion. In addition, a number of other parts of the central nervous system are associated with the visual system including the **posterior parietal cortex** (see Chapter 34); **the frontal cortex and frontal eye fields** (see Chapters 34 and 56); and the subcortical structures of the **hypothalamus** (see Chapter 23) and **upper brainstem** (see Chapter 25).

Often these projections are grouped together into a *ventral stream* which passes through the temporal lobe and is important in object recognition and a *dorsal stream* passing through the parietal lobe that is more concerned with object location.

Did you know?

People born blind have a large amount of inborn visual data stored in their brains. Depth perception is a good example of this, as an image from a single eye carries plenty of three-dimensional information about the objects contained within it.

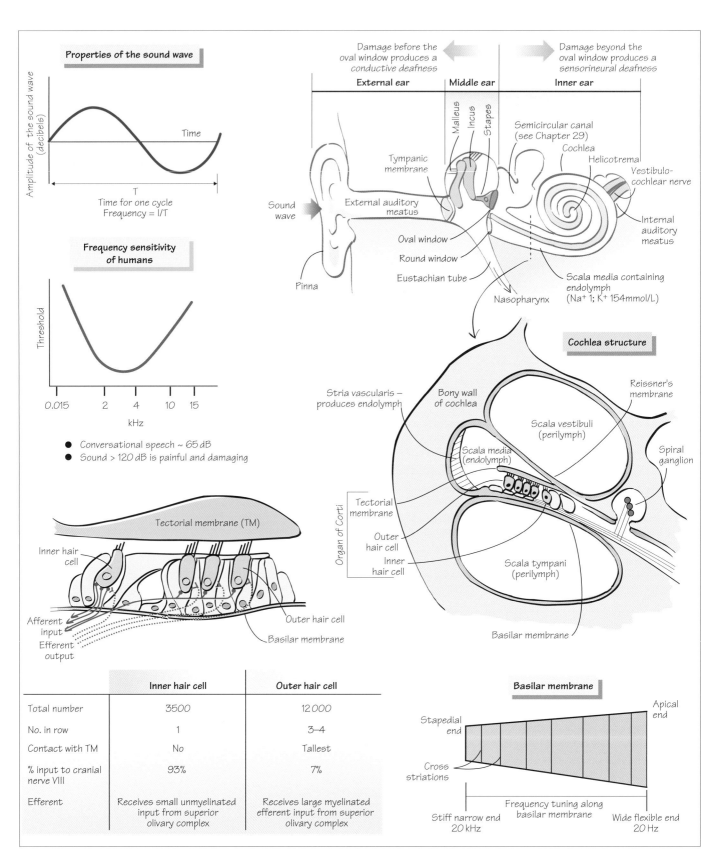

	Inner hair cell	Outer hair cell
Total number	3500	12 000
No. in row	1	3–4
Contact with TM	No	Tallest
% input to cranial nerve VIII	93%	7%
Efferent	Receives small unmyelinated input from superior olivary complex	Receives large myelinated efferent input from superior olivary complex

Neuroanatomy and Neuroscience at a Glance, Fourth Edition. Roger A. Barker, Francesca Cicchetti, Michael J. Neal.

62 © 2012 John Wiley & Sons, Ltd. Published 2012 by John Wiley & Sons, Ltd.

The **auditory system** is responsible for sound perception. The receptive end-organ is the cochlea of the inner ear, which converts sound waves into electrical signals by mechanotransduction. The electrical signal generated in response to a sound is passed (together with information from the vestibular system; see Chapter 29), via the eighth cranial nerve (vestibulocochlear nerve) to the brainstem where it synapses in the cochlear nuclear complex (see Chapter 28).

Although the auditory system as a whole performs many functions, the primary site responsible for frequency discrimination is at the level of the cochlea.

Properties of sound waves

A **sound wave** is characterized by:
- **amplitude** or **loudness** (measured in decibels [dB]);
- **frequency** or **pitch** (measured in hertz [Hz]);
- **waveform**;
- **phase** and
- **quality** or **timbre**.

The intensity of sound can vary enormously but in general we can discriminate changes in intensity of around 1–2 dB. The arrival of a sound at the head creates phase and intensity differences between the two ears unless the sound originates from the midline. The degree of delay and intensity change between the two ears as a result of their physical separation is useful but probably not necessary for the localization of sounds (see Chapter 28).

External and middle ear

On reaching the ear the sound passes down the **external auditory meatus** to the **tympanic membrane or eardrum**, which vibrates at a frequency and strength determined by the impinging sound. This causes the **three ear ossicles** in the **middle ear** to move, displacing fluid within the **cochlea** as the stapedial foot process moves within the oval window of the cochlea. This process is essential in reducing the acoustic impedance of the system and in enhancing the response to sound, because a sound hitting a fluid directly is largely reflected.

There are two small muscles associated with the ear ossicles, which protect them from damage by loud noises as well as modifying the movement of the stapedial foot process in the oval window. Damage to the ear ossicles (e.g. *otosclerosis*), middle ear (e.g. infection or *otitis media*) or external auditory meatus (e.g. blockage by wax) all lead to a reduction in hearing or *deafness* that is **conductive** in nature.

Inner ear and cochlea

The displacement of the stapedial foot process in the **oval window** generates waves in the perilymph-filled **scala vestibuli** and **tympani** of the cochlea. These two scalae are in communication at the apical end of the **cochlea**, the **helicotrema**, but are separated for the rest of their length by the **scala media**, which contains the transduction apparatus in the **organ of Corti**.

The organ of Corti sits on the floor of the scala media on a structure known as the **basilar membrane** (**BM**), the width of which increases with distance from the stapedial end. This increase in width coupled to a decrease in stiffness of the BM means that sounds of high frequency maximally displace the BM at the stapedial end of the cochlea while low-frequency sounds maximally activate the apical end of the BM. Thus, frequency tuning is, in part, a function of the BM although it is greatly enhanced and made more selective by the hair cells of the organ of Corti that lie on this membrane.

The **organ of Corti** is a complex structure that contains the cells of **auditory transduction**, the **hair cells** (see Chapter 23), which are of two types in this structure:
- a single row of **inner hair cells** (IHCs) – which provide most of the signal in the eighth cranial nerve;
- 3–4 rows of **outer hair cells** (OHCs) – which have a role in modulating the response of IHCs to a given sound.

These two types of hair cell are morphologically and electrophysiologically distinct:
- While the IHCs receive little input from the brainstem, the OHCs do so from the superior olivary complex, which has the effect of modifying the shape and response properties of these cells.
- Some of the OHCs make direct contact with the overlying **tectorial membrane** (**TM**) in the organ of Corti which may be important in modifying the response of the IHCs to sound, as these cells do not contact the TM but provide 93% of the afferent input of the cochlear nerve.
- One afferent fibre receives from many OHCs, but a single IHC is associated with many afferent fibres.

In addition to these differences between OHCs and IHCs, there are subtle alterations in the hair cells themselves with distance along the scala media. These alterations in shape modify their tuning characteristics, which adds a degree of refinement to frequency tuning beyond that imparted by the resonance properties of the BM.

Deafness

Damage to the cochlea, hair cells or cochlear part of the vestibulocochlear nerve leads to *deafness* that is described as being **sensorineural** in nature. Trauma, ischaemia and tumours of the eighth cranial nerve can lead to this. Certain hereditary causes of deafness have been associated recently with defects in the proteins found in the stereocilia of hair cells (see also Chapter 23).

Did you know?

Eating too much can actually reduce your ability to hear.

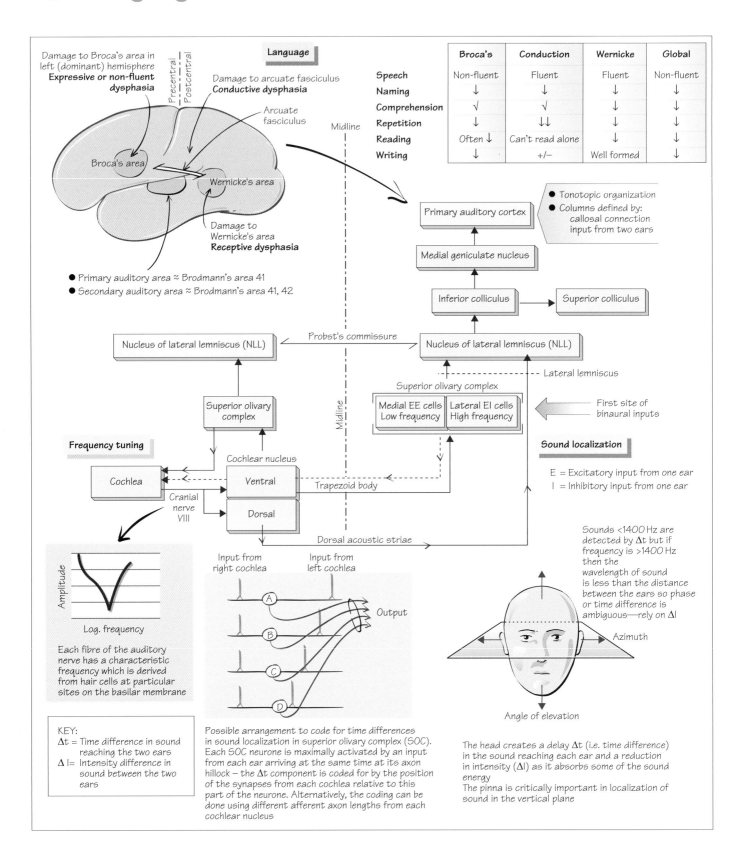

Language

	Broca's	Conduction	Wernicke	Global
Speech	Non-fluent	Fluent	Fluent	Non-fluent
Naming	↓	↓	↓	↓
Comprehension	√	√	↓	↓
Repetition	↓	↓↓	↓	↓
Reading	Often ↓	Can't read alone	↓	↓
Writing	↓	+/−	Well formed	↓

Damage to Broca's area in left (dominant) hemisphere **Expressive or non-fluent dysphasia**

Precentral / Postcentral

Damage to arcuate fasciculus **Conductive dysphasia**

Arcuate fasciculus

Midline

Broca's area

Wernicke's area

Damage to Wernicke's area **Receptive dysphasia**

- Primary auditory area ≈ Brodmann's area 41
- Secondary auditory area ≈ Brodmann's area 41, 42

● Tonotopic organization
● Columns defined by: callosal connection input from two ears

Primary auditory cortex

Medial geniculate nucleus

Inferior colliculus → Superior colliculus

Nucleus of lateral lemniscus (NLL) — Probst's commissure — Nucleus of lateral lemniscus (NLL)

Lateral lemniscus

Superior olivary complex

Midline

Medial EE cells Low frequency | Lateral EI cells High frequency

First site of binaural inputs

Frequency tuning

Cochlear nucleus

Superior olivary complex

Sound localization

E = Excitatory input from one ear
I = Inhibitory input from one ear

Cochlea

Cranial nerve VIII

Ventral

Dorsal

Trapezoid body

Dorsal acoustic striae

Sounds <1400 Hz are detected by Δt but if frequency is >1400 Hz then the wavelength of sound is less than the distance between the ears so phase or time difference is ambiguous—rely on ΔI

Amplitude / Log. frequency

Each fibre of the auditory nerve has a characteristic frequency which is derived from hair cells at particular sites on the basilar membrane

Input from right cochlea / Input from left cochlea

A B C D

Output

Azimuth

Angle of elevation

KEY:
Δt = Time difference in sound reaching the two ears
Δ I= Intensity difference in sound between the two ears

Possible arrangement to code for time differences in sound localization in superior olivary complex (SOC). Each SOC neurone is maximally activated by an input from each ear arriving at the same time at its axon hillock – the Δt component is coded for by the position of the synapses from each cochlea relative to this part of the neurone. Alternatively, the coding can be done using different afferent axon lengths from each cochlear nucleus

The head creates a delay Δt (i.e. time difference) in the sound reaching each ear and a reduction in intensity (ΔI) as it absorbs some of the sound energy
The pinna is critically important in localization of sound in the vertical plane

Neuroanatomy and Neuroscience at a Glance, Fourth Edition. Roger A. Barker, Francesca Cicchetti, Michael J. Neal.

The **vestibulocochlear or eighth cranial nerve** transmits information from both the cochlea and vestibular apparatus. Each fibre of the cochlear nerve is selectively tuned to a characteristic frequency, which is determined by its site of origin within the cochlea (see Chapter 27). These fibres are then arranged according to the location of their innervating hair cells along the basilar membrane (BM), and this tonotopic organization is maintained throughout the auditory pathway.

On entering the brainstem the cochlear nerve synapses in the cochlear nuclear complex of the medulla.

Auditory pathways

• The **cochlear nucleus** is divided into a **ventral (VCN)** and **dorsal (DCN)** part. The VCN projects to the **superior olivary complex (SOC)** bilaterally. The DCN projects via the dorsal acoustic striae to the contralateral **nucleus of the lateral lemniscus** and **inferior colliculus**.

• The **SOC** contains spindle-shaped neurones with a lateral and medial dendrite, which receive an input from each ear. It is the first site of binaural interactions and so is important in sound localization. In the **medial part of the SOC** this input is excitatory from each ear (**EE cells**) whereas in the **lateral SOC** the neurones have an excitatory input from one ear and an inhibitory input from the other (**EI cells**).

• The EE cells by virtue of their input are important in the localization of sounds of low frequency (<1.4 kHz) where the critical factor is the delay (Δt) in the sound reaching one and then the other ear. One possible arrangement relies on the differential localization of the synaptic inputs to a single SOC neurone from the two ears.

• The EI cells are important in the localization of higher frequency sounds where the difference in intensity (ΔI) of sound between the two ears is important (ΔI being generated as a result of the head acting as a shield). Sounds of frequencies greater than 1.4 kHz (in the case of humans) rely on ΔI for localization. In the case of sounds originating in the midline, there will be no Δt and no ΔI, and there is some confusion in localization which can be overcome to some extent by moving the head or using other sensory cues.

• The localization of sound within the vertical plane is dependent in some way on the pinna.

• The SOC not only projects rostrally to the **inferior colliculus (IC)**, but also has an important input to the cochlea where it primarily controls the OHCs and by so doing the response properties of the organ of Corti (see Chapter 27). The projection to the IC is tonotopic, and this structure also receives an input from the **primary auditory cortex (A1)** and other sensory modalities. In this respect it interacts with the superior colliculus and is involved in the orienting response to novel audiovisual stimuli (see Chapters 25 and 56).

• The IC projects to the **medial geniculate nucleus of the thalamus (MGN)**, which projects to the **A1** in the superior temporal gyrus. This area corresponds to Brodmann's areas 41 and 42, with the thalamic afferent input synapsing in layers III and IV of the cortex. The columnar organization of A1 is poorly defined, but the tonotopic map is maintained so that low-frequency sounds are located posteriorly and high-frequency sounds anteriorly.

Language

Language is organized in the dominant, typically left hemisphere and is best developed and most studied in the human brain.

• The localization and network subserving language is controversial as much of the early work used lesion studies, which of late has been refined using functional imaging studies.

• Language dysfunction typically occurs in the context of stroke but can be affected in isolation in some neurodegenerative conditions – such as primary progressive aphasia.

• Developmentally abnormalities in language can occur in isolation or be part of a more widespread problem such as autism, learning disabilities, and importantly can also be seen with hearing problems.

Did you know?

Children who learn two languages before the age of 5 years have altered brain structure while adults who do this have more dense grey matter.

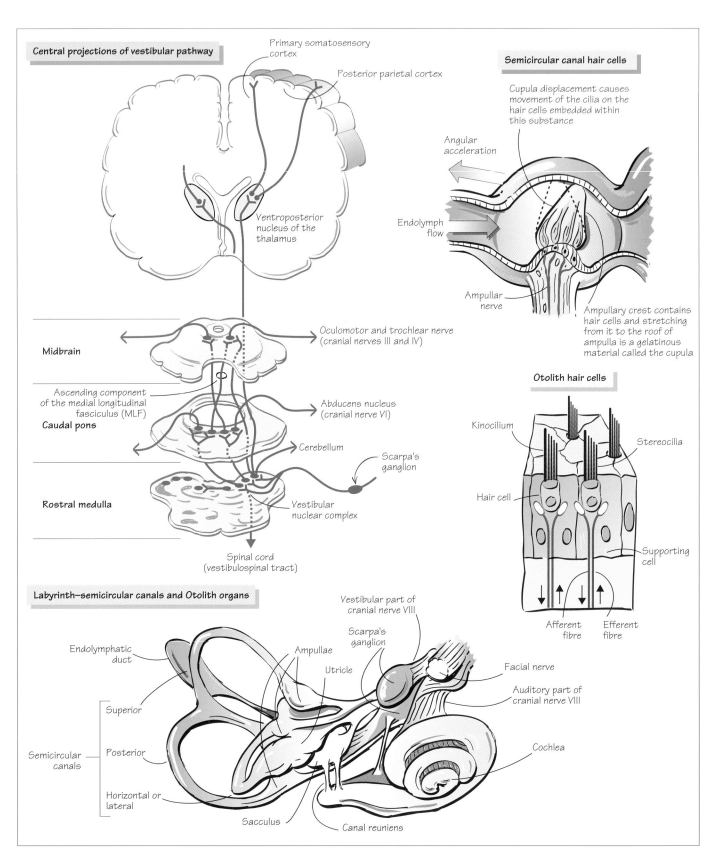

Central projections of vestibular pathway

Primary somatosensory cortex

Posterior parietal cortex

Ventroposterior nucleus of the thalamus

Midbrain

Oculomotor and trochlear nerve (cranial nerves III and IV)

Ascending component of the medial longitudinal fasciculus (MLF)

Caudal pons

Abducens nucleus (cranial nerve VI)

Cerebellum

Scarpa's ganglion

Rostral medulla

Vestibular nuclear complex

Spinal cord (vestibulospinal tract)

Semicircular canal hair cells

Cupula displacement causes movement of the cilia on the hair cells embedded within this substance

Angular acceleration

Endolymph flow

Ampullar nerve

Ampullary crest contains hair cells and stretching from it to the roof of ampulla is a gelatinous material called the cupula

Otolith hair cells

Kinocilium

Stereocilia

Hair cell

Supporting cell

Afferent fibre

Efferent fibre

Labyrinth–semicircular canals and Otolith organs

Endolymphatic duct

Ampullae

Vestibular part of cranial nerve VIII

Scarpa's ganglion

Utricle

Facial nerve

Auditory part of cranial nerve VIII

Superior

Posterior

Semicircular canals

Horizontal or lateral

Cochlea

Sacculus

Canal reuniens

Neuroanatomy and Neuroscience at a Glance, Fourth Edition. Roger A. Barker, Francesca Cicchetti, Michael J. Neal.

The vestibular system is concerned with balance, postural reflexes and eye movements, and is one of the oldest systems of the brain. It consists of a peripheral transducer component which projects to the brainstem (including the oculomotor nuclei), and from there to the thalamus and sensory cortex as well as to the cerebellum and spinal cord. Disruption to the system (e.g., *vestibular neuronitis/labyrinthitis*) results in the symptoms of dizziness, vertigo, nausea with or without blurred vision with signs of eye movement abnormalities (typically nystagmus; see Chapter 56) and unsteadiness. In the comatose patient, clinical testing of the vestibular system can provide useful information on the integrity of the brainstem, as it is associated with a number of primitive brainstem reflexes (see Chapter 44).

Vestibular transduction

The peripheral transducer component consists of the: **labyrinth**, which is made up of two **otolith organs** (the **utricle** and the **sacculus**) together with the **ampullae** located in the three **semicircular canals**.

The otolith organs are primarily concerned with static head position and linear acceleration while the semicircular canals are more concerned with rotational (angular) acceleration of the head.

Hair cells are found in both the otolith organs and the ampullae and are similar in structure to those found in the cochlea (see Chapters 23 and 27). As in the cochlea, deflection of the **stereocilia** towards the kinocilium depolarizes the cell and allows transmitter to be released from the hair cell, leading to activation of the associated afferent fibre. The converse is true if the stereocilia are deflected in the opposite direction.

Movement of the cilia is associated with rotational movement of the head (ampullae receptors in the semicircular canals) and acceleration or tilting of the head (otolith organs in utricle), as although head movement causes the **endolymph** bathing the hair cells to move, it 'lags behind' and so distorts the stereocilia.

Spontaneous activity in the afferent fibres is high, reflecting the spontaneous leakage of transmitter from the cell at the synapse. Hyperpolarization of the hair cell therefore results in a reduced afferent discharge, while depolarization is associated with an increase in firing. Efferent fibres from the brainstem terminating on the hair cells can change the sensitivity of the receptor end-organ.

Peripheral disorders of the vestibular system

Damage to the peripheral vestibular system is not uncommon. Examples include:
• *Benign paroxysmal positional vertigo* (*BPPV*) commonly occurs after trauma or infection of the vestibular apparatus with the deposition of debris (e.g. otolith crystals or otoconia) typically in the posterior semicircular canal. This condition, which is characterized by paroxysms of vertigo, nausea and ataxia induced by turning the head into certain positions (such as lying down or rolling over in bed), is therefore the consequence of distortion of endolymph flow in this canal secondary to the debris. It is diagnosed using Hallpike's manoeuvre, which seeks to manipulate the head in such a way as to provoke the episode of vertigo. Treatment and cure can be effective by undertaking a series of head manoeu-

vres (classically Epley's manoeuvre), which allows the debris to fall out of the semicircular canal and into the ampullae.
• Viral infections of the vestibular apparatus are common (*labyrinthitis*) and can be severely disabling with profound dizziness and vomiting without any head movement. Such infections are usually self-limiting.
• Bilateral failure of the vestibular apparatus can result in *oscillopsia*, a symptom describing an inability to visually fixate on objects especially with head movements (see Chapter 56). In contrast, powerful excitation of the vestibular system, such as that encountered during motion sickness produces dizziness, vomiting, sweating and tachycardia, caused by discrepancies between vestibular and visual information.

Vestibular function can be tested by introducing water into the external meatus (**caloric testing**).

When warm water is applied to a seated subject whose head is tilted back by about 60°, nystagmus towards the treated side is observed.

Cold water produces nystagmus towards the opposite side.
These effects reflect the changes in the temperature of the endolymph and an effect resembling head rotation away from the irrigated side.

Central vestibular system and vestibular reflexes

Afferent vestibular fibres in the eighth cranial nerve have their cell bodies in the vestibular (**Scarpa's**) **ganglion** and terminate in one of the **four vestibular nuclei** in the medulla, which also receive inputs from neck muscle receptors and the visual system.

The vestibular nuclei project to:
• the spinal cord (see Chapters 9, 37 and 40);
• the contralateral vestibular nuclei;
• the cerebellum;
• the oculomotor nuclei;
• and the ipsilateral and contralateral thalamus.

Some of these structures are important in reflex eye movements, such as the ability to maintain visual fixation while moving the head – the vestibulo-ocular reflex (VOR; see Chapters 40, 49 and 56). Other projections of the vestibular nuclei are important in maintaining posture and gait. The cortical termination of the vestibular input to the CNS is the **primary somatosensory cortex (SmI)** and the **posterior parietal cortex** (see Chapter 34). Very rarely, *epileptic* seizures can originate in this area and give symptoms of vestibular disturbance.

Disorders of central vestibular pathways

Caloric testing of the vestibular system examines the integrity of the vestibular apparatus and its brainstem connections. Therefore, it can be useful in comatosed patients when the degree of brainstem function needs to be ascertained. Less severe central damage to the vestibular apparatus can occur in a number of conditions including *multiple sclerosis* (see Chapter 62) and vascular insults (see Chapter 64). In most cases other structures are involved and so there are other symptoms and signs on examination.

Did you know?

The vestibular system in man can detect changes in head orientation of as little as of 0.5° from the upright.

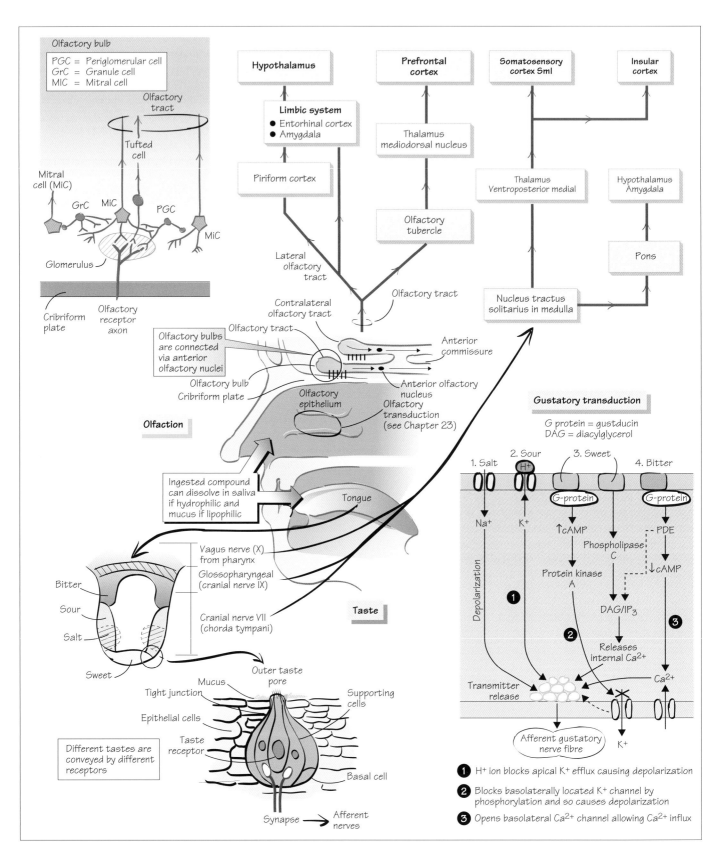

Neuroanatomy and Neuroscience at a Glance, Fourth Edition. Roger A. Barker, Francesca Cicchetti, Michael J. Neal.

The **olfactory** or **first cranial nerve** contains more fibres than any other sensory nerve projecting to the CNS, while **taste** is relayed via the seventh, ninth and tenth cranial nerves (see Chapter 7).

Olfaction

The olfactory system as a whole is able to discriminate a great diversity of different chemical stimuli or odours, and this is made possible through thousands of different **olfactory receptors**. These receptors are located in the apical dendrite of the olfactory receptor cell and the axon of this cell projects directly into the central nervous system (CNS) via the **cribriform plate** at the top of the nose to the olfactory bulb.

The **olfactory stimulus or odour**, on binding to the olfactory receptor, depolarizes it (see Chapter 23) which, if sufficient, leads to the generation of action potentials at the cell body which are then conducted down the olfactory nerve axons to the olfactory bulb.

The **olfactory nerve** passes through the roof of the nose through a bone known as the cribriform plate. Damage to this structure (e.g. head trauma) can shear the olfactory nerve axons causing a loss of smell or *anosmia*, although the most common cause of a loss of smell is local trouble within the nose, usually infection and inflammation. The olfactory receptor axons then synapse in the olfactory bulb that lies at the base of the frontal lobe. Damage to this structure, as occurs in frontal *meningiomas*, produces anosmia that can be unilateral.

The **olfactory bulb** contains a complex arrangement of cells. The axons from the olfactory nerve synapse on the apical dendrites of mitral and, to a lesser extent, tufted cells, both of which project out of the olfactory bulb as the olfactory tract. The olfactory bulb contains a number of inhibitory interneurones (granule and periglomerular cells), which are important in modifying the flow of olfactory information through the bulb. Some of these neurones are replaced throughout life, with the neural precursor cells for them originating in the subventricular zone and then migrating to the olfactory bulb via the rostral migratory stream, a structure that has been shown to exist in the adult mammalian brains including in humans. This system may be important in olfactory learning.

The **olfactory tract** projects to the temporal lobe where it synapses in the **piriform cortex** and **limbic system**, which projects to the **hypothalamus**. This projection is important in the behavioural effects of olfaction, which are perhaps more evident in other species. In humans, lesions in these structures rarely produce a pure anosmia, but activation of this area of the CNS as occurs in *temporal lobe epilepsy* (see Chapter 61) is associated with the abnormal perception of smells (e.g. olfactory hallucinations).

The projection of the olfactory system to the thalamus is small and is mediated via the olfactory tubercle to the mediodorsal nucleus, which projects to the prefrontal cortex. The role of this pathway is not clear.

Taste

The **taste** or **gustatory receptors** are located in the tongue. They are clustered together in fungiform papillae with supportive stem cells; the latter dividing to replace damaged gustatory receptors. The apical surface of the gustatory receptor contains microvilli covered in mucus, which is generated by the neighbouring goblet cells. Any ingested compound can therefore reach the gustatory receptor; hydrophilic substances are dissolved in saliva while lipophilic substances are dissolved in the mucus. Taste is traditionally classified according to four modalities – salt, sour, sweet and bitter – which correlate well with the different transduction processes that are now known to exist for these different tastes. A fifth taste (umami) has also recently been described.

• **Salt stimuli** cause a direct depolarization of the gustatory receptors by virtue of the fact that Na^+ passes through an amiloride-sensitive apical membrane channel. The depolarization leads to the release of neurotransmitter from the basal part of the cell which activates the afferent fibres in the relevant cranial nerve.

• **Sour stimuli**, in contrast, probably achieve a similar effect by blocking apical voltage-dependent H^+ channels.

• **Sweet stimuli** bind to a receptor that activates the G protein, gustducin, which then through adenylate cyclase leads to cyclic adenosine monophosphate (cAMP) production. The rise in cAMP activates a protein kinase that phosphorylates and closes basolateral K^+ channels and by so doing depolarizes the receptor.

• **Bitter stimuli** similarly rely on receptor binding and G-protein activation. One pathway involves gustducin but, in this instance, it leads to activation of a cAMP phosphodiesterase, which reduces the level of cAMP (and so the phosphorylating protein kinase) leading to opening of the basolateral Ca^{2+} channels and so transmitter release. An alternative pathway for both sweet and bitter tastes involves the activation of a phospholipase C and the production of inositol triphosphate (IP_3) and diacylglycerol (DAG), which can release Ca^{2+} from internal stores within the receptor. The increased Ca^{2+} concentration promotes neurotransmitter release.

The receptors relay their information via the **chorda tympani** (anterior two-thirds of the tongue) and **glossopharyngeal nerve** (posterior third of the tongue) to **the nucleus of the solitary tract** in the medulla (see Chapters 7 and 8). The structure projects rostrally via the thalamus to the primary somatosensory cortex (SmI) and the insular cortex, with a possible additional projection to the hypothalamus and amygdala. Some patients with *temporal lobe epilepsy* have an aura of an abnormal taste in the mouth which may relate to ictal electrical activity within the temporal lobe (see Chapter 61).

Did you know?

It is possible for the human nose to identify and discriminate more than 50 000 smells.

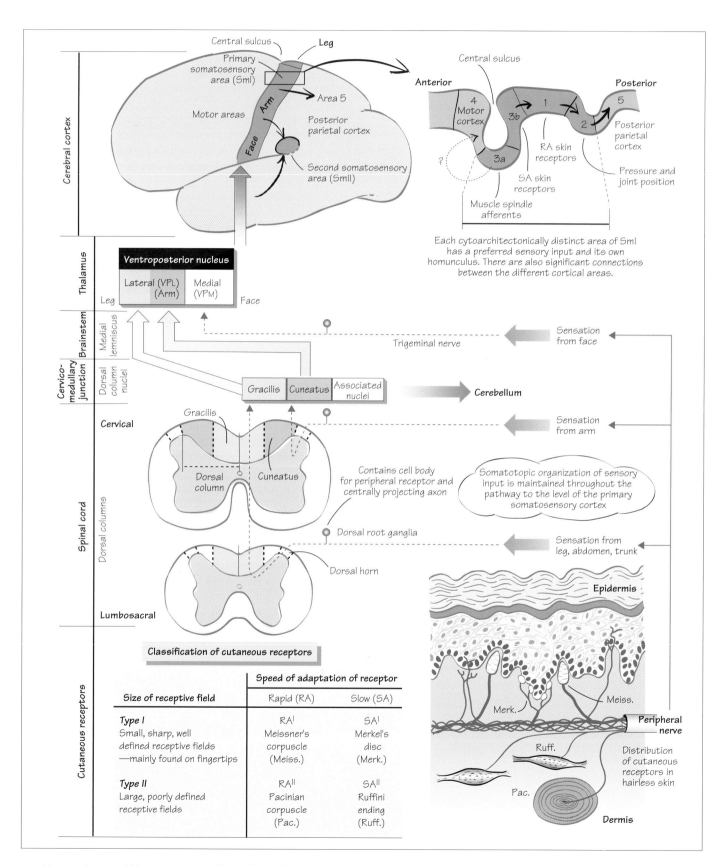

Each cytoarchitectonically distinct area of SmI has a preferred sensory input and its own homunculus. There are also significant connections between the different cortical areas.

Somatotopic organization of sensory input is maintained throughout the pathway to the level of the primary somatosensory cortex

Contains cell body for peripheral receptor and centrally projecting axon

Classification of cutaneous receptors

Size of receptive field	Speed of adaptation of receptor	
	Rapid (RA)	Slow (SA)
Type I Small, sharp, well defined receptive fields —mainly found on fingertips	RA^I Meissner's corpuscle (Meiss.)	SA^I Merkel's disc (Merk.)
Type II Large, poorly defined receptive fields	RA^{II} Pacinian corpuscle (Pac.)	SA^{II} Ruffini ending (Ruff.)

Distribution of cutaneous receptors in hairless skin

Neuroanatomy and Neuroscience at a Glance, Fourth Edition. Roger A. Barker, Francesca Cicchetti, Michael J. Neal.

The somatosensory system is the part of the nervous system that is involved in the processes of touch, pressure, proprioception (or joint position sense; see also Chapter 36), pain and temperature perception (see Chapters 32 and 33).

Sensory receptors

The **receptors for touch** are specialized nerve endings located in the skin with their cell bodies in the dorsal root ganglia. They are found at particularly high density in the fingertips, while those for proprioception are found not only in the skin but also in the muscle and joints (see Chapter 36).

Skin receptors can best be characterized by their structure, location, receptive fields and speed of adaptation.

• Type I receptors with very small, sharply demarcated receptive fields (**Meissner's corpuscles** and **Merkel's discs**) are packed in high density at the fingertips. In particular, Meissner's corpuscles convey information about objects slipping or moving across the skin, while Merkel's discs are more involved with fine touch (i.e. sensory detail).

• In contrast, the rapidly adapting (RA) **Pacinian corpuscles** convey vibration perception as they quickly stop firing to continuous sensory stimulus.

• The more slowly adapting (SA) **Ruffini endings** sense the magnitude, direction and rate of change of tension in the skin and deeper tissues (i.e. skin stretch).

Dorsal column–medial lemniscal pathway

The sensory receptors are specialized nerve endings and the fast conducting, large diameter axons associated with them are found in peripheral nerves and project into the **dorsal horn** of the spinal cord. The **trigeminal sensory system** for the face has a similar organization.

Each class of receptor has a specific pattern of passage through the dorsal horn, but all ultimately end up in the **dorsal column** (with the exception of the trigeminal system), where they are organized according to receptor type and body location (somatotopy; see Chapter 9). They then project ipsilaterally up to the dorsal column nuclei at the cervicomedullary junction (consisting of the gracile and cuneate nuclei), where they make their first synapse, although it should be understood that many dorsal column axons synapse at other spinal sites.

• The **dorsal column nuclei (DCN)** are a complex series of structures that lie at the cervicomedullary junction and send axons which immediately decussate to form the **medial lemniscus**, which projects to the thalamus. The DCN also project to other brainstem structures, as well as receiving input from the primary somatosensory cortex (SmI).

• The medial lemniscus projects to the **ventroposterior (VP) nucleus of the thalamus**, connecting with the trigeminal system as it ascends. This latter projection synapses in the medial part of the VP nucleus (VPM) with the remainder of the tract terminating in the lateral nucleus (VPL). This medial lemniscal termination is in the form of an anteroposterior thalamic rod, where all the cells within the rod have a similar modality and peripheral location (e.g. index finger,

RA type I receptors). The thalamic rod subsequently projects to layer IV of the SmI and forms the basis of the cortical column (see also Chapter 10).

• The **SmI** consists of four different areas (Brodmann's areas 3a, 3b, 1 and 2), each of which has a separate representation of the contralateral body surface, with the tongue being represented laterally and the feet medially. The cortical representation is proportional to the receptor density in the skin so, for example, the hand has a much greater representation than the trunk (the **sensory homunculus**).

Primary and secondary sensory cortices

Each cortical area within SmI has slightly different response properties with respect to the neurones found in these areas. As one moves towards the posterior parietal cortex the response properties of the neurones become more complex, implying a higher level of cortical analysis. SmI projects not only back to the dorsal column nuclei but to the **posterior parietal cortex** and **second somatosensory area (SmII)**. This latter area is found in the lateral wall of the Sylvian sulcus and is important in tactile object recognition, while the posterior parietal cortex input from SmI is important in the attribution of significance to a sensory stimulus (see Chapter 34).

The primary somatosensory pathway has developed during evolution with the corticospinal tract (CoST), which has a selective role in the control of fine finger movements (see Chapters 35–39). These two systems act together in the process of 'active touch' by which we explore our environment. Both systems display a degree of plasticity even in adult life (see Chapters 39 and 49). This is in part made possible by somatotopic organization of the sensory pathway: adjacent areas of skin are represented in neighbouring parts of the sensory system, at least as far as SmI.

Clinical disorders of the somatosensory system

Damage to the receptors and their afferent fibres can occur in a large number of *peripheral neuropathies*. Patients typically complain of both paraesthesiae and numbness, often in association with alterations in proprioception especially if the dorsal root ganglion is involved (see Chapter 54).

Damage to the somatosensory pathway above the level of the DCN produces a contralateral sensory loss that will involve the face if the lesion lies at or above the level of the upper brainstem. Lesions to the dorsal columns in the spinal cord are described in Chapter 54.

Did you know?

Tickling involves both pain and touch fibres. You tickle mostly because of surprise. Even if you know you are about to be tickled, you do not necessarily know where, so you react by being ticklish. When you try to tickle yourself, it usually does not work because your brain already knows how you are going to do it. In other words, you cannot tickle yourself because you cannot surprise yourself.

32 Pain systems I: nociceptors and nociceptive pathways

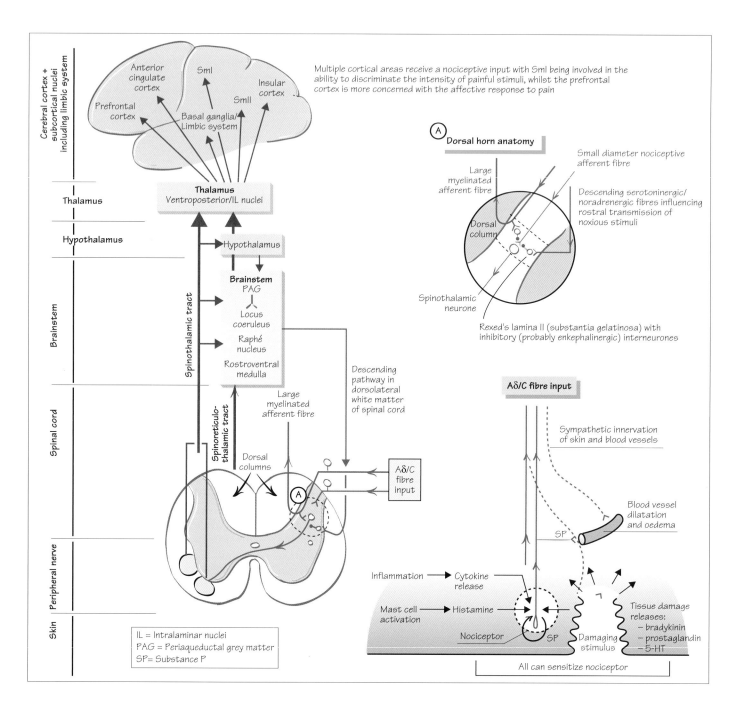

Multiple cortical areas receive a nociceptive input with SmI being involved in the ability to discriminate the intensity of painful stimuli, whilst the prefrontal cortex is more concerned with the affective response to pain

IL = Intralaminar nuclei
PAG = Periaqueductal grey matter
SP= Substance P

All can sensitize nociceptor

Pain is defined as an unpleasant sensory or emotional experience associated with actual or potential tissue damage. Much of what is known about pain mechanisms has derived from animal-based research where the affective component is unclear. For this reason neuroscientists prefer to use the term **nociception**, which defines the processing of information about damaging stimuli up to the point where perception occurs. This is an important distinction because tissue damage is not inevitably linked to pain and vice versa.

Nociceptors

Nociceptors are found in the skin, visceral organs, skeletal and cardiac muscle and in association with blood vessels. They conduct information about noxious events to the dorsal horn of the spinal cord where the primary afferents synapse.

There are basically two types of nociceptor, distinguished by the diameter of the afferent fibre and the stimulus required to activate it.

Neuroanatomy and Neuroscience at a Glance, Fourth Edition. Roger A. Barker, Francesca Cicchetti, Michael J. Neal.

- The **high-threshold mechanoreceptor (HTM)** is activated by intense mechanical stimulation and innervated by **thinly myelinated Aδ fibres** conducting at 5–30 m/s.
- **Polymodal nociceptors (PMN)** respond to intense mechanical stimulation, temperatures in excess of about 42 °C and irritant chemicals. These receptors are innervated by **unmyelinated C fibres** conducting at 0.5–2 m/s.

Sharply localized pain is thought to be conducted in the faster conducting fibres whereas poorly localized pain is conducted in the C fibres.

Although nociceptors are histologically simple free nerve endings, the process of **transduction** at the receptor ending is complex and is associated with some of the chemical mediators of inflammation and tissue damage. Thus, adenosine triphosphate (ATP), bradykinin, histamine and prostaglandins all either activate or sensitize the receptor ending. Indeed, some of the transmitters in the nociceptive pathway are themselves released peripherally **(e.g. substance P)** to produce further sensitization of the receptor ending. Nociceptor receptor sensitization helps explain the perception of heightened pain **(primary hyperalgesia)** in areas of tissue damage and is essentially a peripheral phenomenon usually of relatively short duration.

Chronic and referred pain

Pain that lasts many months is known as chronic pain. It is often disabling and resistant to treatment. It may arise following damage to either the peripheral or central nervous system or chronic inflammatory states (e.g. osteoarthritis). Changes in peripheral nociceptor sensitivity does not explain *secondary hyperalgesia*, in which light touch outside the immediate area of cutaneous damage can lead to pain.

A more serious problem associated with peripheral or central nerve damage is *allodynia*. In this condition light stroking of the skin can give rise to severe pain. Disturbed patterns of sensory input to the dorsal horn (e.g. following compression or sectioning of a peripheral nerve trunk) can lead to long-term changes in the processing of noxious information in the dorsal horn. At these sites, the arrival of axonally conducted substance P in the superficial layers of the dorsal horn leads to both an increase in receptive field sizes and the sensitivity of some dorsal horn neurones. These functional changes are mediated in part by the synaptic release of glutamate acting on postsynaptic *N*-methyl-D-aspartate (NMDA) receptors and may contribute to some chronic pain states.

In addition, allodynia and secondary hyperalgesia are linked to increased activity in microglia and astrocytes, and the release of a number of agents (interleukin-1 and -6, tumour necrosis factor [TNF], nitric oxide [NO], ATP and prostaglandins).

Damage to peripheral nerve trunks can lead to *complex regional pain syndrome* (*CPRS*). One form is associated with disturbances to the sympathetic nervous system (SNS) (CRPS-1, of which reflex sympathetic dystrophy is an example). Severing a peripheral nerve trunk leads to the formation of a neuroma which acts as a generator of ectopic action potentials (ectopic foci) sending barrages of action potentials to the spinal cord. This activity is thought to explain the development of phantom limb pain with the neuroma being sensitive to both mechanical stimulation and SNS activity (i.e. noradrenaline).

Visceral nociceptors project into the spinal cord via the small-diameter myelinated and unmyelinated fibres of the autonomic nervous system (ANS), and synapse at the spinal level of their embryological origin. The development of pain in an internal organ can therefore produce the perception of a painful stimulus in the skin rather than the organ itself, at least in the early stages of inflammation – a phenomenon known as referred pain. For example, inflammation of the appendix initially leads to pain being perceived at the umbilicus.

Nociceptive pathways

The majority of nociceptors and thermoreceptors project into the spinal cord via the dorsal root, although some pass through the ventral horn. On reaching the spinal cord these sensory nerves synapse in a complex fashion in the dorsal horn.

- The postsynaptic cell conveying nociceptive information projects up the spinal cord as the **spinothalamic**, **spinoreticulothalamic** and **spinomesencephalic** tracts (latter not shown on figure), with the axons crossing at the spinal level by passing around the central canal of the cord. This crossing of fibres often occurs a few levels above where the nociceptive fibres enter the cord, and thus damage in the region of the central canal as seen in *syringomyelia* results in a loss of pain and temperature sensibility (see Chapter 54).
- The postsynaptic cell and presynaptic nociceptive nerve terminal receive synapses from other peripherally projecting somatosensory systems, descending projections from the brainstem and interneurones intrinsic to the dorsal horn. Many of these interneurones contain **endogenous opioid substances** known as enkephalins and endorphins which activate opioid receptors of which there are three main subtypes (μ, κ, δ). There is therefore enormous potential for modifying the transfer of nociceptive information at the level of the dorsal horn (see Chapter 33).
- The **ascending nociceptive pathways** synapse in a number of different central nervous system (CNS) sites. Information concerning noxious events ascends in either the spinothalamic tract (providing accurate localization) or the spinoreticulothalamic system (transmitting information concerning the affective components of pain). However, some of the nuclei in the brainstem to which these pathways project (e.g. the raphé nucleus and locus coeruleus) in turn send axons back down the spinal cord to the dorsal horn, and can be exploited in the control of chronic pain syndromes (see Chapter 33).
- The thalamic termination of the spinothalamic pathway is in the ventroposterior and intralaminar nuclei (IL) (including the posterior group), which in turn project to multiple cortical areas but especially the primary and secondary somatosensory area (SmI and SmII) and the anterior cingulate cortex. Lesions to any of these sites alter the perception of pain but do not produce a true and complete loss of pain or analgesia, and indeed may even produce a chronic pain syndrome. Such syndromes are not uncommonly seen with small thalamic cerebrovascular accidents.

The thermoreceptors, and to a lesser extent the nociceptors, also project to the hypothalamus, which has an important role in thermoregulation and the autonomic response to a painful stimulus (see Chapters 3 and 11).

Did you know?

Men and women react differently to pain, which may explain why the two sexes discuss pain differently.

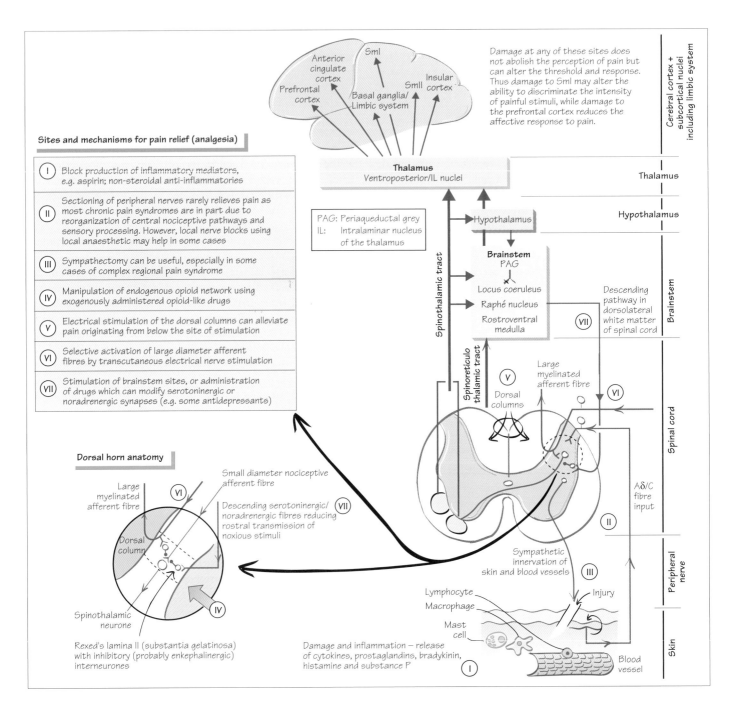

Sites and mechanisms for pain relief (analgesia)

- (I) Block production of inflammatory mediators, e.g. aspirin; non-steroidal anti-inflammatories
- (II) Sectioning of peripheral nerves rarely relieves pain as most chronic pain syndromes are in part due to reorganization of central nociceptive pathways and sensory processing. However, local nerve blocks using local anaesthetic may help in some cases
- (III) Sympathectomy can be useful, especially in some cases of complex regional pain syndrome
- (IV) Manipulation of endogenous opioid network using exogenously administered opioid-like drugs
- (V) Electrical stimulation of the dorsal columns can alleviate pain originating from below the site of stimulation
- (VI) Selective activation of large diameter afferent fibres by transcutaneous electrical nerve stimulation
- (VII) Stimulation of brainstem sites, or administration of drugs which can modify serotoninergic or noradrenergic synapses (e.g. some antidepressants)

Damage at any of these sites does not abolish the perception of pain but can alter the threshold and response. Thus damage to Sml may alter the ability to discriminate the intensity of painful stimuli, while damage to the prefrontal cortex reduces the affective response to pain.

PAG: Periaqueductal grey
IL: Intralaminar nucleus of the thalamus

Dorsal horn anatomy

The development of pain is a common experience and the treatment for it is important, not only where it is caused by injury or inflammation, but also in cases where the nerves themselves are damaged. In these latter cases the pain can arise from a site of previous injury (e.g. *allodynia*) or may develop for more obscure reasons, now renamed *complex regional pain syndrome*. In all cases, pain is both disabling and depressing, and a multidisciplinary approach to management is often needed. However, it should also be realized that some patients with affective disorders, such as depression and anxiety, may complain of pain in the absence of any obvious tissue damage.

Management of pain

Pain relief or analgesia can be approached using a number of different strategies.

Neuroanatomy and Neuroscience at a Glance, Fourth Edition. Roger A. Barker, Francesca Cicchetti, Michael J. Neal.

Site I

Many analgesic therapies work by reducing the peripheral inflammatory response, which is also responsible for receptor sensitization (**site I** on figure). Non-steroidal anti-inflammatory drugs (NSAIDs) are the most widely used analgesics. These drugs have analgesic, antipyretic and, at higher doses, anti-inflammatory actions. *Aspirin* was the first NSAID but has been largely replaced by drugs that are less toxic to the gastrointestinal tract, e.g. paracetamol, ibuprofen, naproxen. NSAIDs produce their effects by inhibiting cyclo-oxygenase (COX), a key enzyme in the production of prostaglandins (PGs). PGs are one of the mediators released at sites of inflammation. They do not themselves cause pain but they potentiate the pain caused by other mediators, e.g. bradykinin, 5-hydroxytryptamine (5-HT), histamine (**site I** on figure).

NSAIDs are not effective in the treatment of visceral pain, which usually requires opioid analgesics.

Site II

The interruption of peripheral nerve conduction by injection of local anaesthetics can be helpful in some pain states, but lesioning of the peripheral nerve is usually without effect in ameliorating neuropathic pain (**site II**), unless it is to remove a neuroma.

Site III

This site involves blocking aberrant sympathetic innervation/activation of peripheral nociceptors as occurs in some patients in response to nerve/limb injury (see below).

Sites IV–VII

The organization of the nociceptive input to the dorsal horn has been explored clinically in pain management. For example, stimulation of non-nociceptive receptors can inhibit the transmission of nociceptive information in the dorsal horn, which means that painful stimuli can be 'gated' out by counter-irritation using non-painful stimuli. This is the basis of the **gate theory** of Wall and Melzack and is exploited clinically in the use of transcutaneous nerve stimulation (TENS) in areas of pain (**site VI**), as well as the stimulation of the dorsal columns themselves in some cases of chronic pain (**site V**).

Similarly, the supraspinal input can also gate out noxious stimuli when activated (**site VII**), as occurs in stressful situations, when attending to a painful stimulus would not necessarily be useful (e.g. war injuries). These supraspinal nuclei can also be manipulated pharmacologically, with the administration of drugs that are usually used in the treatment of depression (see Chapter 57). These antidepressant drugs with a presumed action at the noradrenergic and serotoninergic synapses have been used to treat pain states, irrespective of any antidepressant action they might have (**site VII**). The most commonly used agents are amine uptake inhibitors, such as imipramine and amitriptyline (tricyclic antidepressants). These agents appear to alter the pain threshold but are not without side effects (see Chapter 57).

Furthermore, the recognition that one of the major transmitters in the nociceptive pathway is substance P (SP) has led to the development of other analgesic medications. For example, capsaicin (the active ingredient of red chilli), which initially releases SP from nociceptors and subsequently inactivates the SP-containing C fibres, can be used topically in some pain syndromes such as *post-herpetic neuralgia*. However, perhaps the most common exploitation of this system is the manipulation of the enkephalinergic interneurone and opioid receptors by the exogenous administration of morphine and its analogues to control pain (**site IV**).

Opioid analgesics are drugs that mimic endogenous opioid peptides by causing a prolonged activation of opioid receptors (usually μ-receptors). This reduces pain transmission at synapses in the dorsal horn of the spinal cord by an inhibitory action on the relay neurones. Opioids also stimulate noradrenergic, serotoninergic and enkephalinergic neurones in the brainstem that descend in the spinal cord and further inhibit the relay neurones of the spinothalamic tract. Opioid analgesics are widely used to relieve dull, poorly localized (visceral) pain. Repeated doses can cause dependence so that the sudden termination of opioid analgesics may precipitate a withdrawal syndrome.

- **Morphine** is the most widely used analgesic in severe pain but, like all strong opioids, may cause nausea and vomiting.
- **Diamorphine (heroin)** is more lipid soluble than morphine and therefore has a more rapid onset of action when given by injection and is widely used for postoperative pain.
- **Fentanyl** can be given transdermally in patients with chronic stabilized pain. The patches are very useful in patients with intractable nausea or vomiting when taking oral opioids.
- **Methadone** has a long duration of action and is less sedative than morphine. It is given orally for the maintenance treatment of heroin or morphine addicts. The methadone prevents the 'buzz' of intravenous drugs and so reduces the point of taking them.
- **Buprenorphine** is a partial agonist at the μ-receptors. It has a slow onset of action. It has a much longer duration of action than morphine (6–8 hours), but may cause prolonged vomiting.
- **Tramadol** is a weak μ-agonist and its analgesic action is mainly a result of enhanced serotoninergic neurotransmission.
- **Codeine** and **dextropropoxyphene** are weaker drugs used in mild to moderate pain.
- **Naloxone** is an antagonist at opioid receptors and is used to reverse the effects of opioid overdose.

Although pain typically arises from tissue damage, it can also occur with damage to the peripheral and central nervous systems. One such example is *trigeminal neuralgia* (see Chapter 50). It can be treated surgically by lesioning of the appropriate nerve root, although most patients respond to the antiepileptic agent **carbamazepine** or gabapentin (see Chapter 61).

More recently there has been interest in using deep brain stimulation for managing some patients with chronic pain. Whether this works or not is currently unresolved. The main targets for the stimulator are motor cortical areas for reasons that are not clear.

Did you know?

Young people with aggressive behaviours that include inflicting pain on others demonstrate abnormal patterns of activation on functional magnetic resonance imaging (fMRI) when viewing others in pain.

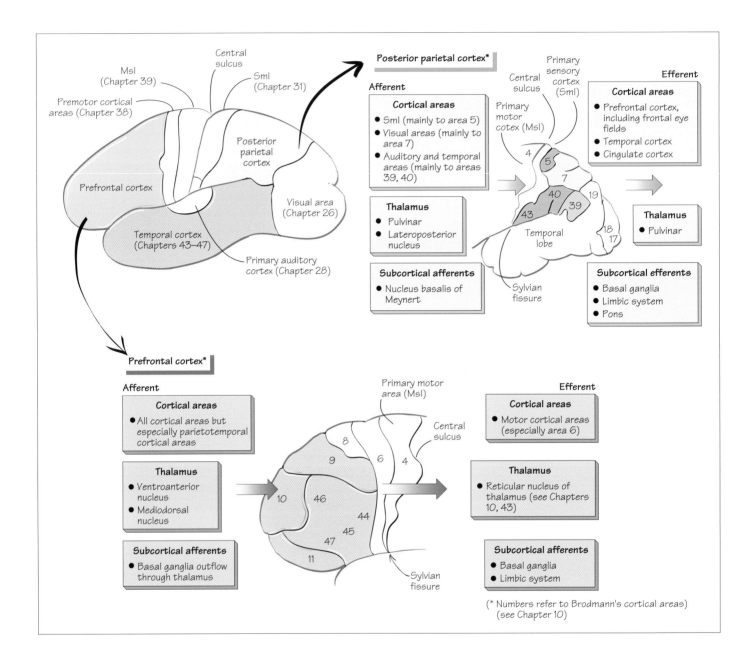

The **association cortices** are parts of the cerebral cortex that do not have a primary motor or sensory role, but instead are involved in the higher order processing of sensory information necessary for perception and movement initiation. These association areas include:

• the posterior parietal cortex (PPC; defined in monkeys as corresponding to Brodmann's areas 5 and 7, and in humans including areas 39 and 40);
• the prefrontal cortex (corresponding to Brodmann's areas 9–12 and 44–47);

• the temporal cortex (corresponding to Brodmann's areas 21, 22, 37 and 41–43). The temporal cortex is involved in audition and language, complex visual processing (such as face recognition) and memory (discussed in Chapters 26–28, 45–47).

Posterior parietal cortex

This area has developed greatly during evolution and relates to specific forms of human behaviour, such as the extensive use of tools, collaborative strategic planning and the development of language. It has two main subdivisions:

Neuroanatomy and Neuroscience at a Glance, Fourth Edition. Roger A. Barker, Francesca Cicchetti, Michael J. Neal.

- one involved mainly with somatosensory information (centred on area 5);
- the other with visual stimuli (centred on area 7).

Neurophysiologically, **area 5** contains many units with a complex sensory input often with a convergence of different sensory modalities, such as proprioceptive and cutaneous stimuli. These units with such a dual input are probably involved in the sensory control of posture and movements. Other units with multiple cutaneous inputs are probably more involved in object recognition. However, in addition to having these complex sensory inputs, units in this area are often only maximally activated when the sensory stimulus is of interest or behavioural significance. Clinical features of lesions in area 5 of the posterior parietal cortex include:

- a contralateral sensory loss that is often subtle, e.g. a failure to recognize objects on tactile manipulation (*astereognosis*).
- an *inattention* to stimuli received on the contralateral side of the body. This can be so severe that the patient denies the existence of that part of his or her body, which can then interfere with the actions of the normal non-neglected side (intermanual conflict or alien limb). More commonly, the patient fails to perceive sensory stimuli contralaterally when stimuli are simultaneously applied to both sides of the body (extinction).

In contrast, **area 7** is more involved in complex visual processing, with many of the units in this area responding to stimuli of interest or behavioural significance (e.g. food). Many different units are found in this cortical area some of which maximally respond to the visual fixation and tracking, while others are more involved in the process of switching attention from one visual object of interest to another (light sensitive or visual space neurones). There are individual neurones in area 7 that respond to both sensory and visual stimuli. Some of these neurones are maximally activated when a stimulus is moved towards the neurone's cutaneous receptive field from extrapersonal (distant) space, while others are maximally activated during visual fixation of a desired object in which there is concomitant movement of the arm towards that object.

Clinical features of lesions in area 7 of the posterior parietal cortex include:
- a neglect of visual stimuli in the contralateral hemifield;
- defects in eye movement and the visual control of movement.
In some patients, more striking deficits occur in the realm of complex visual processing such as route finding, the construction of complex shapes and the copying of motor actions/gestures (*dyspraxia*).

Finally, in humans, and to a lesser extent in other primates and animals, some units in the posterior parietal cortex are maximally activated by vestibular and auditory inputs (see Chapters 28 and 29). Therefore damage to this area in humans can lead to complex difficulties in vision and visually guided movements, balance and language processing, including arithmetic skills. This includes an inability to write (*agraphia*), to read (*alexia*) and calculate simple sums (*acalculia*).

Prefrontal cortex

This cortical area has increased in size with phylogenetic development and has its greatest representation in humans. It is involved in the purposeful behaviour of an organism and thus is intimately involved in the planning of responses to stimuli that include a motor component (see Chapter 35). Within this structure are specialized cortical areas such as the frontal eye fields (FEF; see Chapter 56) and Broca's area (see Chapter 28). Although the prefrontal cortex is treated as a functional whole, this is a gross simplification.

Many different types of units are encountered neurophysiologically in this area of cortex, but they generally respond to complex sensory stimuli of behavioural relevance, which can then be translated into a cue for movement.

Damage to this site in animals leads to increased distractibility with corresponding deficits in working memory (the ability to retain information for more than a few seconds) and a change in locomotor activity and emotional responsiveness. A patient with frontal lobe damage anterior to the motor areas has a characteristic syndrome without insight (as occurs in frontal variant *frontotemporal dementia* (*FTD*)).

The patient:
- is often disinhibited, which results in him or her behaving in an atypical, often childish fashion;
- has very poor attention and is easily distractible, cannot retain information and is sometimes unable to form new memories, with a tendency to perseverate (the repetition of words or phrases and actions) and pursue old patterns of behaviour even in the face of environmental change;
- is unable to formulate and pursue goals and plans, to generalize and deduce, and may have difficulties in judging risk;
- displays a marked reduction in verbal output, which is also reflected in motor behaviour as evidenced by a lack of spontaneous movement;
- has a change in food preference, typically favouring sweet over savoury foods;
- can become apathetic with severe blunting of his or her emotional responses, although in some cases the converse is true with the patient becoming aggressive;
- show overall changes in their personality and it is typically others who bring the patient to medical attention, as the patient usually denies there is any problem (no insight).

The reliance on the clinical symptomatology to describe the function of the prefrontal cortex relates to the fact that this part of the cortex is most developed in humans. However, extensive damage of the frontal lobes can also affect the cortical motor areas (see Chapter 38), eye movements (see Chapter 56), the ability to talk (an expressive dysphasia; see Chapter 28) and the control of micturition.

Did you know?

There is some evidence that permanent traumatic damage to the frontal lobes can occur in footballers through repeated heading of the old leather footballs.

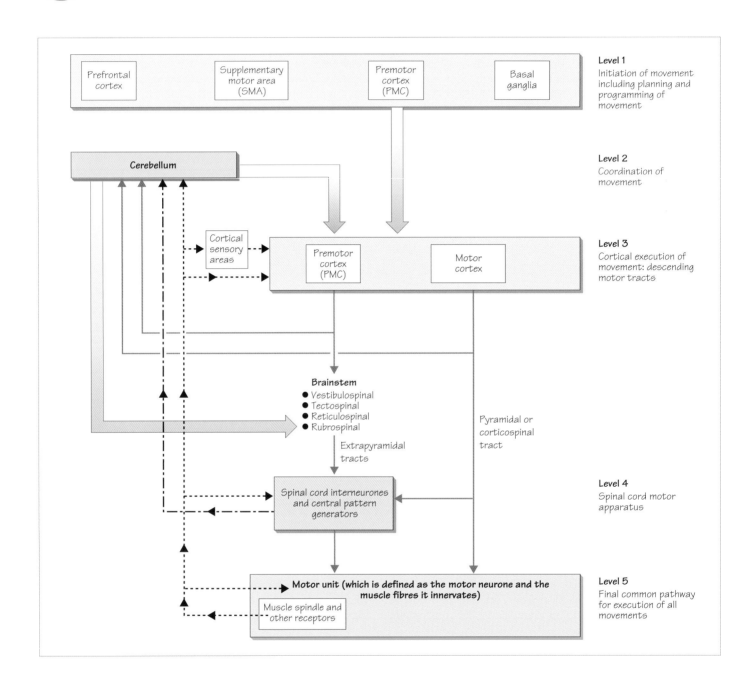

The **motor systems** are those areas of the nervous system that are primarily responsible for controlling movement. The movement can either be:
• guided by inputs from the sensory systems (**closed-loop** or **reflex controlled**); or
• triggered by a sensory cue or some internal desire to move (**open-loop** or **volitional** movement).

In practice, most motor acts involve both types of movement. Closed-loop movements predominantly involve the axial or proximal muscles responsible for balance, posture and locomotion, while the open-loop movements are typically associated with the distal musculature concerned with the control of fine skilled movements.

The organization of the motor structures is best viewed in terms of a hierarchy.

Neuroanatomy and Neuroscience at a Glance, Fourth Edition. Roger A. Barker, Francesca Cicchetti, Michael J. Neal.

Level	Function	Structures involved	Clinical features of lesions
Level 1	The highest level of motor control is concerned with the **initiation, planning and programming of movements**	This desire probably originates in the **limbic system** (see Chapter 47) and **posterior parietal cortex** (see Chapter 34), while the structures primarily responsible for translating that desire into a movement are the **basal ganglia** (see Chapters 41 and 42) and their cortical projection areas to the frontal lobe (see Chapters 37 and 38). These cortical areas include the **supplementary motor area (SMA)** and **premotor cortex (PMC)**	Damage to the basal ganglia and their cortical projection sites leads to a range of complex movement disorders, which includes *Parkinson's disease*, *chorea*, *dystonia* and *ballismus* (see Chapter 42 for the definition of these terms). Damage to these areas does *not* produce any specific weakness or changes in the monosynaptic tendon reflexes (see Chapter 42)
Level 2	This level is involved with the **coordination of movement**	The **cerebellum**; it achieves this by comparing the intended movement descending from the motor areas in the cerebral cortex with the actual movement as detected by the activity of muscle afferents and interneurones (INs) in the spinal cord. It is also capable of storing motor information	Damage to this structure leads primarily to a breakdown in the coordination of movement, without any specific weakness (see Chapter 40).
Level 3	This level is involved with the supraspinal execution and control of movement and to a lesser extent INs	The middle level is concerned with the control of the lower motor neurones (MNs) by the supraspinal **descending motor pathways**. This can broadly be divided into two sets of pathways: (1) the corticospinal (CoST) or pyramidal tract which originates in the motor, premotor and somatosensory cortices and synapses directly on to the MNs in the brainstem cranial nerve nuclei and ventral (or anterior) horn of the spinal cord and to a lesser extent the Ins; and (2) the extrapyramidal tracts, which originate from subcortical structures and have a more complex distribution of synaptic contacts with both MNs and INs.	Damage in the CNS is rarely specific to a single tract but interruption of the descending motor pathways produces a pattern of weakness in the limbs that is more pronounced in the extensor muscles in the arms and flexor muscles in the legs – the so-called (but misnamed) **pyramidal distribution of weakness**. In association with the weakness, there is increased tone in the muscles and brisk reflexes; all three features characterizing an *upper MN lesion* (see Chapter 37). This is the first level where damage is actually associated with weakness.
Level 4	The coordination of movement within the spinal cord by the integration of descending pathways with intrinsic networks of neurones and afferent inputs from peripheral receptors	A low level of motor organization is found in the **spinal cord** itself. The descending motor pathways synapse not only on the MNs but also the INs, and while some of these mediate the spinal cord **reflexes**, others are capable of generating their own outputs to MNs independently of any descending or peripheral sensory input – **central pattern generators**. These are important in locomotion (see Chapter 37), although their existence and role in humans is still unresolved	Damage to structures within the spinal cord causes a mixture of deficits as it will affect both descending motor pathways, ascending sensory pathways and lower MNs. However, there is a series of rare conditions where the pathology is restricted to spinal cord motor pathways such as in *stiff man* syndrome and *hyperekplexia*. In stiff man syndrome there is spinal cord hyperexcitability due to a functional loss of γ-aminobutyric acid (GABA)ergic inhibition, causing the muscles to be stiff when activated (e.g. walking); in hyperekplexia there is an excessive startle response due in some cases to mutations in the glycine receptor.
Level 5	The actual execution of the movement	The lowest level or **final common pathway of the motor system** is the output neurone of the central nervous system (CNS) to the muscle (the MN). The MN not only receives information from the brain and spinal cord INs but also has an important input from sensory organs in the periphery, especially the **muscle spindle** and **Golgi tendon organ** that are found in the muscle and tendon, respectively (see Chapter 36).	Damage to the MN or its axon to the muscle produces a *lower* (as opposed to upper) *MN lesion*, characterized by weakness and wasting, hypotonia and reduced or absent reflexes (see Chapters 36 and 37)

A cautionary note

It is important to remember that the division of the central nervous system into motor and sensory functions is a gross simplification as all the motor areas have some sensory input. It is difficult to know the point at which a highly processed sensory input becomes the impulse for the initiation of a movement. It should also be realized that the division of the motor systems into various levels and different motor pools is a convenient but not strictly accurate device for understanding the control of movement and the pathophysiology of disorders of the motor system.

Did you know?

Cheetahs can run as fast as 120 km/h, and one of the reasons for this is that their spine is so flexible that it provides an additional 'spring' to their movement.

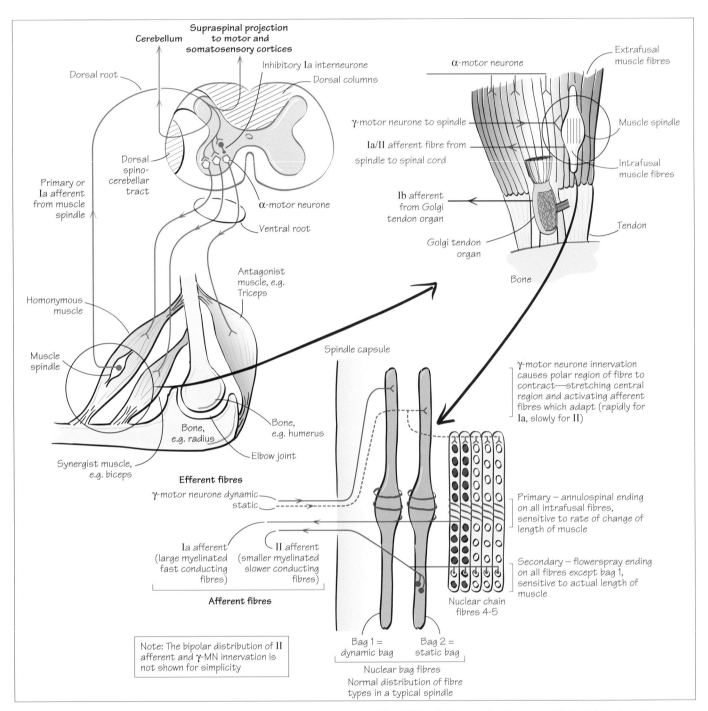

Efferent fibres

γ-motor neurone dynamic static

Ia afferent (large myelinated fast conducting fibres)

II afferent (smaller myelinated slower conducting fibres)

Afferent fibres

Note: The bipolar distribution of II afferent and γ-MN innervation is not shown for simplicity

Spindle capsule

γ-motor neurone innervation causes polar region of fibre to contract—stretching central region and activating afferent fibres which adapt (rapidly for Ia, slowly for II)

Primary – annulospinal ending on all intrafusal fibres, sensitive to rate of change of length of muscle

Secondary – flowerspray ending on all fibres except bag 1, sensitive to actual length of muscle

Nuclear chain fibres 4-5

Bag 1 = dynamic bag

Bag 2 = static bag

Nuclear bag fibres
Normal distribution of fibre types in a typical spindle

Lower motor neurone

The **lower motor neurone (LMN)** is defined as the neurone whose cell body lies in either the anterior or ventral horn of the spinal cord or cranial nerve nuclei of the brainstem and which directly innervates the muscle via its axon. The number of muscle fibres innervated by a single axon is termed the **motor unit**. The smaller the number of fibres per motor neurone (MN) axon, the finer the control (e.g. the extraocular muscles).

The MNs of the anterior horn are divided into two types:
- **α-MNs** (70 μm in diameter) – which innervate the muscle itself (the force generating extrafusal fibres);
- **γ-MNs** (30 μm in diameter) – which innervate the intrafusal fibres of the muscle spindle.

The **muscle spindle** is an encapsulated sense organ found within the muscle, which is responsible for detecting the extent of muscle contraction by monitoring the length of muscle fibres. It is the

Neuroanatomy and Neuroscience at a Glance, Fourth Edition. Roger A. Barker, Francesca Cicchetti, Michael J. Neal.

muscle spindle and its connections to the spinal cord that mediates the **tendon reflexes**:

• sudden stretching of a muscle by a sharp tap of a tendon hammer transiently activates the **Ia afferent nerve endings** which, via an excitatory monosynaptic input to the MN, causes that muscle (the **homonymous muscle**) to contract briefly (e.g. the knee jerk).

• In addition, the Ia afferent input from the muscle spindle, while activating other **synergistic muscles** with a similar action to the homonymous muscle, also inhibits muscles with opposing actions (**antagonist muscles**) through a **Ia inhibitory interneurone (IN)** in the spinal cord.

However, it must be stressed that tendon jerks reflect not only the integrity of this circuit but the overall excitability of the MN, which is increased in cases of an upper MN (UMN) lesion (see Chapter 37).

Muscle spindle

Structure

The **muscle spindle** lies in parallel to the extrafusal muscle fibres and consists of the following:

• **nuclear bag and chain fibres** – which have different morphological properties: the bag 1 or dynamic fibres are very sensitive to the rate of change in muscle length, while the bag 2 or static bag fibres are like the nuclear chain fibres in being more sensitive to the absolute length of the muscle;

• γ-**MN** – which synapses at the polar ends of the intrafusal muscle fibres and which can be one of two types: **dynamic or static**, with the latter innervating all but the bag 1 fibres. Both types of γ-MN are usually coactivated with the α-MN so that the intrafusal fibres contract at the same time as do the extrafusal fibres, thus ensuring that the spindle maintains its sensitivity during muscle contraction. Occasionally, the γ-MN can be activated independently of the α-MN, typically when the animal is learning some new complex movement, which increases the sensitivity of the spindle to changes in length;

• two types of afferent fibres and nerve endings – a **Ia afferent fibre** associated with an annulospiral nerve ending winding around the centre of all types of intrafusal fibres (**primary ending**); and a slower conducting **type II fibre** which is associated with flower-spray endings on the more polar regions of the intrafusal fibres (with the exception of the bag 1 fibres; the **secondary ending**). The stretching of the intrafusal fibre activates both types of fibre. However, the Ia fibre is most sensitive to the rate of change in fibre length, while the type II fibres respond more to the overall length of the fibre rather than the rate of change in fibre length.

Connections

The spindle relays via the dorsal root to a number of sites in the central nervous system (CNS) including:

• MNs innervating the homonymous and synergistic muscles (the basis of the stretch reflex);

• INs inhibiting the antagonist muscles;

• the cerebellum via the dorsal spinocerebellar tract;

• the somatosensory cortex;

• the primary motor cortex via the dorsal column–medial lemniscal pathways.

Thus, the muscle spindle is responsible for mediating simple stretch or tendon reflexes as well as muscle tone, and it is also involved in the coordination of movement, the perception of joint position (proprioception) and the modulation of long–latency or transcortical reflexes (see Chapter 39).

Effects of damage to this structure

Damage to the spindle afferent fibres (e.g. in large-fibre *neuropathies*) produces hypotonia (as the stretch reflex is important in controlling the normal tone of muscles), incoordination, reduced joint position sense and, occasionally, tremor with an inability to learn new motor skills in the face of novel environmental situations.

In addition, large fibre neuropathies disrupt other somatosensory afferent inputs (see Chapters 31 and 54).

Golgi tendon organ

The **Golgi tendon organ** is found at the junction between muscle and tendon and thus lies in series with the extrafusal muscle fibres. It monitors the degree of muscle contraction in terms of the muscular force generated and relays this to the spinal cord via a **Ib afferent fibre**. This sensory organ, in addition to providing useful information to the CNS on the degree of tension within muscles, serves to prevent excessive muscular contractions (see Chapter 37). Thus, when activated it inhibits the agonist muscle.

Motor neurone recruitment and damage

The **principle of recruitment** corresponds to the order in which different types of muscle fibres are activated. The smallest α-MNs, which are those most easily excited by any input, innervate type 1 (*not* to be confused with the bag 1 intrafusal fibres found in the spindle) or slow-contracting fibres (which are responsible for increasing and maintaining the tension in a muscle).

The next population of MNs to be activated are those that innervate the type 2A or fast-contracting/resistant to fatigue fibres, which are responsible for virtually all forms of locomotion. Finally, the largest MNs are only activated by maximal inputs, which innervate type 2B or fast-contracting/easily fatigued fibres that are responsible for running or jumping.

The order of recruitment of MNs to a given input follows a simple relationship known as the **size principle**, which allows muscles to contract in a logical sequence.

Lower motor neurone lesions

The α-MN itself can be damaged in a number of different conditions but in all cases the clinical features are the same:

• wasting of the denervated muscles;

• weakness of the same muscles;

• reduced or absent reflexes (an LMN lesion).

In some cases one can also see fasciculations (muscle twitchings), as the loss of the motor neuronal input to the muscle leads to a more random redistribution of the acetylcholine receptors away from sites of the old neuromuscular junction.

The features of an LMN lesion are *very* different from a UMN lesion (see Chapter 37). Causes of a LMN lesion including infection (poliomyelitis); neurodegenerative disorders (motor neurone disease) as well as entrapment as the nerves exit the spine (radiculopathies) and in the limb itself (e.g. carpel tunnel syndrome).

Did you know?

The human masseter muscle contains 114 spindles.

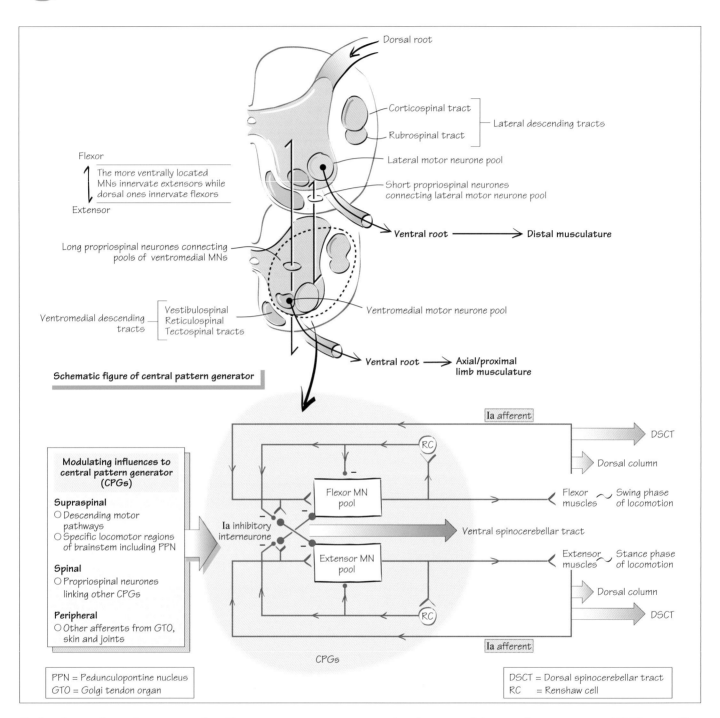

Flexor
The more ventrally located MNs innervate extensors while dorsal ones innervate flexors
Extensor

Schematic figure of central pattern generator

Modulating influences to central pattern generator (CPGs)

Supraspinal
○ Descending motor pathways
○ Specific locomotor regions of brainstem including PPN

Spinal
○ Propriospinal neurones linking other CPGs

Peripheral
○ Other afferents from GTO, skin and joints

PPN = Pedunculopontine nucleus
GTO = Golgi tendon organ

DSCT = Dorsal spinocerebellar tract
RC = Renshaw cell

Spinal cord motor organization

In addition to containing the **α- and γ-motor neurones (MNs)**, the spinal cord also contains a large number of **interneurones (INs)**.

These INs can form networks that are intrinsically active and whose output governs the activity of MNs, **central pattern generators (CPGs)**. These CPGs, which may underlie locomotion, are modulated by both central and peripheral inputs (see Chapters 36 and 38). Such CPGs are not unique to locomotion as they can be seen in other parts of the central nervous system (CNS) controlling rhythmical motor activities, e.g. respiration and the brainstem respiratory network.

Descending motor pathways (see Table 37.1)

The **descending motor pathways** can be classified according to:
• their site of origin, namely pyramidal or extrapyramidal tracts (although clinically **extrapyramidal disorders** refer to diseases of the basal ganglia; see Chapter 42);

Neuroanatomy and Neuroscience at a Glance, Fourth Edition. Roger A. Barker, Francesca Cicchetti, Michael J. Neal.

• their location within the cord and the muscles they ultimately innervate.

Thus, the **pyramidal (corticospinal)** and **rubrospinal tracts** are associated with a **lateral MN pool** that innervates the distal musculature, while the **vestibulo-, reticulo- and tectospinal tracts** are more associated with a **ventromedial MN pool** that innervates the axial and proximal musculature.

These latter MNs are linked by long **propriospinal neurones**, while the converse is true for the lateral MN pool. Thus, the **lateral motor system** is more involved in the control of fine distal movements, while the **ventromedial system** is more concerned with balance and posture.

The MNs of the anterior horn are further organized such that the most ventral MNs innervate the extensor muscles, while the more dorsally located MNs innervate the flexor musculature.

Locomotion

The control of **locomotion** is complex, as it requires the coordinated movement of all four limbs in most mammals. Each cycle in locomotion is termed a **step** and involves a **stance** and a **swing** phase – the latter being that part of the cycle when the foot is not in contact with the ground.
• Each cycle requires the correct sequential activation of flexors and extensors. The simplest way to achieve this is to have **two CPGs (half centres)** which activate flexors and extensors, respectively, and which mutually inhibit each other.
• This mutual inhibition can perhaps best be modelled using the **inhibitory Ia IN** and **Renshaw cells**.
• Renshaw cells are INs that, when activated by MNs, inhibit those same MNs (see Chapter 17). Thus, the activation of a MN pool by a CPG leads to its own inhibition and the removal of an inhibitory input to the antagonistic CPG, thus switching the muscle groups activated.
This half centre model for locomotion can be modulated by a range of descending and peripheral inputs. The Golgi tendon organ can switch the CPGs, while a range of cutaneous inputs can cause the cycle to be modified when an obstacle is encountered. These afferents, termed **flexor reflex afferents**, cause the limb to be flexed so stepping over or withdrawing from the noxious or obstructive object.
• CPGs within the spinal cord communicate with each other through propriospinal neurones.

• In contrast, supraspinal communication of information from and about the CPGs is relayed indirectly in the form of muscle spindle Ia afferent activity via the dorsal spinocerebellar tract (DSCT) and dorsal columns and spinal cord interneuronal activity via the ventral spinocerebellar tract (VSCT).

Clinical disorders of spinal cord motor control and locomotion

Although experimental animals can locomote in the absence of any significant supraspinal inputs (**fictive locomotion**), this is not the case in humans. However, clinical disorders of gait are relatively common and may occur for a number of reasons.
• Disorders of spinal cord INs such as in *stiff person syndrome* are rare and present with increased tone or rigidity in the axial muscles with or without spasms caused by the continuous firing of the MNs as a result of the loss of an inhibitory interneuronal input primarily to the ventromedial MNs. This condition is associated with antibodies against the synthetic enzyme for γ-aminobutyric acid (GABA), glutamic acid decarboxylase (GAD).
• **Damage to the descending pathways** can produce a range of deficiencies. The most devastating is that seen with extensive brainstem damage when the patient adopts a characteristic *decerebrate posture* with arching of the neck and back and rigid extension of all four limbs. In contrast, a more rostrally placed lesion in one of the cerebral hemispheres produces weakness down the contralateral side (hemiplegia or hemiparesis) with increased tone (hypertonia) and increased tendon reflexes (hyperreflexia) which may produce spontaneous or stretch–induced rhythmic involuntary muscular contractions (clonus) (an upper motor neurone lesion). This situation is also seen with interruption of the descending motor pathways in the spinal cord (see Chapters 9, 35 and 55). The pattern of weakness in such lesions characteristically involves the extensors more than the flexors in the upper limb and the converse in the lower limb. This is misleadingly termed a **pyramidal distribution of weakness**, as damage confined to the pyramidal tract in monkeys leads only to a deficiency in fine finger movements with a degree of hypotonia and hypo- or areflexia.

Did you know?

It is well known that chickens can still walk when they have lost most of their head but the longest reported case for this is 18 months!

Table 37.1 Descending motor tracts

Tract	Corticospinal or pyramidal tract (CoST)	Rubrospinal tract (RuST)	Vestibulospinal tract (VeST)	Reticulospinal tract (ReST)
Site of origin	Primary motor cortex (40%) Premotor cortex (30%) Somatosensory cortex (30%)	Magnocellular part of red nucleus in midbrain	Deiter's nucleus in the medulla (part of the vestibular nuclear complex)	Caudal reticular formation in pons and medulla
Major actions	Important in independent fractionated finger movements A role in sensory processing (see Ch 31)	Projects to a similar population of MNs as CoST Experimentally lesions of this tract produce little deficit unless combined with lesions of the CoST Its existence and significance in humans is debated	Innervates predominantly the extensor and axial muscles, and is important in the control of posture and balance	The ReST has both an excitatory and inhibitory input to the spinal cord interneurones and to a lesser extent MNs and is important in damping down activity within the spinal cord such that a loss of this pathway produces profound extensor tone

The tectospinal tract is a relatively minor tract originating from the tectum in the midbrain.

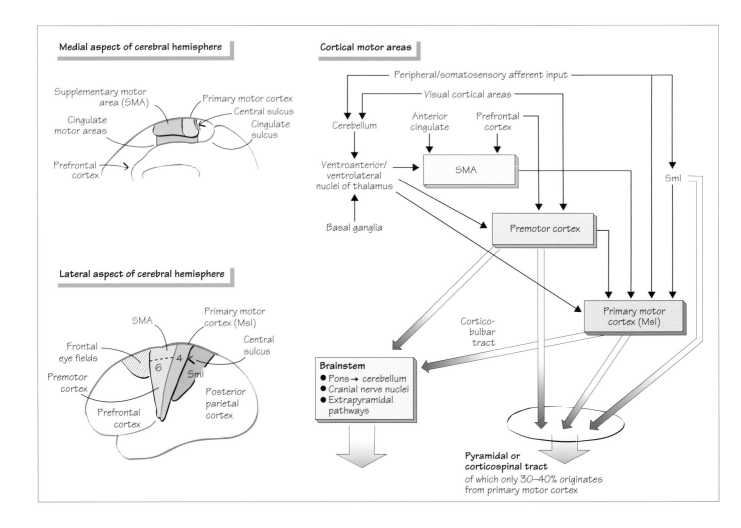

Medial aspect of cerebral hemisphere

Supplementary motor area (SMA)
Primary motor cortex
Central sulcus
Cingulate motor areas
Cingulate sulcus
Prefrontal cortex

Lateral aspect of cerebral hemisphere

SMA
Primary motor cortex (MsI)
Frontal eye fields
Central sulcus
Premotor cortex
4
6
Sml
Prefrontal cortex
Posterior parietal cortex

Cortical motor areas

Peripheral/somatosensory afferent input
Visual cortical areas
Cerebellum
Anterior cingulate
Prefrontal cortex
SMA
Sml
Ventroanterior/ ventrolateral nuclei of thalamus
Basal ganglia
Premotor cortex
Cortico-bulbar tract
Primary motor cortex (MsI)

Brainstem
● Pons → cerebellum
● Cranial nerve nuclei
● Extrapyramidal pathways

Pyramidal or corticospinal tract
of which only 30–40% originates from primary motor cortex

A number of cortical areas are involved with the control of movement, including the primary motor cortex (see Chapter 39), premotor cortex (PMC), supplementary motor area (SMA) and several adjacent areas in the anterior cingulate cortex. In addition, there are other areas that play specific roles in the cortical control of movement, including the frontal eye fields (see Chapter 56) and posterior parietal cortex (see Chapter 34). This chapter briefly discusses the organization of the motor cortical areas and their relative roles in movement control, while the next chapter concentrates on the primary motor cortex.

Primary motor cortex

The **primary motor cortex (MsI)** is that part of the cerebral cortex that produces a motor response with the minimum electrical stimulation. It corresponds to Brodmann's area 4 and lies just in front of the central sulcus and projects to the motor neurones (MNs) of the brainstem via the **corticobulbar tracts** and to the MNs of the spinal cord directly via the **corticospinal tract (CoST)** and indi-

rectly via the subcortical extrapyramidal tracts. Indeed, MsI is closely associated with the pyramidal tract (even though 60–70% of it originates in other cortical areas) and so has a role in the control of distal musculature and fine movements (see Chapter 37).

Other cortical areas

A range of other cortical areas are involved in the control of movement, including the **PMC** (corresponding to the lateral part of Brodmann's area 6); the **SMA** (corresponding to the medial aspect of Brodmann's area 6); a number of motor areas centred on the **anterior cingulate cortex** on the medial aspect of the frontal lobe; the **frontal eye fields** (corresponding to Brodmann's area 8); and the **posterior parietal cortex** (especially Brodmann's area 7).

Some of these areas have specialist functions such as the frontal eye fields with eye movement control (see Chapter 56) and the posterior parietal cortex with the visual control of movement (see Chapter 34). The remaining areas in the frontal lobe are involved with more complex aspects of movement. Most of these other

Neuroanatomy and Neuroscience at a Glance, Fourth Edition. Roger A. Barker, Francesca Cicchetti, Michael J. Neal.

84 © 2012 John Wiley & Sons, Ltd. Published 2012 by John Wiley & Sons, Ltd.

Table 38.1 Cortical motor areas: connections and functions

Cortical area	Afferent input	Efferent output	Neurophysiology	Function
Primary motor cortex (MsI)	SMA PMC SmI Cerebellum via thalamus (VA–VL nuclei) Dorsal column–medial lemniscal system (via VP nucleus of thalamus)	Corticospinal or pyramidal tract Brainstem: • pons to cerebellum • cranial nerve nuclei • extrapyramidal tracts	Lesion of MsI results in a loss of placing, hopping reactions and skilled manipulative movements	Control of distal musculature and fine skilled movements Role in reflex control of movement (transcortical reflexes)
Premotor cortex (PMC)	SMA Prefrontal cortex Somatosensory and visual cortices Cerebellum via thalamus (VA–VL nuclei) Basal ganglia via thalamus (VA–VL nuclei)	MsI Corticospinal or pyramidal tract Brainstem: • pons to cerebellum • extrapyramidal pathways	Lesion of PMC produces a mild paresis and impairment of skilled movements; deficits in executing visuomotor tasks Regional blood flow studies show it is activated during tasks requiring directional guidance of a movement from sensory information	Control of proximal musculature Control of movement sequence and preparation for movement
Supplementary motor area (SMA)	Prefrontal cortex Basal ganglia via thalamus (VA–VL nuclei) Anterior cingulate cortex Contralateral SMA	SMA (contralateral) PMC MsI	Lesion of SMA produces a severe reduction in spontaneous motor activity with forced grasping and failure of bimanual coordination Stimulation of SMA produces vocalization and complex bilateral arm movements Activity in SMA precedes any changes in MsI Units in SMA respond maximally to sensory cues being used as an instruction for a movement Regional blood-flow studies have shown an increased flow with the planning or thinking of a motor act	Role in the initiation and planning of movement Role in bimanual coordination

cortical areas therefore occupy a higher level in the motor hierarchy than MsI, and their connections and functions are summarized in the figure and Table 38.1 (see also Chapter 35).

The PMC refers to a specific area of Brodmann's area 6, and like the primary motor cortex has an input directly to the spinal MNs via the corticospinal or pyramidal tract. This area therefore occupies two levels of the motor hierarchy as it also has a role in the planning of movement (see Chapter 35). In contrast, the SMA lies medial to the PMC, and has a much more clearly defined role in the planning of movements especially in response to sensory cues. Furthermore, it is now clear that the SMA is part of a much larger number of higher order motor cortical areas that lie along the medial side of the frontal cortex and which are involved in the planning of movements more than their execution. It is these cortical areas that receive the predominant outflow of the basal ganglia

(see Chapter 41), which helps explain the abnormal movements that are seen with diseases of this area of the brain (see Chapter 42). For example, in **Parkinson's disease** there is a slowness and poverty of movement that is associated with underactivation of these cortical areas, a situation that is rectified by the administration of antiparkinsonian medication or successful neurosurgical interventions.

Did you know?

Transcranial magnetic stimulation (TMS) is a technique for stimulating cortical areas by placing a magnet on the outside of the skull, which modifies ongoing activity in the brain. TMS is emerging as a possible therapy for patients with neurological disorders.

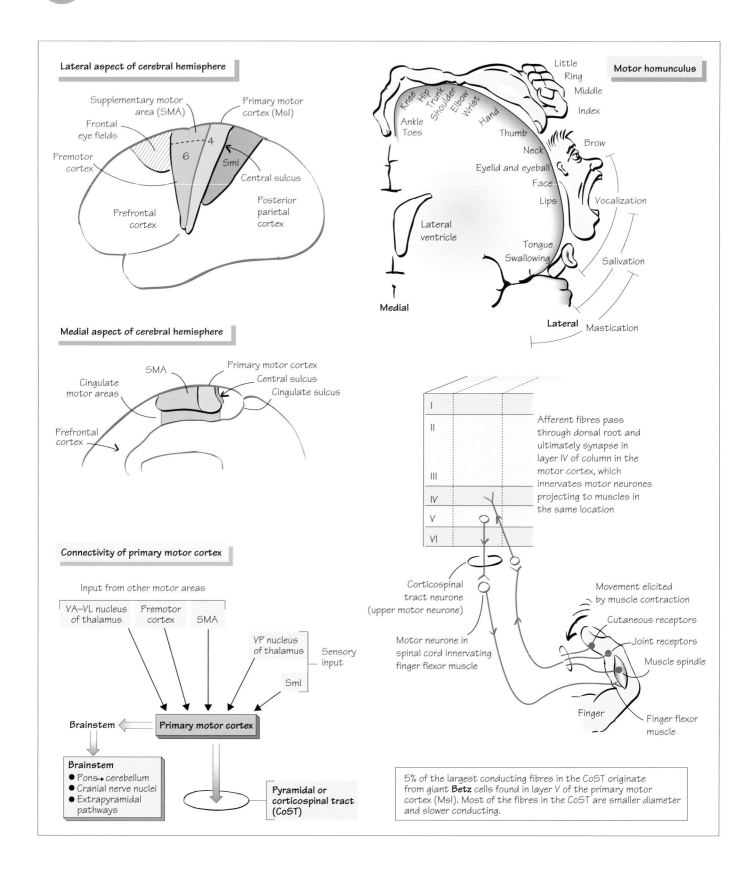

Lateral aspect of cerebral hemisphere

Supplementary motor area (SMA)
Frontal eye fields
Premotor cortex
Primary motor cortex (MsI)
4
6
SmI
Central sulcus
Prefrontal cortex
Posterior parietal cortex

Motor homunculus

Little
Ring
Middle
Index
Knee Hip Trunk Shoulder Elbow Wrist Hand
Ankle Toes
Thumb
Neck
Eyelid and eyeball
Face
Lips
Brow
Vocalization
Lateral ventricle
Tongue
Swallowing
Salivation
Medial
Lateral
Mastication

Medial aspect of cerebral hemisphere

SMA
Primary motor cortex
Central sulcus
Cingulate sulcus
Cingulate motor areas
Prefrontal cortex

I
II
III
IV
V
VI

Afferent fibres pass through dorsal root and ultimately synapse in layer IV of column in the motor cortex, which innervates motor neurones projecting to muscles in the same location

Connectivity of primary motor cortex

Input from other motor areas

VA–VL nucleus of thalamus | Premotor cortex | SMA
VP nucleus of thalamus
SmI
Sensory input

Brainstem ← Primary motor cortex

Brainstem
- Pons → cerebellum
- Cranial nerve nuclei
- Extrapyramidal pathways

Pyramidal or corticospinal tract (CoST)

Corticospinal tract neurone (upper motor neurone)

Motor neurone in spinal cord innervating finger flexor muscle

Movement elicited by muscle contraction
Cutaneous receptors
Joint receptors
Muscle spindle
Finger
Finger flexor muscle

5% of the largest conducting fibres in the CoST originate from giant **Betz** cells found in layer V of the primary motor cortex (MsI). Most of the fibres in the CoST are smaller diameter and slower conducting.

Neuroanatomy and Neuroscience at a Glance, Fourth Edition. Roger A. Barker, Francesca Cicchetti, Michael J. Neal.

The primary motor cortex (MsI) receives afferent information from the cerebellum (via the thalamus) and more anteriorly placed motor cortical areas such as the supplementary motor area (SMA) and a sensory input from the muscle spindle as well as cortical sensory areas. This latter sensory input emphasizes the artificial way in which the central nervous system (CNS) is divided up into motor and sensory systems. In order to acknowledge this, the primary motor cortex is termed the MsI while the primary somatosensory cortex is termed the SmI (see Chapter 31).

Investigation of the **organization of MsI** has shown that the motor innervation of the body is represented in a highly topographical fashion, with the cortical representation of each body part being proportional to the degree of motor innervation – so, for example, the hand and orobuccal musculature have a large cortical representation. The resultant distorted image of the body in MsI is known as the **motor homunculus**, with the head represented laterally and the feet medially. This organization may manifest clinically in patients with *epilepsy* that originates in the motor cortex. In such cases, the epileptic fit may begin at one site, typically the hand, and then spread so that the jerking marches out from the site of origin (**Jacksonian march**, named after the neurologist, Hughlings Jackson). This is in contrast to the clinical picture seen with seizures arising from the SMA, in which the patient raises both arms and vocalizes with complex repetitive movements suggesting that this area has a higher role in motor control (see Chapter 38).

These studies on the motor homunculus by Penfield and colleagues in the 1950s revealed the macroscopic organization of MsI, but subsequent microelectrode studies in animals showed that MsI is composed of **cortical columns** (see Chapter 10). The inputs to a column consist of afferent fibres from the joint, muscle spindle and skin which are maximally activated by contraction of those muscles innervated by that same area of cortex. So, for example, a group of cortical columns in MsI will receive sensory inputs from a finger when it is flexed – that input being provided by the skin receptors on the front of the finger, the muscle spindles in the finger flexors and the joint receptors of the finger joints. That same column will also send a projection to the motor neurones (MNs) in the spinal cord that innervate the finger flexors. Activation of the corticospinal neurone from that column will ultimately activate the receptors that project to that same column, and vice versa.

Thus, each column is said to have **input–output coupling** and this may be important in the more complex reflex control of movement as, for example, with the **long–latency or transcortical reflexes**. These reflexes refer to the delayed and smaller electromyographical (EMG) changes that are seen following the sudden stretch of a muscle – the first EMG change being the M1 response of the monosynaptic stretch reflex (see Chapter 36). The afferent limb of the transcortical reflex is from the muscle spindle input via the Ia fibre (relayed via the dorsal column–medial lemniscal pathway) and the efferent pathway involves the corticospinal tract (CoST). The exact role of this reflex is not known but it may be important in controlling movements precisely, especially when unexpected obstacles are encountered which activate the muscle spindle.

There has been great controversy as to whether MsI controls individual muscles, simple movements or some other aspect of movements. Neurones within MsI fire before any EMG changes and appear to **code for the direction and force of a movement**, although this activity is dependent on the nature of the task being performed. Therefore, as a whole, the motor cortex controls movement by its innervation of populations of MNs, as individual corticospinal axons innervate many different MNs.

MsI is capable of being remodelled after lesions or changes in sensory feedback, implying that it maintains a flexible relationship with the muscles throughout life. Thus, cells in a region of MsI can shift from the control of one set of muscles to a new set. Within given areas of cortex there is some evidence that synaptic strengths can be altered with long–term potentiation (see Chapter 45), which suggests that the MsI may be capable of learning new movements, a function traditionally ascribed to the cerebellum (see Chapter 40).

Damage to MsI in isolation is rare and experimentally tends to produce deficiencies similar to those seen with selective pyramidal tract lesions. However, damage to both MsI and adjacent premotor areas, as occurs in most *cerebrovascular accidents* (*CVAs*) involving the middle cerebral artery (see Chapter 6), produces a much more significant deficiency, with marked hemiparesis.

Did you know?

Scientists have now developed brain–computer interfaces so that patients can move paralysed parts of their body simply by thinking about it.

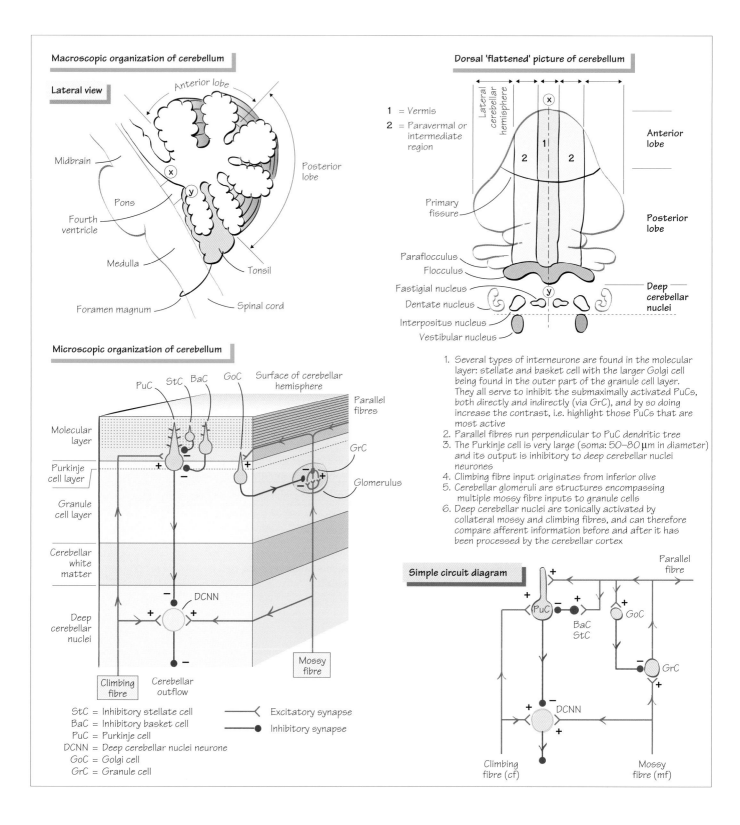

Macroscopic organization of cerebellum

Lateral view

Anterior lobe
Midbrain
x
Pons
Fourth ventricle
Medulla
Foramen magnum
Posterior lobe
y
Tonsil
Spinal cord

Dorsal 'flattened' picture of cerebellum

1 = Vermis
2 = Paravermal or intermediate region

Lateral cerebellar hemisphere
x
1
2   2
Anterior lobe
Primary fissure
Posterior lobe
Paraflocculus
Flocculus
Fastigial nucleus
Dentate nucleus
Interpositus nucleus
Vestibular nucleus
y
Deep cerebellar nuclei

Microscopic organization of cerebellum

PuC StC BaC GoC Surface of cerebellar hemisphere
Parallel fibres
Molecular layer
Purkinje cell layer
Granule cell layer
Cerebellar white matter
Deep cerebellar nuclei
GrC
Glomerulus
DCNN
Climbing fibre
Cerebellar outflow
Mossy fibre

StC = Inhibitory stellate cell
BaC = Inhibitory basket cell
PuC = Purkinje cell
DCNN = Deep cerebellar nuclei neurone
GoC = Golgi cell
GrC = Granule cell

Excitatory synapse
Inhibitory synapse

1. Several types of interneurone are found in the molecular layer: stellate and basket cell with the larger Golgi cell being found in the outer part of the granule cell layer. They all serve to inhibit the submaximally activated PuCs, both directly and indirectly (via GrC), and by so doing increase the contrast, i.e. highlight those PuCs that are most active
2. Parallel fibres run perpendicular to PuC dendritic tree
3. The Purkinje cell is very large (soma: 50–80 μm in diameter) and its output is inhibitory to deep cerebellar nuclei neurones
4. Climbing fibre input originates from inferior olive
5. Cerebellar glomeruli are structures encompassing multiple mossy fibre inputs to granule cells
6. Deep cerebellar nuclei are tonically activated by collateral mossy and climbing fibres, and can therefore compare afferent information before and after it has been processed by the cerebellar cortex

Simple circuit diagram

Parallel fibre
PuC
BaC StC
GoC
GrC
DCNN
Climbing fibre (cf)
Mossy fibre (mf)

Neuroanatomy and Neuroscience at a Glance, Fourth Edition. Roger A. Barker, Francesca Cicchetti, Michael J. Neal.

Organization of the cerebellum

The **cerebellum (CBM)** is a complex structure found below the tentorial membrane in the posterior fossa and connected to the brainstem by three pairs of (cerebellar) peduncles (see Chapter 8). It is primarily involved in the coordination and learning of movements, and is best thought of in terms of three functional and anatomical systems:
• spinoCBM – involved with the control of axial musculature and posture ▨ + ▨;
• pontoCBM – involved with the coordination and planning of limb movements ▢;
• vestibuloCBM – involved with posture and the control of eye movements ▨.

These three systems have their own unique pattern of connections (see Table 40.1).
• The spinoCBM can be divided into a vermal and paravermal (intermediate) region with the former having a close association with the axial musculature. It is therefore associated with the ventromedial descending motor pathways and motor neurones (MNs) while the paravermal part of the spinoCBM is more concerned with the coordination of the limbs.
• The pontoCBM has a role in this coordination but is associated with the visual control of movement and relays information from the posterior parietal cortex to the motor cortical areas.
• The vestibuloCBM has no associated deep cerebellar nucleus and is phylogenetically one of the oldest parts of the cerebellum. Like the vermal part of the spinoCBM, it is involved with balance through its connections with the ventromedial motor pathways but also has a role in the control of eye movements (see Chapter 56).

Long-term depression (LTD) and motor learning

In general, the CBM compares the intended movement originating from the motor cortical areas with the actual movement as relayed by the muscle afferents and spinal cord interneurones, while receiving an important input from the vestibular and visual system. The comparison having been made, an error signal is relayed via descending motor pathways, and the correction factor stored as part of a motor memory in the synaptic inputs to the Purkinje cell (PuC). This modifiable synapse at the level of the PuC is an example of **long-term depression (LTD**; see Chapters 45 and 49). It describes the reduced synaptic input of the parallel fibre (pf) to PuC when it is activated in phase and at low frequency with the climbing fibre input to that same PuC and persists at least for several hours. In other words, at times of new movements the climbing fibre input to the PuC increases which has a modifying effect on the pf input to that same PuC. As the movement becomes more routine, the climbing fibre (cf) lessens but the modified (reduced) pf input persists: it is this modification that is thought to underlie the learning and memory of movements.

This modifiable synapse was first proposed by Marr in 1969 and subsequently has been verified, especially with respect to the vestibulo-ocular reflex (see Chapter 49). The biochemical basis of LTD in the CBM is unknown but appears to rely on the activation of different glutamate receptors in the PuC and the subsequent influx of calcium and the activation of a protein kinase. The presence of a modifiable synapse implies that the CBM is capable of learning and storing information in a motor memory (see Table 40.1).

The microscopic organization of the cerebellum

The microscopic organization of the cerebellum, which allows for the generation of LTD, is well characterized even if the biochemical basis for it remains obscure. The excitatory input to the cerebellum is provided by a mossy and climbing fibre input. The mossy fibre indirectly activates PuC through parallel fibres that originate from granule cells (GrC). In contrast, the climbing fibre directly synapses on the PuC and, as with the mossy fibre input, there is an input to the deep cerebellar nuclei neurones (DCNNs). These neurones are therefore tonically excited by the input fibres to the cerebellum, and are inhibited by the output from the cerebellar cortex (the PuC). The PuC in turn are inhibited by a number of local interneurones, while Golgi cells (GoC) in the outer granule cell layer provide an inhibitory input to the GrC. All of these interneurones have the effect of inhibiting submaximally activated PuC and GrC, and by so doing highlight the signal to be analysed.

The final output of the cerebellum from the deep cerebellar nuclei to various brainstem structures is also inhibitory.

Functional and anatomical systems of the cerebellum

System	SpinoCBM or paleoCBM: vermal region ■	SpinoCBM or paleoCBM: paravermal or intermediate region ▨	PontoCBM or neoCBM	VestibuloCBM or archeoCBM ■
Major afferent connections	Vestibular nucleus	Ia/Ib afferents from distal limb via DSCT	Posterior parietal cortex	Semicircular canals via vestibular nucleus
	Proximal limb Ia/Ib afferents and interneuronal activity relayed via DSCT and VSCT respectively	Interneuronal activity from distal spinal motor pools relayed in VSCT	Primary motor and premotor cortical areas	Visual information from superior colliculus, lateral geniculate nucleus and primary visual cortex relayed via pontine nuclei
	Visual and auditory information to posterior lobe only	Primary motor and somatosensory cortex	*Both* relayed via pontine nuclei	
Associated deep cerebellar nucleus	Fastigial	Interpositus (globose and emboliform)	Dentate	–
Major efferent projections	Reticular formation → ReST	Red nucleus (magnocellular part) → RuST	VA–VL nuclei of thalamus → Areas 4 and 6 → corticospinal tract	Vestibular nucleus → VeST
	Vestibular nucleus → VeST (ventromedial descending motor pathways)	VA–VL nuclei of the thalamus → PMC (Brodmann's area 6) and MsI (Brodmann's area 4) → corticospinal tract (Dorsolateral descending motor pathways)	Red nucleus (parvocellular part) → inferior olive → CBM (Mollaret's triangle)	Vestibular nucleus → oculomotor nuclei
Specific role	Control of axial musculature	Distal limb coordination	Motor planning	Posture
	Regulate muscle tone	Regulate muscle tone	Visual control of movement Minor role in distal limb coordination	Eye movement control

Colour shading at the top of the table refers to the figure.

Clinical features of cerebellar damage

Much that can be deduced about the function of the CBM is derived from the clinical features of patients with cerebellar damage.

Dysfunction of the CBM is found in a large number of conditions, and the clinical features of cerebellar damage are as follows:
• *Hypotonia or reduced muscle tone.* This is caused by a reduced input from the DCNN via the descending motor pathways to the muscle spindle (see Chapter 36).
• *Incoordination/ataxia.* There are a number of manifestations of this including: asynergy (an inability to coordinate the contraction of agonist and antagonist muscles); dysmetria (an inability to terminate movements accurately which can result in an intention tremor and past pointing); and dysdiadochokinesis (an inability to perform rapidly alternating movements). Ataxia is often used to describe incoordinated movements. In cases where the vermis is predominantly involved, as occurs in alcoholic cerebellar degeneration, this results in a staggering, wide-based, 'drunk-like' character to the gait. When there is involvement of the more lateral parts of the cerebellar hemisphere the incoordination involves the limbs.
• *Dysarthria.* This is an inability to articulate words properly caused by incoordination of the oropharyngeal musculature. The words are slurred and spoken slowly (scanning dysarthria).

• *Nystagmus.* This describes rapid jerky eye movements caused by a breakdown in the outflow from the vestibular nucleus and its connections with the oculomotor nuclei (see Chapters 29 and 56).
• *Palatal tremor or myoclonus.* This is a rare condition in which there is hypertrophy of the inferior olive, with damage in a triangle bounded by this structure, the dentate nucleus of the CBM and the red nucleus in the midbrain (Mollaret triangle). The patient characteristically has a low-frequency tremor of the palate, which oscillates up and down.

Finally, there is a recent suggestion that the cerebellum may also subserve some cognitive function, as subtle deficits can be seen in this domain in some patients with cerebellar disease.

Function of the cerebellum

The **role of the CBM** can be defined by area and correlates well with the localizing signs of cerebellar disease. Exactly how the CBM achieves these functions is unknown, but the repetition of the same elementary circuitry in all parts of the cerebellar cortex implies a common mode of function. Three possibilities exist which are not mutually exclusive.
• *By acting as a comparator.* The CBM compares the descending supraspinal motor signals (efference copy, intended movement) with the ascending afferent feedback information (actual move-

ment), and any discrepancy is corrected by the output of the CBM through descending motor pathways. This allows the CBM to coordinate movements so that they are achieved smoothly and accurately.

• *By acting as a timing device.* The CBM (especially the pontoCBM) converts descending motor signals into a sequence of motor activation so that movement is performed in a smooth and coordinated fashion, with balance and posture maintained by the vestibulo- and spinoCBM.

• *By initiating and storing movements.* The existence of a modifiable synapse at the level of the PuC means that the CBM is capable of storing motor information and updating it. Therefore, under the appropriate circumstances, the right sequence for a movement can be accessed and fed through the supraspinal motor pathways, and by so doing an accurate learnt movement is initiated (see also Chapter 35).

Did you know?

The adult human cerebellum weighs 150 g and contains in excess of 20 million Purkinje cells.

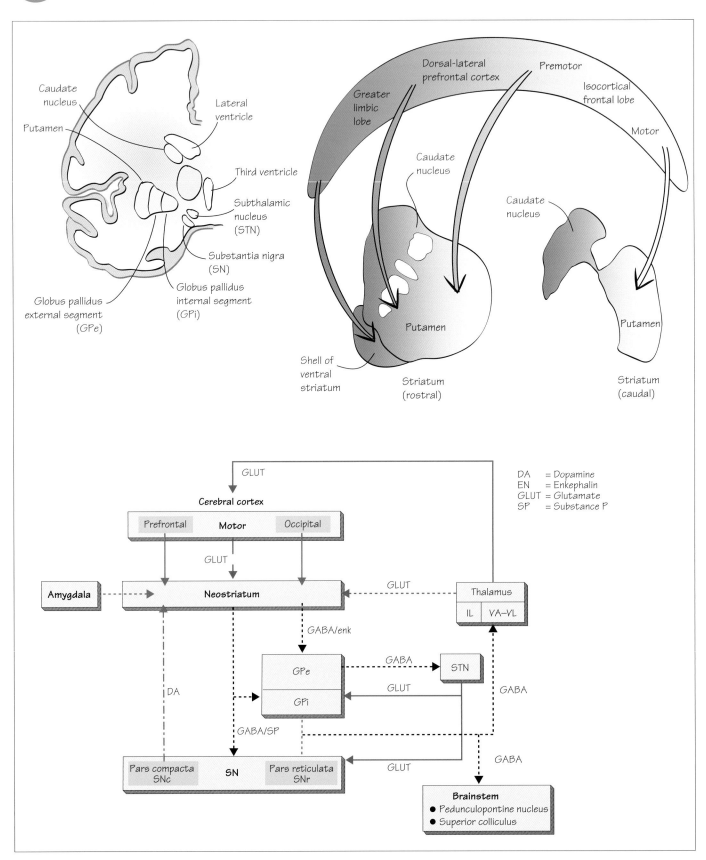

Neuroanatomy and Neuroscience at a Glance, Fourth Edition. Roger A. Barker, Francesca Cicchetti, Michael J. Neal.

The basal ganglia consist of the **caudate and putamen** (dorsal or neostriatum; NS), the **internal and external segments of the globus pallidus** (GPi and GPe, respectively), the **pars reticulata and pars compacta of the substantia nigra** (SNr and SNc, respectively) and the **subthalamic nucleus** (STN).

• The NS is the main receiving area of the basal ganglia and receives information from the whole cortex in a somatotopic fashion as well as the intralaminar nuclei of the thalamus (IL). The major outflow from the basal ganglia is via the GPi and SNr to the ventroanterior–ventrolateral nuclei of the thalamus (VA–VL) which in turn project to the premotor cortex (PMC), supplementary motor area (SMA) and prefrontal cortex. In addition, there is a projection to the brainstem, especially to the pedunculopontine nucleus (PPN), which is involved in locomotion (see Chapter 37), and to the superior colliculus, which is involved with eye movements (see Chapters 25 and 56).

• The basal ganglia also have a **number of loops** within them that are important. There is a striato–nigral–striatal loop with the latter projection being dopaminergic (DA) in nature. There is also a loop from the GPe to the STN which then projects back to the GPi and SNr. This pathway is excitatory in nature and is important in controlling the level of activation of the inhibitory output nuclei of the basal ganglia to the thalamus. However, although a marked degree of convergence and divergence can be seen throughout the basal ganglia, the projections do form parallel pathways, which at the most simplistic level divide into a motor pathway through the putamen and a non-motor pathway through the caudate nucleus.

• The NS consists of **patches or striosomes** that are deficient in the enzyme acetylcholinesterase (AChE). These are embedded in an otherwise AChE-rich striatum, which forms the large extrastriosomal **matrix**. In general, the striosomes are closely related to the dopaminergic nigrostriatal pathway and prefrontal cortex and amygdala, while the matrix is more involved with sensorimotor areas. However, the relationship of these two components of the neostriatum to any parallel pathways is not clear.

• This non-motor role of the basal ganglia is perhaps more clearly seen with the **ventral extension of the basal ganglia** which consists of the **ventral striatum (nucleus accumbens)**, ventral pallidum and substantia innominata (not shown in the figure). It receives a dopaminergic input from the ventral tegmental area that lies adjacent to the SNc in the midbrain, and projects via the thalamus to the prefrontal cortex and frontal eye fields. These structures are intimately associated with motivation and drug addiction (see Chapter 47).

• The **neurophysiology** of the basal ganglia shows that many of the cells within it have complex properties that are not clearly sensory or motor in terms of their response characteristics. For example, some units in the NS respond to sensory stimuli but only when that sensory stimulus is a trigger for a movement. In contrast, many units in the pallidum respond maximally to movement about a given joint before any electromyographic (EMG) changes. Thus, from a neurophysiological point of view, the basal ganglia take highly processed sensory information and convert it into some form of motor programme. This is supported by the clinical disorders that affect the basal ganglia (see Chapters 42 and 55).

Did you know?

Marijuana has actions at many sites in the central nervous system (CNS), and this includes the basal ganglia as they have high levels of the receptors for the active ingredient δ-9-tetrahydrocannabinol (THC). Chronic use of this drug may cause long-term changes to the brain including the basal ganglia.

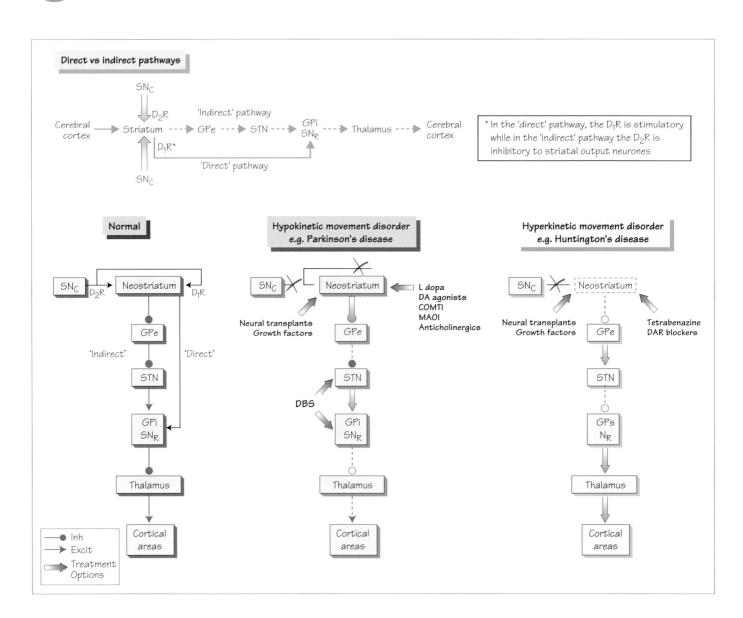

Parkinson's disease

Parkinson's disease is a degenerative disorder that typically affects people in the sixth and seventh decades of life. The primary pathological event is the loss of the dopaminergic nigrostriatal tract, with the formation of characteristic histological inclusion bodies, known as Lewy bodies. In the vast majority of cases the disease develops for reasons that are not clear (idiopathic Parkinson's disease; see Chapter 60). However, in some cases clear aetiological agents are identified, such as vascular lesions in the region of the nigrostriatal pathway, administration of the antidopaminergic drugs in schizophrenia (see Chapter 59) or genetic abnormalities in young patients and some rare families.

Over 50–60% of the dopaminergic nigrostriatal neurones need to be lost before the classical clinical features of idiopathic Parkinson's disease are clearly manifest: slowness to move (bradykinesia); increased tone in the muscles (cogwheel rigidity); and rest tremor. However, most patients also display a range of cognitive, affective and autonomic abnormalities, which relates to pathological changes at other sites.

Neurophysiologically, these patients have increased activity of the neurones in the GPi with a disturbed pattern of discharge, which results from increased activity in the STN secondary to the loss of the predominantly inhibitory dopaminergic input to the neostriatum (NS). The increased inhibitory output from the GPi

Neuroanatomy and Neuroscience at a Glance, Fourth Edition. Roger A. Barker, Francesca Cicchetti, Michael J. Neal.

and SNr to the ventroanterior–ventrolateral nuclei of the thalamus (VA–VL) results in reduced activation of the supplementary motor area (SMA) and other adjacent cortical areas. Thus, patients with Parkinson's disease are unable to initiate movement because of their failure to activate the SMA.

Antiparkinsonian drugs

Currently, no drugs have been shown to slow the progression of Parkinson's disease. For most patients, **dopamine replacement therapy** with **levodopa** (L-dopa) or dopamine agonists is the treatment of choice (dopamine itself does not pass the blood–brain barrier).

• L-dopa is the immediate precursor of dopamine and is converted in the brain by decarboxylation to dopamine. Orally administered L-dopa is largely metabolized outside the brain and so it is given with an extracerebral decarboxylase inhibitor (carbidopa or benserazide), which greatly reduces the effective dose and peripheral adverse effects (e.g. hypotension, nausea). L-dopa frequently produces adverse effects that are mainly caused by widespread stimulation of dopamine receptors. After five years' treatment about half of the patients will experience some of these complications. In some the akinesia gradually recurs producing so-called wearing off effects, while in others various dyskinesias may appear in response to L-dopa (so-called L-dopa-induced dyskinesias). These latter problems may lead to rapid changes in the motor state of the individual ('on–off' problems) and are found in all cases of advanced PD.

• **Selegiline** and **rasagiline** are selective monoamine oxidase type B (MAO$_B$) inhibitors that reduce the metabolism of dopamine in the brain and potentiate the action of L-dopa. They may be used in conjunction with L-dopa to reduce 'end of dose' deterioration.

• Catecholamine-*O*-methyltransferase (COMT) inhibitors such as **entacapone** reduce the peripheral (and also central in the case of tolcapone) metabolism of L-dopa and by so doing increase the amount that can enter the brain.

• **Dopamine agonists** (e.g. ropinirole, pramipexole) are also used often as first-line treatment in young patients or in combination with L-dopa in the later stages of Parkinson's disease. Dopamine agonists directly bind to the dopamine receptors in the striatum (and substantia nigra) and by so doing activate the postsynaptic output neurones of the striatum.

• Other drugs that can be used in Parkinson's disease include **antimuscarinic drugs** (e.g. trihexyphenidyl [benzhexol], procyclidine) in the early stages where tremor predominates and in some young patients with PD. These drugs are believed to correct a relative overactivity of central cholinergic activation that results from the progressive decrease of (inhibitory) dopaminergic activity. Adverse effects are common.

Surgical therapies

Although most patients with Parkinson's disease are best treated with drugs, surgical approaches have been undertaken in advanced disease. Initially this took the form of lesions of the GPi (pallidotomy) but more recently the insertion of electrodes for deep-brain stimulation especially into the STN. This latter approach may work by generating a temporary lesion, possibly by inducing a conduction blocks, although this is not proven.

An alternative surgical approach is the implantation of dopamine-rich tissue into the striatum to replace and possibly restore the damaged nigrostriatal pathway. The efficacy of this approach is still debatable, as is the use of growth factors such as glial cell line derived neurotrophic factor (GDNF).

Huntington's disease

Huntington's disease is an inherited autosomal dominant disorder associated with a trinucleotide expansion in the gene coding for the protein huntingtin on chromosome 4 (see Chapter 63), and as such affected individuals can be diagnosed with certainty using a simple genetic test on the blood.

The disease presents typically in mid-life with a progressive dementia and abnormal movements which usually take the form of chorea – rapid dance-like movements. This type of movement is described as being hyperkinetic in nature, unlike the hypokinetic deficits seen in Parkinson's disease, and reflects the fact that the primary pathology is the loss of the output neurones of the striatum. This results in relative inhibition of the STN and thus reduced inhibitory outflow from the GPi and SNr, which leads to the cortical motor areas being overactivated, generating an excess of movements.

Treatment of the movement disorder in Huntington's disease is designed to reduce the level of dopaminergic stimulation within the basal ganglia. However, there are no treatments for the cognitive deficits in Huntington's disease, although mood disturbances in this condition often do respond to drugs such as antidepressants (see Chapter 57).

Other disorders of the basal ganglia

• Another example of a hyperkinetic movement disorder is *hemiballismus*, which is the rapid flailing movements of the limbs contralateral to damage to the STN.

• A number of other conditions can affect the basal ganglia including *Wilson's disease* (an autosomal recessive condition associated with copper deposition); *Sydenham's chorea* (a sequela of rheumatic fever); defects in mitochondrial function (*mitochondrial cytopathies*; see Chapter 63); a number of toxins (e.g. carbon monoxide and manganese); and *choreoathetoid cerebral palsy* (athetosis is defined as an abnormal involuntary slow writhing movement).

• The spectrum of movement disorders seen with these diseases is variable because the damage is rarely confined to one structure so patients may exhibit either *parkinsonism*, *chorea* and *ballismus*, or *dystonia*, where a limb is held in an abnormal fixed posture.

• Many of these conditions, including Parkinson's disease and Huntington's disease, have a cognitive impairment – if not frank dementia – and while this relates to additional damage in the cerebral cortex, there is increasing evidence that it may in part be as a direct result of basal ganglia damage. In this respect the ventral extension of the basal ganglia may be important.

• The basal ganglia have a major role in the control of eye movements (see Chapter 56) and so many patients with diseases of the basal ganglia have abnormal eye movements, which may be helpful in establishing their clinical diagnosis.

Did you know?

Patients with severe Parkinson's disease can suddenly move normally when faced by life-threatening situations by using a different motor strategy that bypasses the basal ganglia.

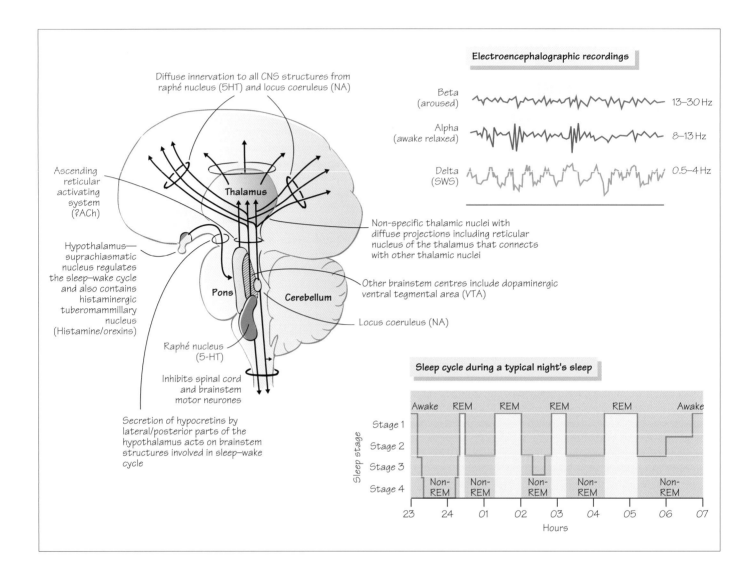

Sleep

Sleep is a characteristic of all mammals and is defined behaviourally as a reduced responsiveness to environmental stimuli, and electrophysiologically by specific changes in electroencephalographic (EEG) activity. In addition, there are a number of changes associated with autonomic nervous system (ANS) function.

Normal patterns of sleep are essential for human wellbeing, although it is still unclear why we need to dream.

EEG patterns during states of consciousness and slow-wave sleep

EEG recordings from normal awake subjects at rest show a characteristic high-frequency (13–30 Hz, β activity) low-voltage pattern. This desynchronized activity changes as the subject closes their eyes and becomes drowsy, with the new EEG pattern having a lower frequency (8–13 Hz, α activity) but slightly higher voltage. This pattern is said to be synchronized and results from the simultaneous firing of many cortical neurones following thalamocortical activity.

EEG studies have revealed that sleep occurs in stages.

1. As the subject falls asleep (stage 1), the EEG is similar to the awake EEG (low-voltage, fast activity).

2. As sleep deepens through stages 2 and 3 to stage 4, the EEG amplitude progressively increases and its frequency falls. Stage 3 and 4 sleep is called collectively slow-wave sleep (SWS) or **non-rapid eye movement** (non-REM) sleep because the eyes are still.

3. After about 90 minutes of sleep, the EEG changes back to a low-voltage, fast pattern that is indistinguishable from stage 1 non-REM sleep. However, during this phase of sleep there are rapid eye movements. This type of sleep is called **rapid eye move-**

Neuroanatomy and Neuroscience at a Glance, Fourth Edition. Roger A. Barker, Francesca Cicchetti, Michael J. Neal.

ment sleep (REM sleep), or paradoxical sleep because although the EEG is similar to that of an awake person, sleepers are difficult to arouse and muscle tone is absent. Most dreaming occurs during REM sleep, although that which takes place during non-REM sleep is said to have a higher emotional content with less detail.

Neural mechanisms of sleep

Sleep is an active process involving a number of neurotransmitter systems.

• Cholinergic neurones in the **ascending reticular activating system** project via two pathways: a dorsal route through the medial thalamus and a ventral one through the lateral hypothalamus, basal ganglia and forebrain. Extensive thalamocortical projections provide the basis for widespread changes in cortical cell excitability. Activity in cholinergic neurones lead to an increase in arousal and cortical desynchrony. Activity in this system is also responsible for the pontine–geniculo–occipital (PGO) waves, at the onset of REM sleep.

• Both noradrenergic neurones in the locus coeruleus and serotoninergic (5-hydroxytryptamine [5-HT]) neurones in the raphé nuclei are involved in controlling the balance between different sleep stages and sleep and arousal.

• Neurones in the ventrolateral preoptic area (VLPA) send an inhibitory γ-aminobutyric acid (GABA)-mediated input to the locus coeruleus, raphé nuclei and tuberomammillary nucleus. The latter contains histaminergic neurones, which are likely to be the substrate for the sedative effects of antihistamine drugs.

• Other brain regions implicated in sleep and arousal patterns include the suprachiasmatic nucleus of the hypothalamus.

• A number of peptides have been identified as being associated with sleep states (e.g. orexins and delta sleep-inducing peptide [DSIP]) and appear to be involved in switching sleep–wake cycles.

Sleep disorders

Insomnia

Insomnia is the most common sleep disorder. It can be defined as the failure to obtain the required amount or quality of sleep to function normally during the day. *Primary insomnia* supposedly brought about by dysfunction of sleep mechanisms in the brain is rare, but these patients may require treatment with hypnotic drugs. Causes of secondary insomnia include psychiatric disease (especially depression and anxiety disorders), physical disorders, chronic pain, drug misuse (e.g. excessive alcohol, caffeine), and old age.

Management of insomnia

Hypnotics are drugs that promote sleep. They include drugs acting at the benzodiazepine receptor (**benzodiazepines** and **Z-drugs**), chloral hydrate, chlormethiazole and barbiturates. Benzodiazepines and the more recent Z-drugs are by far the most widely used hypnotics. They also have anxiolytic, anticonvulsant, muscle relaxant and amnesic actions.

• All the actions of benzodiazepines are believed to be caused by the enhancement of GABA-mediated inhibition in the CNS. GABA$_A$ receptors possess several 'modulatory' sites including one for benzodiazepines, which when activated causes a conformational change in the GABA receptor. This increases the affinity of GABA binding and enhances the actions of GABA on the Cl$^-$ conductance of the neuronal membrane. Any benzodiazepine

given at night will induce sleep but a rapidly eliminated drug (e.g. **temazepam**) is usually preferred to avoid daytime sedation. Adverse effects of benzodiazepines include drowsiness, impaired alertness and ataxia as well as a low-grade dependence after a few weeks' use. Suddenly stopping the drug may cause a physical withdrawal syndrome (anxiety, insomnia) that may last for weeks.

• Some newer drugs do not have the benzodiazepine structure but are benzodiazepine-receptor agonists. These are the so-called Z-drugs, **zopiclone, zolpidem and zaleplon**. The Z-drugs have shorter half-lives than the benzodiazepines and are less likely to cause daytime sedation. They have a reduced propensity to tolerance and withdrawal and are becoming increasingly popular for the management of insomnia.

For many cases of insomnia, psychological strategies may be effective alternatives to drugs.

Hypersomnia (daytime sleepiness)

This is a serious but less common complaint than insomnia. Common causes of persistent daytime sleepiness include narcolepsy, obstructive sleep apnoea, drugs (e.g. benzodiazepines, alcohol) and depression (20% have hypersomnia rather than insomnia).

Narcolepsy

Narcolepsy is characterized by irresistible sleep episodes lasting 5–30 minutes during the day, often in association with cataplexy (loss of muscle tone and temporary paralysis) usually provoked by emotion, e.g. laughter, anger, as well as sleep paralysis and hallucinations at the time of going to or waking up from sleep. It has a very strong histocompatibility locus antigen (HLA) association (DR2/DQW1) and, while no pathological abnormalities have been detected in these patients, it is likely that there are abnormalities in the brainstem structures underlying sleep, as there is evidence of short latency REM sleep during normal waking hours. In addition, deficiencies in **hypocretins or orexins** have recently been described in narcolepsy in some patients. The syndrome has a devastating effect on quality of life, which may be improved by long-term treatment with stimulants, e.g. dexamfetamine, methylphenidate and modafinil. Clomipramine is used to treat the cataplexy.

Obstructive sleep apnoea syndrome

This occurs if the upper airway at the back of the throat collapses when the patient breathes during sleep. This reduces the oxygen in the blood, which arouses the patient causing him or her to momentarily awake and prevents a normal sleep pattern. The patient, usually an overweight man, is often unaware of these awakenings, but the disruption to sleep results in daytime sleepiness and impaired daytime performance. It can be treated by weight loss, positive ventilatory support at night and, occasionally, oropharyngeal surgery. If sleep apnoea is not treated it can lead to long-term cardiorespiratory problems such as pulmonary hypertension and right heart failure. It is also known that sleep apnoea can have a central nervous system origin.

Did you know?

Dolphins can put one hemisphere to sleep while keeping the other awake.

44 Consciousness and theory of mind

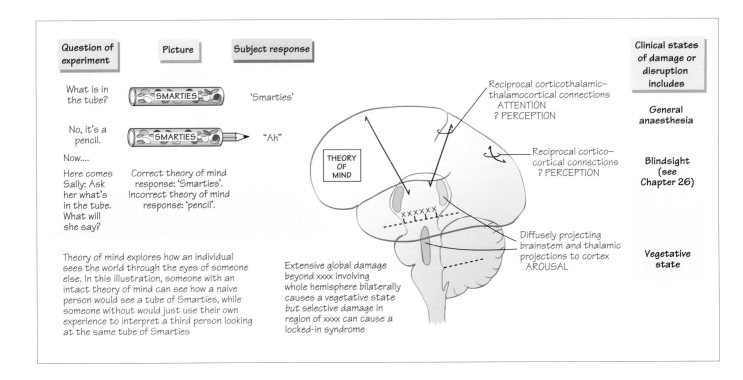

In this chapter we discuss what is meant by consciousness, and how this can be altered in certain pathological conditions. This ability to be aware of what we are doing, namely consciousness, is then discussed further in terms of how we can understand the thought processes of others, so-called theory of mind, disorders of which may underlie a range of conditions, especially *autism*.

Consciousness – what is it?

In thinking about consciousness, it is important to differentiate between the **level** and the **content** of conscious experience. **The level of consciousness** may also be referred to as the level of **arousal** while the **contents of consciousness** refers to the objects and occurrences of which we are aware. Of course, the contents of consciousness will be affected greatly by the level of consciousness but these two phenomena are likely to be at least partly dissociable. For example, people in hyperaroused states may be less aware of surroundings than less-aroused individuals. Conversely, it has recently been shown that individuals in a **vegetative state** may actually show neurophysiological patterns of activity (as measured by functional magnetic resonance imaging [fMRI]; see Chapter 53), indicating a much richer level of awareness than their immobile unresponsive state would suggest.

In general, experimental and clinical access to the contents of consciousness relies on verbal report and certain behavioural indicators. We may ask a subject to tell us or to indicate whether they are aware of a stimulus in the periphery of their visual field. We may assess their memory by requiring them to indicate whether they have an awareness of a particular stimulus that was previously presented to them. We may also attempt to ascertain the richness of their awareness through such measures; with respect to memory, for example, does the subject truly recollect a prior presentation or do they simply have a strong sense that it is familiar?

An important observation with respect to the contents of consciousness is that while our awareness obviously defines our experience of the world, the explanations that they provide for our behaviour is only partial and may be inaccurate. This was shown strikingly in an experiment by Libet and colleagues, who required volunteers to make periodic movements while simultaneously recording cerebral activity. They showed that subjective assessments of becoming aware of an intention to move actually occurred some 500 ms after there had been a brain response. This finding, subsequently replicated, suggests that our brain can indicate what we are about to do before we are aware of wanting to do it.

Further evidence of a discrepancy between what we are aware of and what we actually do comes from work by Castiello and colleagues. These authors showed that when subjects receive incorrect feedback about the trajectory of an arm movement that they are in the process of making, they will correct the movement without actually being aware of doing so, even when the correction made is relatively large. Furthermore, when asked to reproduce

Neuroanatomy and Neuroscience at a Glance, Fourth Edition. Roger A. Barker, Francesca Cicchetti, Michael J. Neal.

the movement that they have just made, subjects will reproduce the one that mirrors the incorrect feedback that they were given, further suggesting that they were unconscious of the control that they have exerted over the movement.

It is also the case that previously experienced events or objects may influence our ongoing actions and decisions without necessarily re-emerging into consciousness. The occurrence of basic processing outside our awareness would seem to be an efficient way of freeing our conscious processing to deal with more complex problems. However, it should be remembered that there are clear instances where the contents of consciousness may have a marked impact on lower level processes. For example, Haggard and colleagues showed that subjects who have made a willed (conscious) movement are likely to link more closely in time that movement with an outcome than when the movement is not felt to be consciously initiated (if it is produced by application of a brief magnetic field over the motor cortex).

Thus, consciousness enables actions to gain greater prominence in our memory, but much of what we do routinely does not require this to happen. As to the precise neurobiological origin of consciousness, this is unknown, but the coordinated activity of the cortex and its reciprocal connections to the thalamus and diffusely projecting brainstem nuclei is important. This is best illustrated in patients in a *vegetative state* (see below) and *blindsight* (see Chapter 26). In this latter condition there is damage to the primary visual cortex such that individuals cannot consciously see but when tested it is clear that their visual system can detect stimuli of different forms including colour and motion. It is thought to arise from the intact extrastriate visual areas, which cannot feedback to the primary visual cortex, as a result of which conscious visual perception is lost.

Consciousness and theory of mind

As humans, we may be unique in being conscious of our consciousness. This "thinking about thinking" has been referred to as 'meta-representation' and it is perhaps the ability to represent our own mental states and those of others that facilitates and shapes our most complex social interactions. To be able to represent the mental states of others has been referred to as having a **theory of mind**. We use this theory of mind to interpret, explain and predict many of the actions and utterances of other people. If someone is being sarcastic or deceitful, they say and do precisely the opposite of what they feel. By understanding these possibilities their behaviour may become more logical and predictable to us.

What happens if we have difficulty with theory of mind processing? It has been suggested that the isolation and very limited social repertoire of individuals with **autism** may arise from the difficulty that they have in understanding the mental states of other people. There is also evidence that people with *schizophrenia* may have deficits in theory of mind abilities and in both cases the abnormality underlying this deficit is thought to reside in the prefrontal cortex (see Chapter 34).

Vegetative state

Some patients who have a major global brain injury (e.g. anoxia secondary to a cardiac or respiratory arrest) can end up in a state of unresponsive wakefulness or a *vegetative state* (which is said to be permanent if it continues for more than six months to a year depending on the nature of the original insult). In this state the patient clearly has periods of sleep and wakefulness, but during the latter time they are unable to respond to any stimuli as there is extensive damage above the level of the arousal systems in the brainstem. In some cases the responses to such stimuli are present, but inconsistently so, and such individuals are deemed to be in a *minimally conscious state* (*MCS*).

It is important that all individuals in a vegetative state or MCS are investigated thoroughly over time using a range of stimuli and functional imaging (see Chapter 53). This is because although some patients appear not to be able to respond there is evidence of cortical activation with sensory stimuli on functional imaging. In these cases, the patient may have had a more focal injury to the upper brainstem that prevents them from being able to make any clear motor responses to stimuli – the so-called *locked-in syndrome*. Once diagnosed, such patients may be able to communicate through the use of eye movements and blinking (see Chapter 56).

Did you know?

Some patients with autism can show *savantism* (as was demonstrated by Dustin Hoffman in the film Rain Man), a condition in which the person shows a remarkable talent that is in striking contrast with their overall limitations. This is thought to relate to the way in which the person uses detail focused processing.

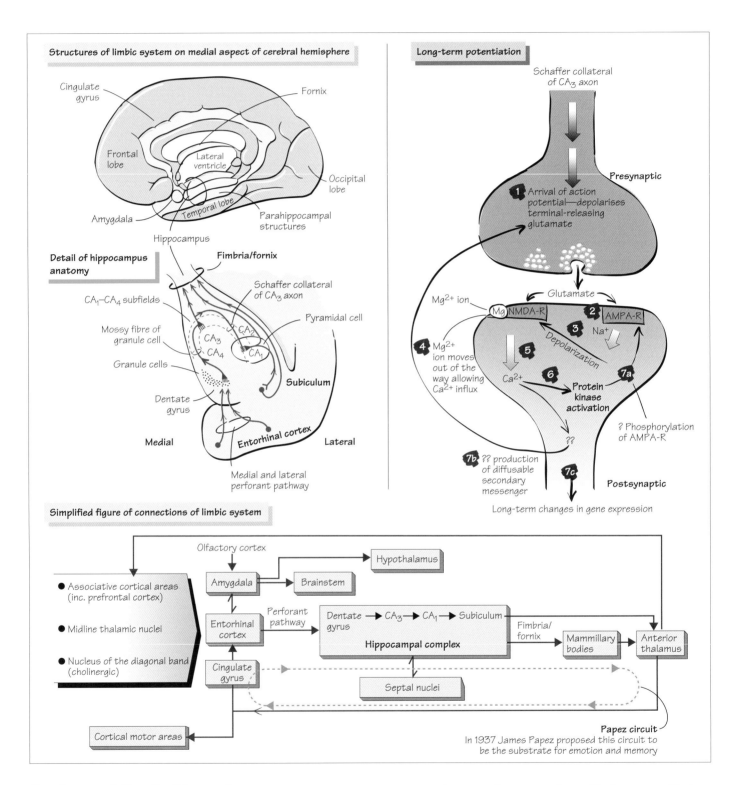

Structures of limbic system on medial aspect of cerebral hemisphere

Cingulate gyrus

Fornix

Frontal lobe

Lateral ventricle

Occipital lobe

Amygdala

Temporal lobe

Parahippocampal structures

Hippocampus

Detail of hippocampus anatomy

Fimbria/fornix

CA₁–CA₄ subfields

Schaffer collateral of CA₃ axon

Mossy fibre of granule cell

Pyramidal cell

Granule cells

Dentate gyrus

Subiculum

Medial

Entorhinal cortex

Lateral

Medial and lateral perforant pathway

Long-term potentiation

Schaffer collateral of CA₃ axon

Presynaptic

1 Arrival of action potential—depolarises terminal-releasing glutamate

Glutamate

Mg^{2+} ion

Mg NMDA-R

2 AMPA-R

3 Na^+

Depolarization

4 Mg^{2+} ion moves out of the way allowing Ca^{2+} influx

5

Ca^{2+}

6

Protein kinase activation

7a

? Phosphorylation of AMPA-R

??

7b ?? production of diffusable secondary messenger

7c

Postsynaptic

Long-term changes in gene expression

Simplified figure of connections of limbic system

Olfactory cortex

Hypothalamus

- Associative cortical areas (inc. prefrontal cortex)
- Midline thalamic nuclei
- Nucleus of the diagonal band (cholinergic)

Amygdala

Brainstem

Entorhinal cortex

Perforant pathway

Dentate gyrus → CA₃ → CA₁ → Subiculum

Hippocampal complex

Fimbria/ fornix

Mammillary bodies

Anterior thalamus

Cingulate gyrus

Septal nuclei

Cortical motor areas

Papez circuit
In 1937 James Papez proposed this circuit to be the substrate for emotion and memory

Anatomy of the limbic system

Many different definitions of the limbic system exist, and in this chapter we will be restricting our definition to structures that lie primarily along the medial aspect of the temporal lobe: **cingulate gyrus, parahippocampal structures (postsubiculum, parasubiculum, presubiculum and perirhinal cortex), entorhinal cortex, hippocampal complex (dentate gyrus, CA1–CA4 subfields and subiculum), septal nuclei** and the **amygdala**. Additional structures closely associated

Neuroanatomy and Neuroscience at a Glance, Fourth Edition. Roger A. Barker, Francesca Cicchetti, Michael J. Neal.

with the limbic system include the mammillary bodies of the hypothalamus, the olfactory cortex and the nucleus accumbens (see Chapters 11, 30, 42 and 47, respectively).

The **anatomical organization** of the limbic system indicates that it performs some high level processing of sensory information, given its input from the associative cortical areas (see Chapter 34). The predominant outflow of the limbic system is to the prefrontal cortex and hypothalamus as well as to cortical areas involved with the planning of behaviour, including motor response (see Chapters 35 and 38). Thus, anatomically the limbic system appears to have a role in attaching a behavioural significance and response to a stimulus, especially with respect to its emotional content. The hippocampal complex has been shown to have both a high degree of susceptibility to hypoxia and yet a remarkable degree of plasticity, which helps explain why this structure is important in the generation of epileptic seizures (see Chapter 61) as well as memory acquisition. It is also one of the major sites for neurogenesis in the adult brain, which may also be important in some forms of memory and mood functions.

Functions of the limbic system

Hippocampal complex and parahippocampal structures (see also Chapter 46)

The original description in the 1950s by Scoville and Milner of patient HM with bilateral anterior temporal lobectomy and a resulting profound amnesic state suggested that this area of the brain had a major role in memory. Subsequently, the hippocampus proper and parahippocampal areas were shown to have a role in the acquisition of information about events (see Chapter 46), although the major role of the hippocampus itself probably relates more to spatial memory.

However, the long-term storage of memories occurs at a distant site, probably within the overlying cerebral cortex – as demonstrated by the pattern of memory loss seen in **dementia of the Alzheimer type** (DAT; see Chapter 60), namely well-preserved retrograde memory (for distant events such as childhood) in the face of severely impaired or absent anterograde memory (inability to remember what the patient has just done).

Amygdala (see also Chapter 47)

The amygdala is a small, almond-shaped structure made up of many nuclei that lies on the medial aspect of the temporal lobe. Damage to this structure experimentally leads to blunted emotional reactions to normally arousing stimuli, and can even prevent the acquisition of emotional behaviour. In humans with selective amygdala damage there appears to be a profound impairment in the ability to recognize facial expressions of fear. Conversely, stimulation of this structure produces a pattern of behaviour typical of fear with increased autonomic activity. This is sometimes seen clinically in **temporal lobe epilepsy**, in which patients complain of brief episodes of fear.

Cingulate gyrus

The cingulate gyrus running around the medial aspect of the whole hemisphere has a number of functions, including a role in complex motor control (see Chapter 38), pain perception (see Chapters 32 and 33) and social interactions. Damage to this structure can produce motor neglect, as well as reduced pain perception, reduced aggressiveness and vocalization, emotional blunting and altered social behaviour which can result in a clinical state of **akinetic mutism** (not talking or moving). Stimulation of this area, either experimentally or during an epileptic seizure, produces alterations in the autonomic outflow and motor arrest, with vocalization and complex movements.

Long-term potentiation

Long-term potentiation (**LTP**) is defined as an increase in the strength of synaptic transmission with repetitive use that lasts for more than a few minutes, and in the hippocampus it can be triggered by less than 1 second of intense synaptic activity and lasts for hours or much longer. It can be induced at a number of CNS sites but especially the hippocampus, and it has therefore been postulated to be important in **memory acquisition**. However, different mechanisms may underlie LTP at different synapses within the hippocampal complex, and most of the work is based on the excitatory glutamate synapse in the CA1 subfield of the hippocampal complex.

The current model of LTP is as follows:

Stage 1 (see figure): An afferent burst of activity leads to the release of glutamate from the presynaptic terminal.

Stages 2 and 3: The released glutamate then binds to both N-methyl-D-aspartate (NMDA) and non-NMDA receptors in the postsynaptic membrane. These latter receptors lead to a Na^+ influx (stage 2) which depolarizes the postsynaptic membrane (stage 3).

Stage 4: The depolarization of the postsynaptic membrane not only leads to an excitatory postsynaptic potential (EPSP), but also removes Mg^{2+} from the NMDA-associated ion channel.

Stage 5: The Mg^{2+} normally blocks the NMDA-R associated ion channel and thus its removal in response to postsynaptic depolarization allows further Na^+ and Ca^{2+} influx into the postsynaptic cell.

Stage 6: The Ca^{2+} influx leads to the activation of a postsynaptic protein kinase, which is responsible for the initial **induction of LTP** – a postsynaptic event.

Stage 7: The **maintenance of LTP**, in addition to requiring a persistent activation of protein kinase activity, the insertion possibly of more postsynaptic glutamate receptors (stage 7a) and changes in gene transcription (stage 7c), may also require a modification of neurotransmitter release (stage 7b), i.e. an increase in transmitter release in response to a given afferent impulse. The presynaptic modification, if necessary in the maintenance of LTP, means that the postsynaptic cell must produce a diffusible secondary signal that can act on the presynaptic terminal such as permeant arachidonic acid metabolites, nitric oxide, carbon monoxide and platelet activating factor.

In some circumstances **long-term depression** (**LTD**) can be induced in the mossy fibre synapses in the CA3 subfield of the hippocampus. This, in contrast to LTP, is thought to be mediated by a presynaptic metabotropic glutamate receptor.

Did you know?

It has been reported that London taxi drivers have bigger hippocampi compared with other people because of the fact that they have to constantly remember complex maps and routes of the city.

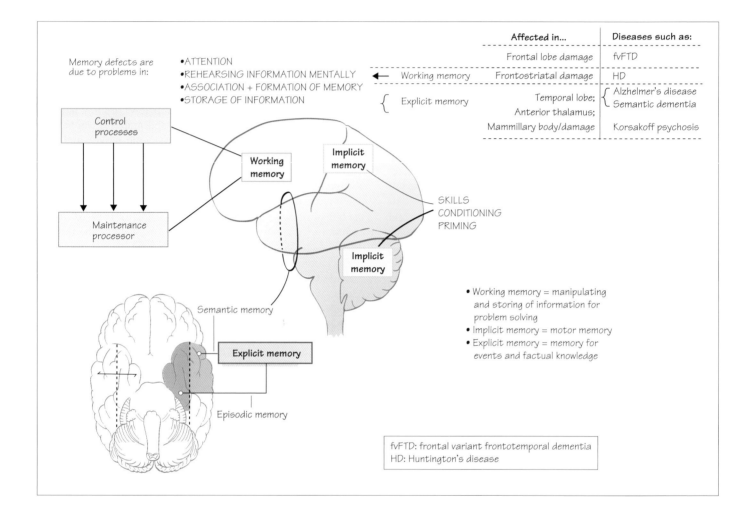

Memory defects are due to problems in:
- ATTENTION
- REHEARSING INFORMATION MENTALLY
- ASSOCIATION + FORMATION OF MEMORY
- STORAGE OF INFORMATION

	Affected in...	Diseases such as:
Working memory	Frontal lobe damage	fvFTD
	Frontostriatal damage	HD
Explicit memory	Temporal lobe;	Alzhelmer's disease / Semantic dementia
	Anterior thalamus;	
	Mammillary body/damage	Korsakoff psychosis

Control processes → Maintenance processor

Working memory
Implicit memory
SKILLS CONDITIONING PRIMING

Semantic memory
Explicit memory
Episodic memory

- Working memory = manipulating and storing of information for problem solving
- Implicit memory = motor memory
- Explicit memory = memory for events and factual knowledge

fvFTD: frontal variant frontotemporal dementia
HD: Huntington's disease

The term memory is commonly used to refer to the ability to remember information but it is important to understand that there are several **different types of memory** that subserve different functions. In the first instance, there is a distinction between motor and non-motor memories – the former is a form of **implicit memory** and typically involves the cerebellum, motor cortical areas and basal ganglia (see Chapters 38–42) and will not be discussed further in this chapter. The other forms of memory are more involved with the taking in, manipulating and storing of information for problem solving (**working memory**), events and factual knowledge (**explicit memory**).

In clinical practice it is not uncommon for patients and their families to complain about disorders of memory when they are referring to a range of different cognitive problems such as a deficit in language (see Chapter 28), attention or perception (see Chapter 34). In this chapter we discuss the different types of memory, their neurobiological basis, and disorders that affect these different systems and their clinical manifestations. In particular it is useful to distinguish between **long-term** and **working memory** (which is often erroneously referred to as short-term memory). While this distinction relates to the duration of a memory, it primarily refers to whether material is maintained in consciousness (**working memory**) or whether it is stored unconsciously and then retrieved into consciousness (**long-term memory**).

Working memory
Definition
Working memory is the limited capacity (around seven items or chunks of information) to store information in consciousness that rapidly disappears when attention is diverted. A distinction is typically made between processes required for maintaining material and the control ('executive') processes required for manipulation of that material. Maintenance processes would typically be engaged by reciting a list of digits and requiring a subject to repeat them immediately (**digit span**). Executive control processes might be tested by requiring the subject to repeat the digits in reverse order.

Neuroanatomy and Neuroscience at a Glance, Fourth Edition. Roger A. Barker, Francesca Cicchetti, Michael J. Neal.

Neurobiological basis and disorders of working memory

Studies in humans and monkeys have unequivocally demonstrated the importance of the lateral prefrontal cortex in working memory processes (see also Chapter 34). It has been suggested that different parts of the prefrontal cortex are important for the maintenance and control processes that constitute working memory. Other brain regions are clearly implicated in working memory processes in a modality-dependent way. Working memory for visuospatial material may rely on occipitotemporal regions (when remembering, for example, the visual properties of an object) or occipitoparietal regions (when remembering spatial properties). On the other hand, holding verbal or phonological material in working memory seems to require the lateral temporal cortex. Whatever the domain, it appears that the efficient flexible use of working memory processes depends upon coordinated interactivity of frontal control processes and modality-dependent 'slave' systems.

Abnormalities in this system typically occur with damage in the sites listed above, especially the prefrontal cortex, as well as in some disorders of the basal ganglia (e.g. *Huntington's* and *Parkinson's disease*) where there is disruption of corticostriatal circuits (see Chapter 42). In these patients there is a difficulty in taking in information and as such the individuals have difficulty solving problems that require the ongoing manipulation of data.

Long-term memory

Definition

Long-term memory is the store of practically unlimited capacity and the memories within this system may persist over a lifetime. Long-term memory is primarily divided in to explicit and implicit components.

• **Explicit memory** refers to memories that are accessible to consciousness. It is divided into **episodic memory** (memory for episodes or events; typically, memory with an autobiographical content) and **semantic memory** (knowledge of facts; memory that is not characterized by an autobiographical content). Thus, an episodic memory of Paris might comprise the memory of a visit there, while a semantic memory is that Paris is the capital of France, situated on the Seine, etc.

• **Implicit memory** refers to memory that is not accessible to consciousness and typically refers to motor memory; it encompasses the acquisition of **motor skills**, **conditioning** (e.g. Pavlov's dogs salivating when hearing a bell), as well as **priming**. This latter process is defined as the subject's ability to provide answers to general questions (e.g. the word 'Paris' when asked to name a city), even when they do not remember this prior exposure.

Neuroanatomical basis and disorders of long-term memory

The famous case of HM, in whom both medial temporal cortices were removed for intractable epilepsy, provided the first clear evidence that the episodic memory system depends on medial regions of the temporal lobe. In addition, his case also highlighted the difference between explicit and implicit memories and that different systems underlie episodic and semantic memory at the neuroanatomical level. Subsequent to his operation, HM was unable to learn or recall new episodes or experiences in his life. However, his ability to learn new motor skills was preserved as was his factual knowledge. While there is a great deal of evidence underpinning the importance of medial temporal structures, especially the hippocampus, in episodic memory processes, it is clear that, as with working memory processes, distributed brain systems, frequently requiring prefrontally mediated control, are necessary for optimum autobiographical memory processes (see Chapters 11 and 34). In this respect, patients with certain forms of neurodegenerative disorders with relatively widespread pathology may have profound disorders of long-term memory, as for example in *Alzheimer's disease* (see Chapter 60). In this condition there is pathology within the hippocampus and related structures (see Chapter 45) as well as temporal and parietal cortices, and patients develop problems of anterograde memory (i.e. the laying down of new memories) followed by progressive problems with retrograde memory (the retrieval of preformed established memories). This distinction in anterograde and retrograde memories is thought to have a basis in transferring information from hippocampal structures to the overlying cortex and thus as the pathology spreads out so the memory processes are affected in a similar fashion. While in Alzheimer's disease the initial memory problem is more of an episodic nature, in some people there are problems within the semantic memory system. These cases of semantic dementia, wherein individuals begin to lose their knowledge of the meanings of words, depends on damage to the inferior and lateral temporal cortices and is seen in some patients with *frontotemporal dementia* (*FTD*).

Did you know?

Henry Gustav Molaison better known as HM, died in 2008 aged 82. He had been studied by neuroscientists for 55 years.

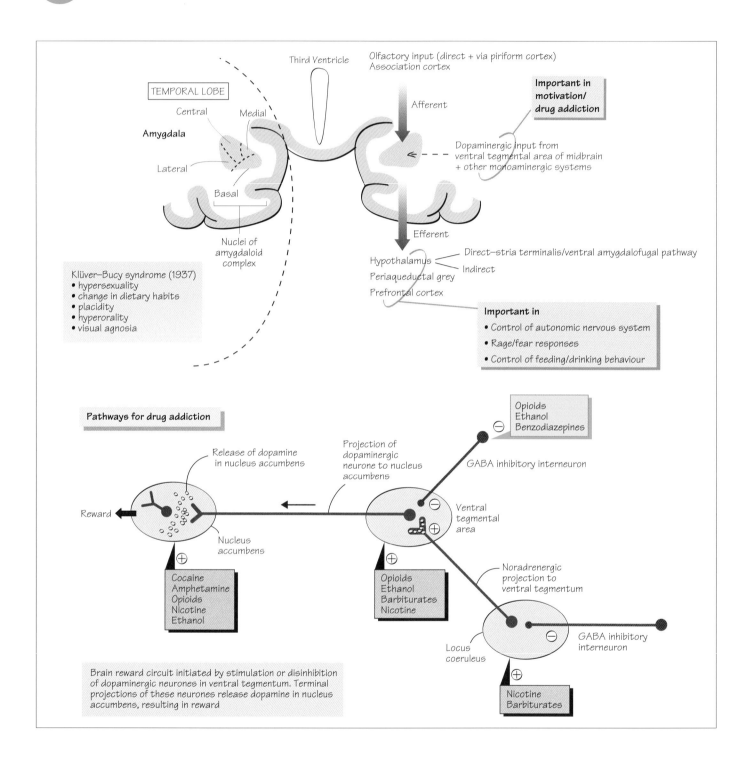

Emotion

Initial attempts to understand the brain bases of emotions focused on the limbic system (see Chapter 45), with the **amygdala** as the key component in the system thought to be central to emotional processing. The evidence to support such an association has already been discussed in part (in Chapter 45), but it is also worth mentioning the *Klüver–Bucy syndrome*. This condition is seen with bilateral amygdala damage and is characterized by, among other phenomena, an apparent absence of the normal fear response and by marked placidity.

Neuroanatomy and Neuroscience at a Glance, Fourth Edition. Roger A. Barker, Francesca Cicchetti, Michael J. Neal.

In addition, functional neuroimaging studies in humans have been consistent with animal studies, implicating the amygdala in the processing of emotional stimuli and, notably, in fear conditioning (wherein a previously neutral stimulus can, through association with an unpleasant outcome, produce a fear response when presented alone). It is proposed that the amygdala is the critical site in which: the necessary associations between the stimuli are formed using a process akin to the long-term potentiation (LTP) seen in the hippocampus (see Chapter 45); and the origin of the broad series of phenomena that constitute a fear response through its efferent projections.

Motivation

Emotions are potentially useful in that they are allied with, and perhaps consist of, behavioural responses. They may be critical in helping us choose between competing behavioural possibilities and to guide behaviours that maximize rewarding and minimize punishing outcomes. The relationship between emotion and motivation is therefore an important one. In this respect, the dopamine systems, most notably the **mesolimbic system** (see also Chapters 19 and 58), which has connections with the amygdala, appear critical. A series of hypotheses have been put forward concerning the dopaminergic contribution to motivation.

• *Hedonia hypothesis*: whilst dopamine has been thought to be critical to the experience of pleasure. There is increasing evidence against this view.

• *Learning hypothesis*: dopamine is critical to learning the relationship between stimuli and rewards. Dopamine acts as a 'teaching signal' for stimuli that predict rewards and thus is the origin of behaviour that makes the reward manifest.

• *Activation hypothesis*: dopamine is required for the actual engagement in work that must be done to obtain the reward. It is important for both the attentional and the locomotor components of the work involved in reward-seeking and consumption.

• *Incentive salience*: dopamine is important in imbuing certain stimuli with motivational or incentive properties.

It would be simplistic to express motivational processes solely in terms of the input of the mesolimbic dopamine system to the amygdala but it is nevertheless a useful model by which to explain drug addiction.

In addition to the motivational properties of specific stimuli, in many circumstances we must consider motivational states that appear stimulus independent. Feeding behaviours, for example, arise not solely from the motivational properties of foods (sight, smell, taste) but also from a drive state (hunger) dependent on a number of homeostatic factors, for example endocrine signals (levels of insulin, and of the hormones leptin and ghrelin which, respectively, reduce and promote feeding behaviour) acting predominantly through the hypothalamus (see Chapter 11). A comprehensive description of a motivational state would require several levels of description together with an understanding of the interactions inherent in the state; for example, the extent to which motivational properties of stimuli themselves influence, and/or are

influenced by, the drive state of the individual. An additional, important concern is when individuals are motivated towards behaviours that are at odds with their homeostatic requirements and consequently detrimental to health, as is the case with addictive behaviours.

Drug addiction

Using some recreational drugs can be rewarding, but the evidence is that addictive behaviours (and associated withdrawal phenomena) are determined by how the brain adapts in response to repeated drug administration rather than as a direct result of the fact that drugs may be intensely pleasurable. Conversely, although the reward properties of the drug are insufficient to explain addictive behaviours, it is simplistic, too, to consider addiction solely as behaviours aimed towards avoiding withdrawal symptoms. In addition to considering addiction in terms of the pursuit of pleasurable states (drug-induced euphoria) or the avoidance of withdrawal states (an array of physical and psychological symptoms which may actually be produced simply by a stimulus or environment that has become associated with previous withdrawal), we must also take into account what may be considered a markedly augmented state of motivation to taking the drug – referred to as *craving*. Important in this respect is the fact that a craving may be precipitated by a drug-related stimulus or environment long after the individual has recovered from the withdrawal symptoms.

Other important phenomena that need to be explained are tolerance (a requirement for increased frequency and/or dose of the drug with repeated usage) and sensitization (in contrast to tolerance effects, some of the consequences of the drug may actually increase with repeated ingestion). Interestingly, neither tolerance nor sensitization are explicable in purely pharmacological terms because both phenomena also show certain features suggesting that they are conditioned responses. One view that has been put forward to account for the simultaneous occurrence of tolerance and sensitization is that while the pleasurable effects of the drug diminish with repeated administration (leading to tolerance), the drug and related environments and paraphernalia become, over time, more likely to capture attention and to precipitate the associated behaviours (sensitization).

While the neurobiological basis of drug addiction is still not fully understood, there is increasing evidence that it involves mesolimbic dopamine systems and genetic susceptibilities, which may in turn affect the normal functioning of this pharmacological system. An example of this is the recent recognition that some patients with *Parkinson's disease* develop abnormal behaviours with their dopaminergic therapies – the so-called **dopamine dysregulation syndrome** which can involve pathological gambling and hypersexuality.

Did you know?

Oestrogens have been shown to promote memory functions.

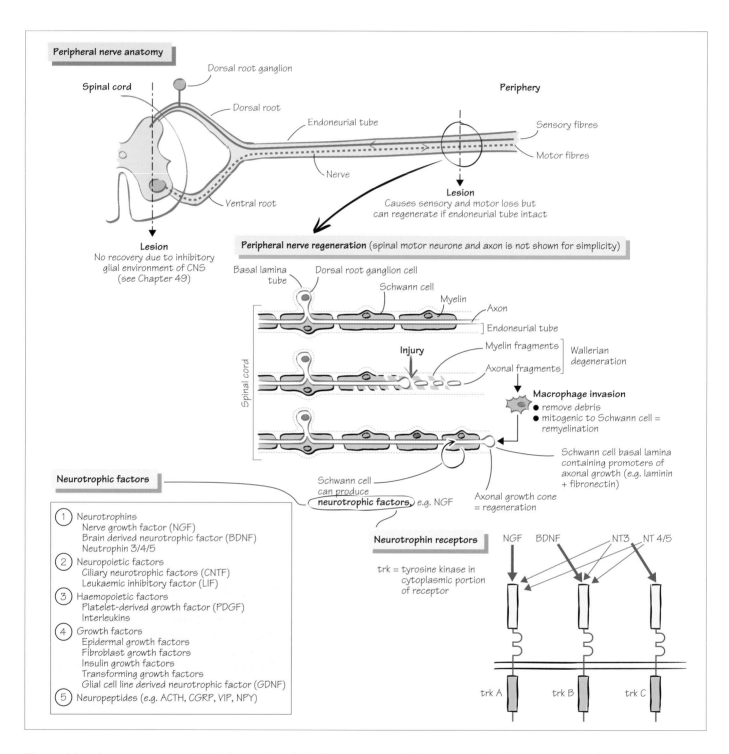

The peripheral nervous system (PNS) is capable of significant repair, to some extent independent of the age at which damage occurs. In contrast, the central nervous system (CNS) has always been thought of as being unable to repair itself, although there is now mounting evidence for considerable plasticity within it even in the adult state and that most, if not all areas of the CNS, are capable of some degree of reorganization (see Chapter 49).

Repair in the peripheral nervous system

Injury to a peripheral nerve if severe enough will cause permanent damage with loss of sensation, loss of muscle bulk and weakness.

Neuroanatomy and Neuroscience at a Glance, Fourth Edition. Roger A. Barker, Francesca Cicchetti, Michael J. Neal.

However, in many cases the nerve is able to repair itself, as the peripheral axon can regrow under the influence of the favourable environment of the Schwann cells. This is in contrast to the CNS where the neuroglial cells (astrocytes and oligodendrocytes) are generally inhibitory to axonal growth, even though most CNS neurones are capable of growing new axons.

When a peripheral nerve is damaged, the distal aspect of the axon is lost by the process of **wallerian degeneration**. Wallerian degeneration leads to the removal and recycling of both axonal and myelin-derived material, but leaves in place dividing Schwann cells inside the basal lamina tube that surrounds all nerve fibres. These columns of Schwann cells surrounded by basal lamina are known as **endoneurial tubes**, and provide the favourable substrate for axonal growth.

Following injury, the degenerating nerve fibre elicits an initial macrophage invasion and this in turn provides the mitogenic input to the Schwann cell. The regenerating axon starts to sprout within hours of injury and contacts the Schwann cell basal laminae on one side, and the Schwann cell membrane on the other. The Schwann cell basal lamina is especially important in the process of axonal sprouting as it contains a number of molecules that are powerful promoters of axonal outgrowth *in vitro* (e.g. laminin and fibronectin).

In addition to providing a substrate for axonal growth, Schwann cells also produce a number of neurotrophic factors, including nerve growth factor (NGF; see below). Thus, the Schwann cell provides a substrate along which the regenerating axon can grow, as well as providing a favourable humoral neurotrophic environment. It also helps direct the regenerating axon back to its appropriate target, by means of the endoneurial tube. Occasionally, the regrowth of the axons is inaccurate or incomplete so, for example, following damage to the third cranial nerve one can have aberrant regeneration such that there is elevation of the eyelid on looking down.

In contrast to axonal damage, the loss of the cell body (in the ventral horn or dorsal root ganglia) leads to an irreversible and permanent loss of axons in the peripheral nerve. Examples of such disorders include *poliomyelitis* and *motor neurone disease* (*MND*) with respect to the α-MN, and a number of inflammatory and *paraneoplastic syndromes* in the case of the dorsal root ganglia (see Chapters 60 and 62). In all these cases the loss of axons is secondary to the loss of the cell body and so no regeneration is possible. Attempts to rescue dying α-MN in *MND* via the peripheral delivery of neurotrophic factors have been made without much success to date (see Chapter 60).

Neurotrophic factors

The number of identified neurotrophic factors has expanded greatly since the original description of the first of these, NGF. These factors, many of which are also found to influence non-neural populations of cells, form discrete families that act through specific types of receptors. Many of these receptors are composed of subunits, one or some of which form common binding domains for a family of neurotrophic factors. For example, the neurotrophin family of neurotrophic factors and the *trk* receptors use a range of cytoplasmic tyrosine kinases as part of their signalling mechanism.

Many populations of neurones respond to neurotrophic factors experimentally both *in vitro* and in the lesioned animal. However, despite these encouraging results, administration of neurotrophic factors to patients in clinical trials of neurodegenerative disorders and neuropathies has met with only limited success. This argues against these disorders being the result of specific neurotrophic factor deficiencies (see Chapter 60). More recently, greater success has been achieved with the direct infusion of neurotrophic factors into the brain parenchyma rather than using the cerebrospinal fluid (CSF) or periphery, e.g. glial cell line derived neurotrophic factor (GDNF) in Parkinson's disease (see Chapters 41 and 42).

Did you know?

Salamanders can regrow their complete limbs over the course of a few weeks.

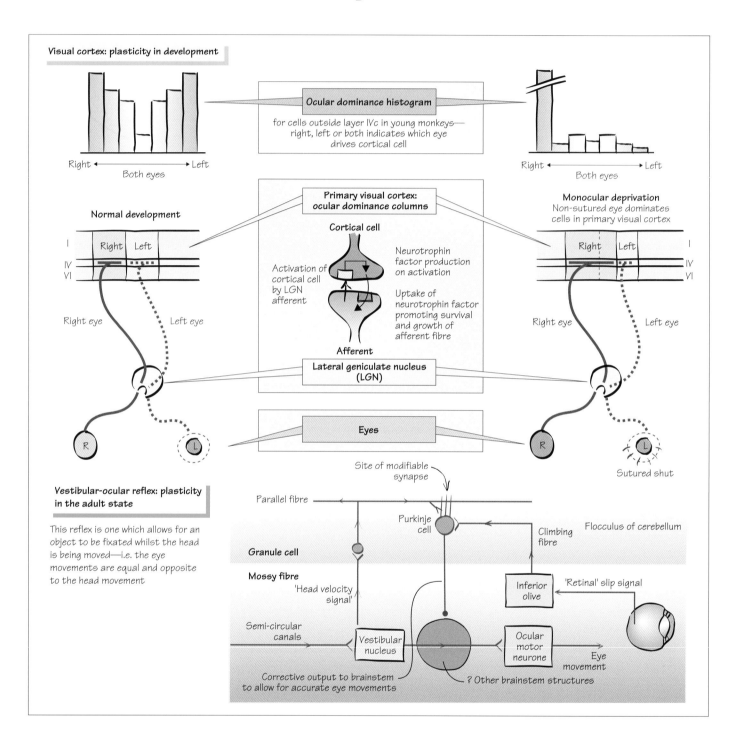

There is now mounting evidence that regeneration and reorganization can occur in the adult central nervous system (CNS). However, plasticity in the CNS is probably not due to a major production of new neurones, as most neurones in the mature CNS are post-mitotic, but to their ability to extend branching new axons. The time at which this is most florid is in the early postnatal period when the systems of the brain are developing, and it is during this time that major modifications can be made.

Neuroanatomy and Neuroscience at a Glance, Fourth Edition. Roger A. Barker, Francesca Cicchetti, Michael J. Neal.

The mechanisms underlying this plasticity are not fully known, but the production and uptake of factors promoting neuronal growth and survival (**neurotrophic factors**) are important.

Plasticity in the developing visual system

In their pioneering studies, Hubel and Wiesel demonstrated that at birth the input to lamina IV of the primary visual cortex (V1) is diffuse, and that it is only during the **critical period** of development (in cats this is up to 3–14 weeks of postnatal life while in humans it may be several years) that these inputs segregate and form the basis of ocular dominance columns (see Chapter 26).

The segregation of input is dependent on the amount and type of activity within the afferent pathway from each eye; the greater this is, the more likely it is that the afferent input will gain control over those cortical neurones. Thus, ocular dominance (OD) columns will form in the absence of competition between the input from the two eyes but will not develop when there is no afferent input from either eye.

Hubel and Wiesel experimentally manipulated the inputs by initially depriving one eye of an input by suturing it shut (**monocular deprivation**) and then reversing the procedure in later experiments ('**reverse suturing**'). Monocular deprivation created an expansion of the thalamic influence from the unsutured eye in layer IV with a subsequent shift in OD columns so that more cortical cells were under the control of the open eye. This pattern could be rapidly changed by 'reverse suturing' during the critical period, which implies that the initial shift in thalamic influence on cortical cells is caused by the activation of synapses that were present but functionally suppressed as there is not enough time for any axonal outgrowth. However, in time, the initially suppressed synapses from the uncompetitive eye would be physically lost as the active thalamic input takes over the control of cortical cells.

The correct segregation of the ocular inputs into V1 as OD columns is important for the generation of many of the other visual functions in V1. However, once outside the critical period the ability to modify the visual cortex in such a fashion is reduced, but not lost.

Plasticity in the adult state

Somatosensory system and the vestibulo-ocular reflex

It is now known that the somatosensory system is capable of being remodelled in the face of alterations in the input from the peripheral receptors. Thus, the loss of input from a digit (e.g. by amputation) does not lead to a permanently silent area of cortex, but instead the adjacent cortical areas with sensory inputs from adjacent digits would sprout axons and exert influence over this initially silent cortical area.

Conversely, increased afferent information in a sensory pathway results in an expansion of the cortical area receiving that input. Simplistically, it can be imagined that the activity in a given afferent induces the production of a neurotrophic factor in the postsynaptic cell, which then binds to the appropriate receptor in the active presynaptic terminal, promoting its growth and survival. In this way the CNS is constantly remodelling itself based on the amount and type of ongoing afferent information.

Subsequently, it was discovered that major sensory deficits, such as the deafferentation of a whole limb, produces similar results, which implies that the reclaiming of cortical areas by adjacent

inputs is not solely achieved by the local sprouting of axons in the cortex.

Occasionally, this plasticity may go awry in certain situations, such as in *dystonia*. In this condition, abnormal plasticity in the primary motor and sensory cortices is thought to cause abnormal activation of muscles, and this results in abnormal posturing of a body (see also Chapter 42). A further example of the plasticity of the mature CNS is seen with the vestibulo-ocular reflex (see Chapters 29 and 40). The vestibular system provides a signal to the CNS on head velocity and this is relayed to the cerebellum via mossy fibres. However, the other input to the cerebellum – the climbing fibre – can provide information on the degree to which the image is slipping across the retina (the degree to which eye movements are compensating or not for head movement). This input from the climbing fibre is not only important in providing a signal on the degree to which the reflex is working or not (i.e. provides an error signal), but also gives a critical input to correct it. Thus, if one alters the relationship between ocular and head movements by having the patient wear prisms, for example, the reflex adapts with time to compensate for the new relationship and this adaptation is possible because the climbing fibre input can modify the parallel fibre (and so indirectly mossy fibre) input to the Purkinje cell (see Chapter 40). The basis for this latter modification at the level of the Purkinje cell is an intracellular process and is termed **long-term depression** (**LTD**; see Chapter 45).

Neural stem cells

In many adult tissues, cell loss occurring through natural attrition or injury is balanced by the proliferation and subsequent differentiation of stem cells. In the adult CNS this was thought not to be the case, but recent evidence has shown that neural precursor cells are to be found in the mature CNS of mammals including humans. These cells are mainly found in the hippocampus and around the ventricles (in the subventricular zone) and appear to be able to form functionally active neurones. However, their role in plasticity and repair is unknown, but in the dentate gyrus of the hippocampus these cells may have a role in memory and mediating the effects of various hormones (e.g. cortisol/corticosterone) and drugs (e.g. antidepressants) on CNS function.

Limits on the regenerative capacity of the adult central nervous system

The regenerative capacity of the CNS is limited by:
• neurones are postmitotic in the mature CNS, and the stem cell population is small and localized to certain sites;
• glial cells in the CNS are generally inhibitory to axonal outgrowth (see Chapter 13).

Astrocytes produce signals that stop axons growing and oligodendrocytes produce a number of factors that repel axons or even cause the approaching axonal growth cone to collapse. Attempts to overcome these inhibitory signals are now entering early clinical trial in patients with spinal cord damage.

Did you know?

Rita Levi Montalcini, who won the Nobel Prize for her co-discovery of neurotrophic factors, did much of her early experimental work in this area in a laboratory she set up in her apartment.

The nervous system	Syndromes	Symptoms	Signs	Chapter
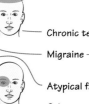	Stroke	Sudden onset weakness/ sensory loss/speech/loss of consciousness	LOC/UMN signs/sensory loss/language difficulties	6, 64
	Meningitis	Headache/photophobia/ phonophobia/stiff neck often subacute onset	LOC/confused/stiff neck, may occasionally have focal signs	5, 62
	Encephalitis	Headache, delirious, odd behaviours, abscences, may be unconscious	Rarely any focal signs. LOC Behavioural/confusional features	62
	Neurodegeneration	Slowly progressive problems typically involving movement and cognition	Cognitive and motor abnormalities such as dementia/parkinsonism/ UMN and LMN signs	42, 60
	Epilepsy	Intermittent episodes typically of altered consciousness and/or odd behavioural attacks	In most cases there are NO abnormal findings between attacks	61
	Multiple sclerosis	Episodes of altered feeling/ movement control, visual upset that initially come and go over days/weeks, developing permanent symptoms with time	Signs are dependent on site of inflammation but typically cause problems with visual acuity; eye movement control; cranial nerves; UMN and sensory sign with ataxia	62
	Myelitis/myelopathy	Can present acutely or subacutely with increasing difficulty in walking +/- use of arms/bladder problems +/- sensory loss	Typically have UMN signs in legs +/- LMN signs in arms with sensory features	54, 62
	Plexopathy	Present with subacute loss of power and sensation in a limb	LMN signs and sensory loss in affected limb	54
	Neuropathy	Present with sensory loss +/- weakness: Can be acute, sub-acute or chronic. Can affect all four limbs if a generalized neuropathy or just part of one if focal	LMN signs and sensory loss – the extent of which depends on the nature/type of neuropathy	54
	Neuromuscular junction disorder	Fatiguable weakness of arms/legs with intermittent diplopia, dysphonia, dysphagia	Examination can be normal but with exercise weakness can be seen. NO sensory signs should be found	16 , 62
	Muscle disease	Typically present with difficulty getting out of chairs/climbing stairs but may on occasions involve face/speech/swallowing and respiration, and can rarely just involve distal musculature	Often show proximal weakness +/- wasting with normal reflexes and no sensory loss	20, 21

Central nervous system – controls all basic bodily functions, and responds to external changes

Peripheral nervous system – provides a complete network of motor and sensory nerve fibres connecting the central nervous system to the rest of the body

LMN = Lower motor neurone
LOC = Loss of consciousness
UMN = Upper motor neurone

Common types of headaches

Chronic tension type headache – typically bifrontal extending over the head, present most of the time and worse as the day goes on. NOT associated with any abnormalities on examination

Migraine – typically comes and goes and is unilateral associated with nausea and vomiting/ photophobia +/– positive visual phenomena (zig-zag lines, etc). Rarely causes weakness or sensory loss. Can be caused by underlying problems to do with coagulation and channelopathies. No abnormalities on examination

Atypical facial pain – covers many symptoms. Typically no abnormal findings on examination and pain is poorly localized on the face

Other causes of headache

Cluster headache – rare, M>F, severe pain around one eye causing the eye to run, redden +/– close. Patient tends to be very agitated and even suicidal during the attack. Pain lasts 15-45 mins but comes and goes in clusters over weeks

Trigeminal neuralgia – paroxysms of pain that radiate down one of the three divisions of the trigeminal nerve. Typically mandibular branch

Raised intracranial pressure – rare, pain worse in morning or on lying down and can be associated with nausea/vomiting/visual problems and evolving neurological signs and decreased levels of consciousness

Giant cell/temporal arteritis – pain over the region of the superficial temporal artery. Can affect ophthalmic arteries, causing blindness and so must be treated urgently with steroids

Sinusitis – can cause headaches and/or facial pain/tenderness

Neuroanatomy and Neuroscience at a Glance, Fourth Edition. Roger A. Barker, Francesca Cicchetti, Michael J. Neal.

The overall aim of the history, examination and investigation of a patient is to establish if there is a neurological problem and if so:

- WHERE is the site of that pathology?
- WHAT is the nature of the abnormality?
- HOW can one best investigate it?
- HOW can one best treat it?

History taking

This may require input from a carer/spouse/relative/friend in the case of disorders of altered consciousness (e.g. epilepsy) or central nervous system (CNS) degenerative processes or major injury (e.g. head injury; Alzheimer's disease), especially if there is frontal lobe damage as this causes patients to lose insight into their problems.

The main elements of the history require the following information:

- What is the primary complaint?
- When did it begin?
- How has it progressed?
- Is it a recurrent problem?
- What associated features are seen with the main complaint?
- Have you had any neurological problems/injuries in the past?
- Is there a family history of neurological problems?
- What medication are you taking?
- What medical illnesses to date do you have or have had?
- What is your occupation?
- Do you smoke/drink/use illicit drugs?
- Any recent travel abroad?

Obviously, further direct questioning can be targeted to try to better define the nature of the problem depending on the initial complaint. It is worth bearing in mind that psychiatric problems can present with neurological symptoms.

Examination

What the patient complains about is a **symptom** and what you find on examination is a **sign**. The process by which one examines the nervous system is detailed in Chapter 51. However on occasions it may be necessary to also do a brief psychiatric assessment, and in cases where the disorder is thought to not be neurological then examination of other systems is mandatory (e.g. cardiovascular system with blackouts).

Investigations (see Chapters 52 and 53)

The number and type of investigations is driven by the answers to the above questions 1–3. Many tests are non-invasive and easy to do, but careful consideration must always be given as to why a test is being done and whether it is necessary.

Blackouts (see also Chapter 61)

This can be due to epilepsy, disturbances of circulation (faints, cardiac dysrhythmias, aortic stenosis) or on occasions due to anxiety/psychiatric problems. It is important to get a clear history of when the attacks occur, what causes them and what happens during them, which typically requires a *witnessed* account.

Dizziness

This is a very common problem and it is often hard to make a diagnosis. It is rarely due to CNS disease. It is more commonly a feature of an inner ear problem (see Chapter 29) or anxiety with hyperventilation.

Sensory symptoms (see Chapter 54)

Many patients complain of focal sensory disturbances – numbness or tingling. If very focal and not associated with weakness then the chances of finding a cause for it are very rare. Indeed if no 'hard' signs can be elicited, again, it is unlikely that a cause will be found.

Fatigue

This is a very non-specific symptom and rarely yields to a diagnosis. It is important to differentiate between fatigue/tiredness and:

- weakness = motor neurone involvement;
- daytime somnolence = sleep problem;
- fatiguable weakness = neuromuscular junction problem.

Fatigue is a common feature of depression but can also be seen in multiple sclerosis (MS) and Parkinson's disease.

Did you know?

The first neurology book in English was written in 1650 by Robert Pemell, an English country physician. It was entitled *De Morbis Capitis* or *Of the Chief Internal Diseases of the Head*.

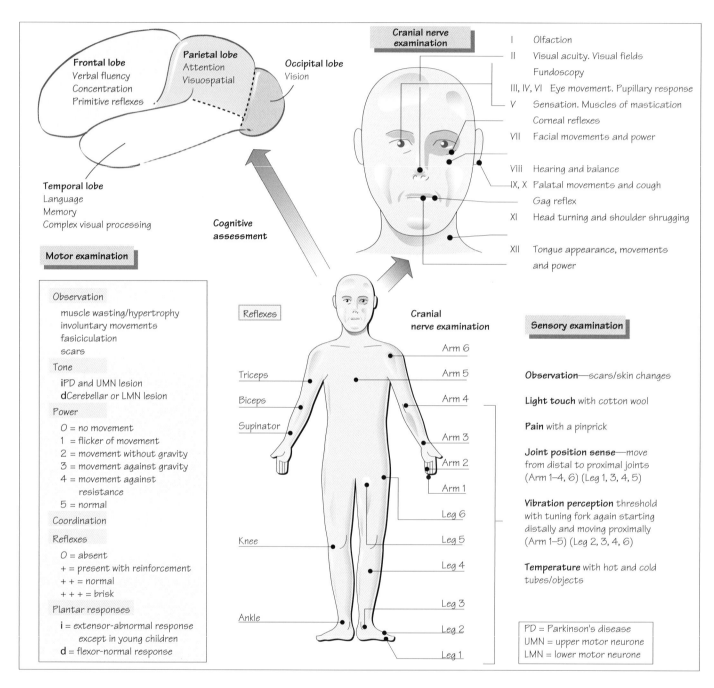

The examination of the nervous system can be broken down into a number of separate assessments.

Cognitive examination

There are a number of widely available assessment tools including the Mini Mental State Examination (MMSE; <25 is taken to indicate dementia) and the revised Addenbrooke's Cognitive Examination (ACE-r). However in clinic, targeted tests of cognition are very helpful at delineating the main site of pathology causing cognitive problems. However, these tests are only useful to do if the patient has a normal level of consciousness, is able to pay attention and has no major problem with language.

General

• **Orientation in time, person and place**: if these cannot be correctly answered (assuming the patient has no major language deficits) then the patient is either acutely confused or severely demented, in which case the remainder of the cognitive examination is unlikely to be helpful.

Neuroanatomy and Neuroscience at a Glance, Fourth Edition. Roger A. Barker, Francesca Cicchetti, Michael J. Neal.

Frontal lobe function

• **Verbal fluency**: number of words generated beginning with a certain letter (e.g. 's') or specific category (e.g. animals) over a 60- or 90-second period.
• **Concentration**: the ability to take in and repeat back immediately a list of objects or a name and address.
• **Primitive reflexes**: including pouting of the lips when they are tapped and grasping the examiner's hand when it is gently moved across the patient's hand.

Parietal lobe function

• **Attention**: or neglect of visual or somatosensory stimuli in the contralateral sensory hemifield.
• **Dyspraxia**: the patient is unable to form, copy or mime gestures and common tasks (e.g. combing hair).
• **Visuospatial function**: the ability to copy drawings (e.g. interlocking pentagons).

Temporal lobe function

• **Anterograde memory**: the ability to remember a standard name and address given to the patient (e.g. Peter Marshall, 42 Market Street, Chelmsford, Essex) 5 minutes after it has been given. It is though important to ensure that the patient has taken in information in the first place.
• **Language**: language assessment involves listening to spontaneous speech for content and fluency, naming objects, repeating phrases (e.g. 'no ifs, ands or buts'), following commands, reading and writing (see also Chapter 28).

Cranial nerves

• **Olfactory nerve**: each nostril is tested separately with a range of standard odours.
• **Optic nerve**: visual acuity for each eye is tested using standard eyesight charts. The visual fields for each eye are then tested with examination of the blind spot if necessary (see Chapter 24). The fundi (back of the eye) are examined with an ophthalmoscope looking for abnormalities of the retina and optic disc, e.g. swollen (papilloedema) or pale and atrophic (optic atrophy). Colour vision (using the Ishihara colour plates) and pupillary responses can also be tested.
• **Oculomotor, trochlear and abducens nerves**: ptosis, pupillary abnormalities and eye movements are looked at (e.g. see Chapters 3, 25 and 56).
• **Trigeminal nerve**: sensation is tested in all three divisions of the trigeminal nerve and the power of the jaw muscles. In some cases, the corneal reflex is tested by lightly touching the cornea with cotton wool.
• **Facial nerve**: the power of facial muscles is tested, e.g. the patient screws up their eyes tightly, blows out their cheeks or purses their lips. The examiner should *not* be able to overcome any of these movements.
• **Vestibulocochlear nerve**: hearing is tested in each ear by gently whispering a number into each. More formal testing can be performed with tuning forks.
• **Glossopharyngeal and vagus nerves**: the patient opens their mouth wide and says 'ahhhhhh' so that the movement of the palate can be assessed. The gag reflex can be tested by gently placing a spatula against the posterior pharyngeal wall and noting any reflex movement of the palate. Testing the strength and character of a cough can also be helpful in some cases.
• **Spinal accessory nerve**: this is tested by getting the patient to turn their head to the right and left and shrug their shoulders. The examiner should not be able to overcome this movement.

• **Hypoglossal nerve**: this is tested by looking at the tongue in the floor of the mouth for wasting or fasciculation; it is then protruded from the mouth and any deviation from the midline noted. Power is tested by getting the patient to push the tongue into each cheek, assuming they do not have any significant facial weakness.

Motor system examination of the limbs

The examination of the motor system includes:
• **Observation**: involuntary movements, wasting, weakness, fasciculation, scars or deformities.
• **Tone**: the limb is gently moved and its stiffness assessed. Stiffness is increased in Parkinson's disease or upper motor neurone (UMN) lesions and decreased in lower motor neurone (LMN) or cerebellar lesions (see Chapters 35–42). Sometimes the tone is increased because the patient cannot relax or is in pain.
• **Power**: movements are assessed and scored according to the Medical Research Council (MRC) rating scale (see figure).
• **Coordination**: the ability to coordinate movements in the upper limb is tested by getting the patient to touch the examiner's finger and then their own nose with the same finger after it has slowly moved about in front of the patient. This may be abnormal if there is weakness, sensory loss or cerebellar disease. In the lower limb, coordination is tested by getting the patient to walk normally, then heel–toe walking and finally by getting the patient to run their right/left heel along their left/right shin, respectively, while lying down.
• **Reflexes**: these are tested by tapping the tendons at certain sites in the upper and lower limb. Reflexes can be absent, reduced, normal or brisk. The latter implies a UMN lesion while reduced or absent reflexes implies a dysfunction in part of the spinal monosynaptic reflex (see Chapter 35).
• **Plantar responses**: the sole of the foot is gently scratched along its lateral aspect and the toes should fan out and the big toe go down (flexor or normal plantar response). If the toes point up and this is not a withdrawal response, it implies a UMN lesion.

Sensory examination

Sensation in the limbs is tested at the extremities and in the dermatomes using a number of tests.
• **Light touch**: cotton wool is gently applied to the skin, having checked that the patient can feel it normally (test on face first, assuming there is no trigeminal sensory loss).
• **Pinprick**: a blunted pin is used.
• **Temperature**: cold and hot tubes or objects are used.
• **Vibration perception threshold** (VPT): a tuning fork is applied to the distal interphalangeal joint or big toe. The patient must feel it vibrating, *not* just feel it being applied to the joint. If it is not felt to vibrate, the fork is moved proximally.
• **Joint position sense** (JPS): this is tested by slightly moving the terminal joint in the hand or toe, having checked that the patient understands what is meant by up and down movements. This movement should be very slight, as JPS is very sensitive in humans. If the movement cannot be detected then larger movements are made at these joints before moving to more proximal joints, in the same way as for VPT.

Did you know?

The plantar response was originally described by Joseph Babinski in 1896, whose brother was a famous cook and engineer.

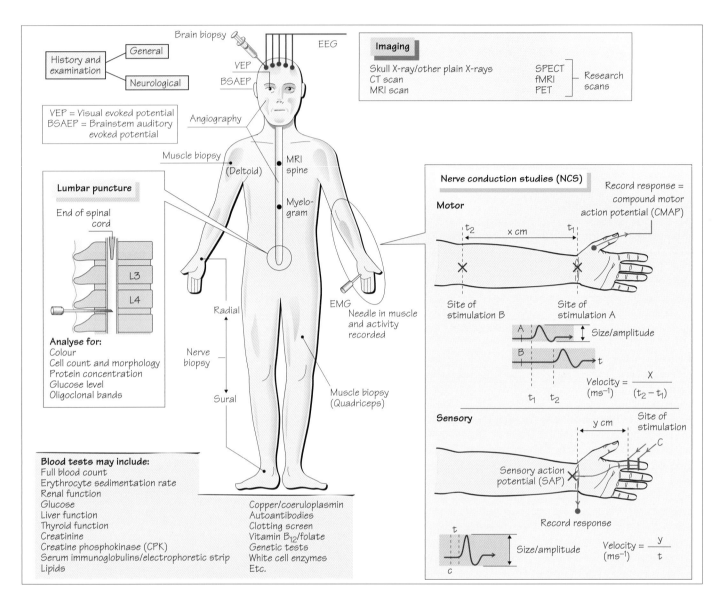

The key to investigating any patient is through their history and examination, as this will highlight the likely nature and site of the problem.

History and examination (see Chapters 50 and 51)

At the end of the history and examination one should have formulated a hypothesis of where the problem lies and what the problem could be, which will then guide investigations.

Blood tests

A large number of tests are available (see figure for examples).

Imaging (see also Chapter 53)

• Plain X-rays are rarely of value in the diagnosis of neurological disease, unless one suspects the patient has a related disease in another site such as the chest (e.g. lung cancer).

• Computed tomography (CT) gives detailed X-ray images of the brain, skull and lower spine. It is useful for diagnosing structural lesions such as tumours, major strokes or skull fractures. It is widely available but has limited resolution especially in the posterior fossa and cervicothoracic spinal cord.

• Magnetic resonance imaging (MRI) is a noisy, claustrophobic procedure which relies on patient cooperation. It provides detailed images of all parts of the brain and spinal cord and the use of different sequences has increased its utility and diagnostic strength. It does not involve any radiation.

• Magnetic resonance angiography and venography (MRA/MRV) scans delineate the major blood vessels to, within and from the brain. They are primarily used to look for significant narrowing (stenosis) of the extracranial carotid arteries in the neck, aneurysms in the brain and blockage of the major venous sinuses in the brain, but are not as sensitive as angiography.

Neuroanatomy and Neuroscience at a Glance, Fourth Edition. Roger A. Barker, Francesca Cicchetti, Michael J. Neal.

- Angiography involves the passing of a small catheter to the origin of the major blood vessels of the brain (both carotid and vertebral arteries), and a small amount of dye is injected. The dye can then be followed using a video and images captured rapidly over time as the dye passes through the vascular tree. The procedure is invasive and carries a small risk of complication, but is useful in accurately delineating any vascular abnormalities (e.g. carotid stenoses, aneurysms, arteriovenous malformations and venous sinus thrombosis). It can also be used to look for specific vascular abnormalities in the spinal cord.
- Myelography is rarely used nowadays to delineate abnormalities in the spinal cord because of the non-invasiveness and resolution of MRI. However, it can be helpful in some circumstances and involves injecting a radio-opaque dye via a lumbar puncture into the subarachnoid space around the spine.
- Single photon emission computed tomography (SPECT) involves radioactive isotopes which typically provide information on perfusion within the brain. It has low resolution.
- Positron emission tomography (PET) detects the release of positrons from specific substances that bind to certain chemical sites within the brain. It is only used to localize small occult tumours in patients with suspected paraneoplastic syndromes at the moment.

Electrical tests

- Electrocardiography (ECG) is an electrical recording from the heart, and is performed in many patients with neurological disease, especially those with muscle disease, blackouts or some genetic disorders (e.g. myotonic dystrophy).
- Electroencephalography (EEG) measures the electrical activity and rhythms of the brain and is helpful in patients with decreased levels of consciousness, epilepsy (see Chapter 61) and some patients with sleep disorders (e.g. narcolepsy; see Chapter 43).
- Nerve conduction studies (NCS) involve stimulating both sensory and motor nerves and measuring the response. The general principle is that one stimulates at one site of the nerve and records at another site or the muscle it innervates. The size and speed of the response are important. Loss of myelin (demyelination) slows the speed of conduction, while a loss of axons gives a smaller response but normal conduction velocity. It is useful in determining whether the patient has a neuropathy, what type (demyelinating versus axonal) and the extent (focal or generalized).
- Electromyography (EMG) involves placing a needle into the muscle and recording the electrical activity within it. It is useful in the diagnosis of muscle disease and in patients with motor neuronal loss as occurs in *motor neurone disease* (*MND*) because EMG can show the extent of denervation, helping in the diagnosis.
- Evoked potentials (EPs) can be recorded from the visual pathway (visual-evoked potential or responses; VEP), auditory pathway (brainstem auditory-evoked potential BSAEP) or peripheral nerves in the arms or legs (somatosensory-evoked potential). The test involves stimulating the peripheral receptor (eye, ear or median/posterior tibial nerve) and measuring the cortical response. This gives a measure of conduction that has both a peripheral and CNS component. The most commonly used test is VEP in *multiple sclerosis* to look for asymptomatic demyelination in visual pathways.
- Central motor conduction time (CMCT) measures the time from stimulating the motor cortex to measuring a muscle response in the periphery such as the hand. It is not routinely available and can be used as a measure of integrity of the descending corticospinal tract assuming that there is no dysfunction within the peripheral motor apparatus.
- Thermal thresholds are a subjective test designed to look at small fibre responses in patients. It relies on the patient detecting changes in temperature in the hands and feet. It is not routinely available.

Cerebrospinal fluid analysis

Cerebrospinal fluid (CSF) can be obtained from a number of sites but is routinely obtained by a lumbar puncture, which involves passing a small needle into the subarachnoid space in the lower lumbar spine. CSF should be clear and sent for analysis to include the following:
- Numbers of certain cell types are typically raised in infections (e.g. **meningitis** and **encephalitis**) as well as in **malignant meningitis** (where cancer cells seed themselves along the meninges).
- Culture of the CSF to look for infective organisms, including Gram staining in meningitis and polymerase chain reaction (PCR) for the causative organism in some infections of the CNS (e.g. herpes simplex virus in herpes encephalitis).
- Glucose levels, which can be low in certain types of infection or meningitis and metastatic tumours growing in the meninges.
- Protein levels, which can be raised in some types of neuropathy, tumour and in lesions blocking spinal CSF flow.
- Oligoclonal bands indicative of immunoglobulin synthesis specifically within the CNS, typically seen in *multiple sclerosis*.

Nerve/muscle biopsy

In cases where there is evidence of nerve or muscle disease, a biopsy may be helpful in identifying the defect more specifically. Typical biopsy sites are the radial and sural nerves and the quadriceps and deltoid muscles.

Brain biopsy

This is routinely performed in patients with brain tumours to confirm the diagnosis and to some extent predict prognosis. In some cases of progressive neurological disease for which no obvious cause can be found, a biopsy looking specifically for inflammation in the blood vessels (vasculitis) as well as prion disease may be considered.

Did you know?

The first documented experiments with EMG were undertaken by Francesco Redi in 1666.

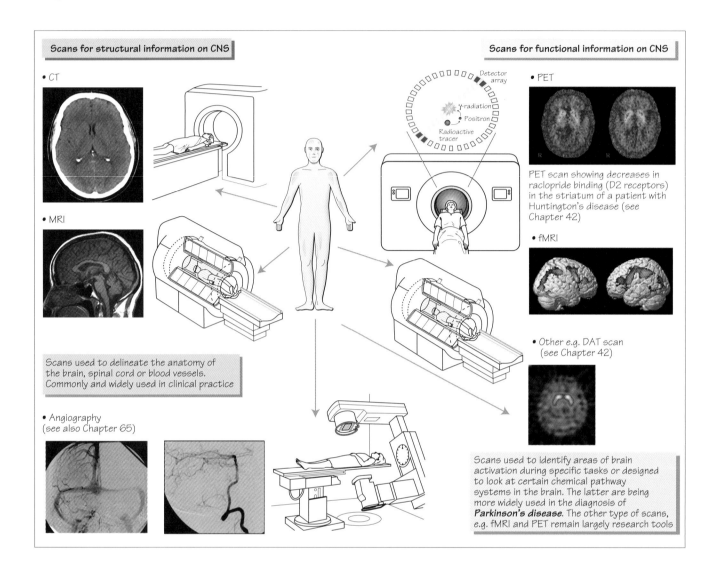

Scans for structural information on CNS

• CT

• MRI

Scans used to delineate the anatomy of the brain, spinal cord or blood vessels. Commonly and widely used in clinical practice

• Angiography (see also Chapter 65)

Scans for functional information on CNS

Detector array

γ-radiation

Positron

Radioactive tracer

• PET

PET scan showing decreases in raclopride binding (D2 receptors) in the striatum of a patient with Huntington's disease (see Chapter 42)

• fMRI

• Other e.g. DAT scan (see Chapter 42)

Scans used to identify areas of brain activation during specific tasks or designed to look at certain chemical pathway systems in the brain. The latter are being more widely used in the diagnosis of **Parkinson's disease**. The other type of scans, e.g. fMRI and PET remain largely research tools

Imaging of the central nervous system (CNS) is essentially designed to look either at structure (computed tomography [CT], magnetic resonance imaging [MRI], angiography) or function (functional MRI [fMRI], positron emission tomography [PET], and single photon emission CT [SPECT]). In clinical practice it is the former that is the mainstay of practice, with the latter tests reserved for patients being investigated for specific problems or as part of a research project.

• In general structural scanning is undertaken to determine if there is any abnormality in the CNS on imaging.

• If there is an abnormality, then where is it and does it fit with the history and clinical examination?

• What is the likely nature of that abnormality pathologically based on its radiological appearance?

This information can be used for the future investigation and management of patients with neurological disorders. This chapter outlines the major imaging modalities used in clinical practice, their indications, value and drawbacks.

Structural imaging
CT imaging

• **Basic principle**: this technique uses X-rays to scan the brain or spine (typically lumbar) and then reconstruct an image of that structure; it can be performed with or without a contrast agent, the latter being used to better define blood vessels and abnormalities in the blood–brain barrier.

• **Use**: imaging of the brain looking for major abnormalities, in particular stroke, head trauma, hydrocephalus or tumour, especially in the acute medical situation. It can also be used to look for skull fractures and prolapsed intervertebral discs in the lumbar spine, and in some cases to look for cerebral aneurysms.

Neuroanatomy and Neuroscience at a Glance, Fourth Edition. Roger A. Barker, Francesca Cicchetti, Michael J. Neal.

- **Advantages**: widely available, and often gives useful and vital information especially in acute situations. It is well tolerated by nearly all patients, even those who cannot fully cooperate, and if general anaesthesia is needed, this is more easily performed with CT than MRI.
- **Disadvantage**: it has poor contrast resolution compared with MRI and as such is not so good at identifying lesions in the posterior fossa and cervicothoracic spine. This is because dental fillings can often result in several artefacts on scans of the posterior fossa. It also involves radiation, which can be an issue in some situations – e.g. pregnancy.

MRI

- **Basic principle**: this technique places the patient in a strong magnetic field which is then subject to a series of magnetic perturbations (scan sequence), which alter the orientation of hydrogen ions, such that their change and subsequent shift back to normal position is detected. Thus, it does not use X-rays and is very sensitive to subtle changes in water content, which makes it a highly sensitive scan.
- **Use**: most patients with neurological problems should have an MRI scan, given its superior spatial resolution compared with CT scanning and the fact that any part of the neural axis can be scanned with it. Thus, it is employed in patients with chronic neurological problems (e.g. *multiple sclerosis*) as well as those with evolving acute disorders (e.g. *herpes encephalitis*). It can also be used with a contrast agent (gadolinium) and to image blood vessels both on the arterial side (magnetic resonance angiography [MRA]) looking for carotid artery disease or intracerebral aneurysms and on the venous side (magnetic resonance venography [MRV]), especially to look for major venous sinus thromboses.
- **Advantages**: high spatial resolution and the fact that any part of the neural axis can be imaged, along with the major vessels, without recourse to X-ray exposure or invasive procedures.
- **Disadvantage**: it is a noisy, claustrophobic experience and requires the patient to be cooperative to some extent. Some patients cannot cope with the claustrophobia while agitated patients will move in the scanner causing major artefacts on the images. It also cannot be used in patients with metallic magnetic materials such as a cardiac pacemaker.

Angiography

- **Basic principle**: this is the imaging of blood vessels and it can be carried out using CT and MRI, but in some cases it requires the direct visualization of blood vessels using a radiolucent contrast agent injected into an artery with video fluoroscopy to follow its course. Thus, the flow of the dye can be followed through the vasculature and X-rays taken to capture various different phases of the injection; this can identify problems on the arterial and venous sides of the circulation.

- **Use**: its main value is the identification of vascular abnormalities such as aneurysms, arteriovenous malformations and venous sinus disease. In all cases angiography is either performed to confirm an equivocal MRA/MRV result or as a prelude to a more invasive procedure to deal with the underlying abnormality such as the obliteration of vascular malformations through intravascular occlusion techniques (gluing or coiling).
- **Advantage**: it is the most high-resolution scan for identifying vascular abnormalities and is essential if intravascular interventional therapies are being considered.
- **Disadvantage**: it is an invasive procedure with a small but nevertheless real complication rate of stroke and local haemorrhage/haematoma at the site at which the catheter is passed into the artery (typically the femoral artery in the groin).

Functional scanning

This embraces SPECT, PET and fMRI. Although there are a number of different types of scan, they can be thought of as looking at either:
- Blood flow/metabolism, using glucose and oxygen markers to reflect neuronal activity and pathology, such that a loss of activity reflects an area that contains dysfunctional or dead neurones. So, for example, in Alzheimer's disease, there will be hypoperfusion in the parietotemporal cortices. Such 'metabolic' scans can be undertaken for diagnostic and therapeutic purposes in some patients in routine clinical practice. Another related approach, which is currently only used in research, relies on looking at oxygen extraction in areas of the brain while the patient is being tested on a particular task while being imaged in the MRI scanner. The resultant scan will show which areas of the brain are activated by that task. This is called fMRI, and has been used, for example, to see which brain areas are activated by specific types of cognitive or visual processing tasks.
- Specific neurochemical markers which are used to identify and label particular aspects of a neurotransmitter pathway. In Parkinson's disease this may involve looking at the dopamine transporter (e.g. DAT scans) or certain types of dopamine receptors (e.g. ^{11}C-raclopride labelling of D2 receptors in PET). The former types of scan are found in many nuclear medicine departments and are widely available, while PET scanning is still only an experimental tool and found in a few research centres. However, [^{18}F]2-fluoro-2-deoxy-D-glucose (FDG)-PET scanning is being increasingly used to find small tumours in patients with suspected paraneoplastic syndromes (see Chapter 62). This is because they can detect small metabolically active tumours that cannot be seen using traditional imaging modalities.

Did you know?

The first PET scanner was built in 1961 and was nicknamed the head shrinker.

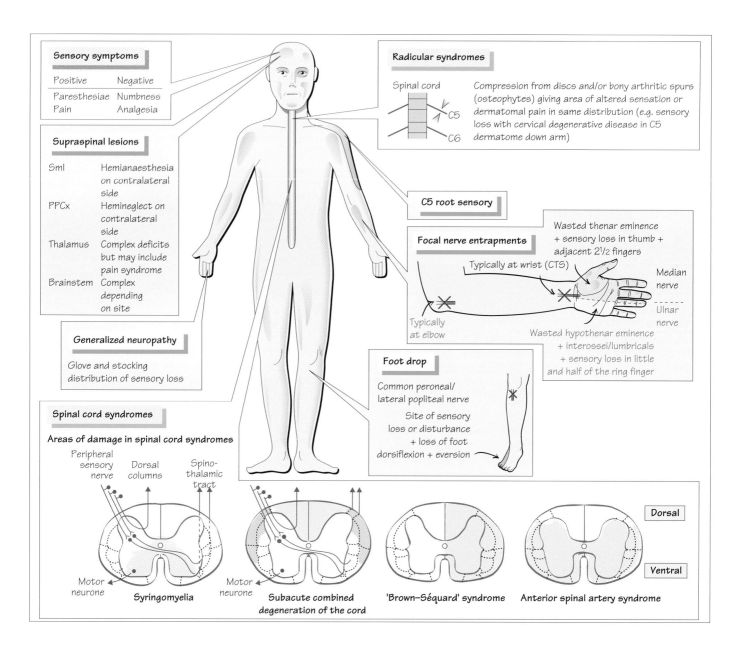

Disturbances in the sensory pathways can produce one of two main symptoms:
• negative ones, with a loss of sensation such as numbness or analgesia;
• positive ones, such as pins and needles (paraesthesiae) or pain.
These symptoms can arise from many different sites along the sensory pathways, but it is often the distribution of sensory change that points towards the likely site of pathology.

In order to determine the nature and cause of the sensory disturbance a full history and examination is needed along with appropriate tests. Most patients with isolated sensory symptoms do not yield to a diagnosis but the most common causes are neuropathies and multiple sclerosis.

A typical screen of tests for patients with sensory symptoms involves blood tests, nerve conduction studies (NCS) and magnetic resonance imaging (MRI) of brain and spinal cord. In all cases it is important to remember that non-neurological causes, e.g. hyperventilation.

Peripheral nerves

Diseases of the peripheral nerves can cause sensory disturbance. This can either be caused by *focal nerve entrapment* or a *generalized neuropathy*, in which case the disease process can target either the large or small fibres or both. Common focal nerve entrapments include:
• The median nerve at the wrist (*carpel tunnel syndrome*). Patients typically present with aching in the forearm especially at night,

Neuroanatomy and Neuroscience at a Glance, Fourth Edition. Roger A. Barker, Francesca Cicchetti, Michael J. Neal.

weakness of some of the thumb muscles and loss of sensation over the thumb and adjacent two and a half fingers. It can resolve spontaneously but in cases where it does not, simple splinting, steroid injection or even surgical decompression is often curative.

• The ulnar nerve at the elbow. Patients present with wasting of most of the intrinsic hand muscles with weakness and loss of sensation in the hand involving the little and half of the ring finger but without involvement of the forearm. It can be treated by surgical transposition of the nerve in some cases.

• The common peroneal (or lateral popliteal nerve) can be trapped around the knee. Patients typically present with foot drop and numbness on the outer aspect of the foot.

Generalized neuropathies may be caused by many disorders and if large fibres are preferentially involved then there is a loss of joint position sense, vibration perception and light touch along with absent or reduced reflexes. These neuropathies are rarely purely sensory and often associated with weakness and wasting. The typical pattern of sensory loss in these neuropathies is 'glove and stocking' which, as the name implies, reflects the symmetrical loss of sensation in all four limbs to the wrist/forearm and to the ankle/shin.

In some cases patients complain of much pain but paradoxically have reduced sensation for pain and temperature. These patients are more likely to have **small fibre neuropathy**. Rarely, the dorsal root ganglion cell (as opposed to the peripheral nerve) is targeted by the disease process. In these instances there is a devastating loss of proprioception which greatly compromises motor function.

Peripheral pain syndromes are discussed in Chapters 32 and 33, but it is always important to remember that pain is more often the result of non-neurological causes such as arthritis or local tissue damage.

The nerves as they emerge out of the spinal column can be trapped typically by bony spurs or intervertebral discs and give sensory disturbance along that nerve root. Patients normally complain of pain radiating down that nerve root with sensory abnormalities confined to that dermatome (see Chapter 2). This commonly happens in the cervical and lumbar region and may require surgical decompression especially in cases where there is weakness, wasting and loss of the appropriate reflexes.

Spinal cord

Syringomyelia
Syringomyelia is the development, for a number of reasons, of a cyst or cavity around or near to the central canal, usually in the cervical region, which tends to spread over time up and down the spinal cord. The lesion typically disrupts the spinothalamic tract (STT) fibres as they cross just ventral to the central canal, resulting in a dissociated sensory loss, i.e. reduced temperature and pain sensation at the level of the lesion but normal light touch, vibration perception and joint position sense (see Chapter 31). In addition, there may be motor involvement because of expansion of the cyst into the ventral horn or dorsolaterally into the descending motor tracts and other ascending sensory pathways.

Subacute combined degeneration of the spinal cord
This is usually associated with pernicious anaemia and a lack of vitamin B_{12}. It is characterized by demyelination and eventually degeneration of the dorsal columns (DCs), the spinocerebellar (SCT) and corticospinal tracts (CoST) as well as damage to peripheral nerves (**peripheral neuropathy**). Patients therefore develop a combination of paraesthesiae and sensory loss (especially light touch, vibration perception and joint position sense) with weakness and incoordination (see Chapter 55). The weakness may be of both an upper *and* lower motor neurone type (see Chapter 55).

Brown–Séquard syndrome
This describes a lesion involving half of the cord such that there is an ipsilateral loss of position and tactile senses (DC sensory information), a contralateral loss of temperature sensation originating from several segments below the lesion (STT sensory information), and ipsilateral spasticity and weakness because of involvement of the CoST pathway (see Chapters 31, 32, 37).

Anterior spinal artery syndrome
This syndrome describes the situation when there is occlusion of the artery providing blood to the anterior two-thirds of the cord. The patient has weakness and sensory loss to temperature and pain with preservation of DC sensory modalities such as joint position sense and vibration perception (see Chapter 6).

Transverse myelitis
Transverse myelitis (not shown in figure) describes a complete lesion of the whole spinal cord at one level that produces a complete sensory loss with weakness from that level down. The weakness is characteristically caused by a disruption of both the descending motor pathways and the spinal motor neurones. It is typically seen as a part of **multiple sclerosis** or a secondary acute demyelinating process in response to infection such as an atypical pneumonia.

Brain
Abnormalities in supraspinal sites can result from a variety of causes and depending on the disease process and site determines the type of sensory disturbance. Typically, hemispheric lesions give a loss of sensation down the contralateral side of the body. Brainstem lesions give rise to a range of sensory deficits depending on the exact level of the lesion. For example, a pontine lesion can give ipsilateral sensory loss of the face but contralateral sensory loss in the limbs.

Cortical lesions can give a loss of sensation if the primary somatosensory cortex is involved, or can give more complex sensory deficits such as astereognosis (an inability to recognize objects by touch) or even sensory neglect or inattention. These latter abnormalities are typically seen with lesions of the posterior parietal cortex (see Chapter 34).

In some cases, irritative lesions of the primary sensory cortex give rise to simple partial seizures (see Chapter 61) in which the patient experiences brief migrating sensory symptoms up one side of the body. This can also be seen in some patients with transient ischaemic attacks (TIAs).

Pain syndromes can also develop with central lesions and this is best seen in small thalamic vascular events, where dysaesthesia is found in the contralateral limb in a typically diffuse distribution (see Chapter 33).

Did you know?

The word paraesthesia derives from the Greek words *para* (meaning beside or abnormal) and *aisthēsis* (meaning sensation) and was first used in 1860.

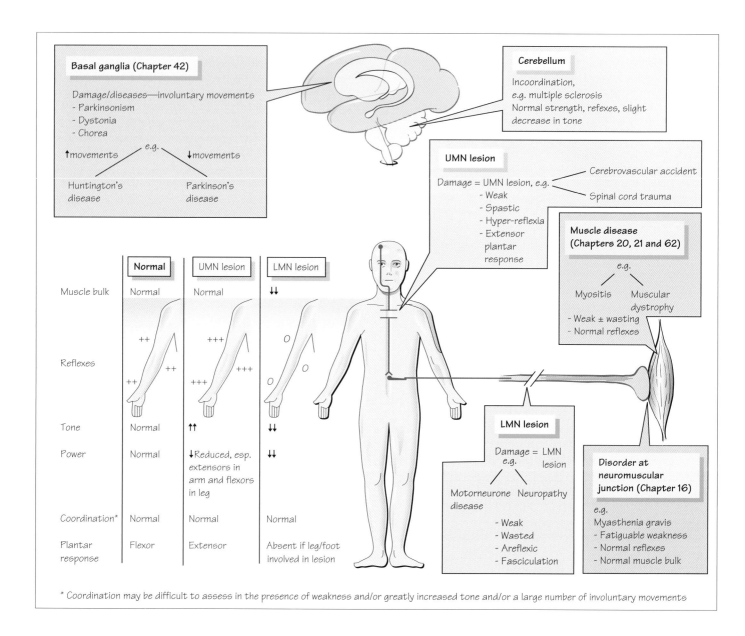

Basal ganglia (Chapter 42)

Damage/diseases—involuntary movements
- Parkinsonism
- Dystonia
- Chorea

↑movements   e.g.   ↓movements

Huntington's disease   Parkinson's disease

Cerebellum

Incoordination,
e.g. multiple sclerosis
Normal strength, refexes, slight
decrease in tone

UMN lesion

Damage = UMN lesion, e.g. — Cerebrovascular accident
- Weak
- Spastic   Spinal cord trauma
- Hyper-reflexia
- Extensor
  plantar
  response

Muscle disease (Chapters 20, 21 and 62)

e.g.

Myositis   Muscular dystrophy
- Weak ± wasting
- Normal reflexes

	Normal	UMN lesion	LMN lesion
Muscle bulk	Normal	Normal	↓↓
Reflexes	++ ++ ++	+++ +++ +++	0 0 0
Tone	Normal	↑↑	↓↓
Power	Normal	↓Reduced, esp. extensors in arm and flexors in leg	↓↓
Coordination*	Normal	Normal	Normal
Plantar response	Flexor	Extensor	Absent if leg/foot involved in lesion

LMN lesion

Damage = LMN lesion
e.g.

Motorneurone   Neuropathy
disease
- Weak
- Wasted
- Areflexic
- Fasciculation

Disorder at neuromuscular junction (Chapter 16)

e.g.
Myasthenia gravis
- Fatiguable weakness
- Normal reflexes
- Normal muscle bulk

* Coordination may be difficult to assess in the presence of weakness and/or greatly increased tone and/or a large number of involuntary movements

Disturbances in the motor pathways can produce a range of disorders of movement. These typically involve:
- the basal ganglia, causing abnormal involuntary movement without any effect on power, reflexes or coordination.
- the cerebellum and its connections, causing problems with coordination without any changes in power or reflexes;
- the motor neurones (lower or upper), causing weakness and changes in muscle tone and reflexes;
- the neuromuscular junction (NMJ), causing fatiguable weakness;
- the muscle, causing weakness;

In order to determine the nature and cause of the motor disturbance a full history and examination should be undertaken along with appropriate tests. The majority of patients with isolated motor symptoms have either Parkinson's or motor neurone disease, although by far the most common clinical scenario is the patient with both motor and sensory abnormalities as a result of strokes or damaged nerves as they emerge or pass along the limb.

A typical screen of tests for patients with motor symptoms involves blood tests, nerve conduction studies (NCS), electromyography (EMG) and magnetic resonance imaging (MRI) of brain and spinal cord.

Neuroanatomy and Neuroscience at a Glance, Fourth Edition. Roger A. Barker, Francesca Cicchetti, Michael J. Neal.

Muscle (see Chapters 20 and 21)

The typical features of a muscle disease are weakness, which may relate to exercise, and, on occasions, muscle pain (myalgia). The age and rate of progression is often helpful in determining the type of muscle disease, e.g. progressive slow weakness without pain from childhood would suggest a degenerative *muscular dystrophy* (see Chapter 20), while a short history of painful weakness in adulthood would suggest an *inflammatory myositis* (see Chapter 62). The distribution of weakness is also helpful in defining the likely type of muscle disease, e.g. proximal arm and leg weakness in *limb girdle muscular dystrophy*. The investigations that are especially useful in muscle disease are blood tests to look at levels of muscle-specific creatine phosphokinase (CPK) – a measure of muscle damage; EMG and muscle biopsy. In some cases genetic testing is of value, especially if the muscle weakness is associated with myotonia and other features of *myotonic dystrophy*.

Neuromuscular junction (see Chapters 16 and 62)

Patients with these disorders present with a history of weakness that gets worse with continued use of the muscle. The most common disorder of the NMJ is *myasthenia gravis*, which typically presents in early or late adulthood with fatiguable diplopia, ptosis, facial and bulbar weakness and proximal limb weakness. The examination confirms weakness that may be present at rest but clearly gets worse with exercise. Patients can present as a neurological emergency if there is bulbar and respiratory failure. Diagnosis typically relies on history and examination, the presence of acetylcholine receptor (AChR) or muscle-specific kinase (MUSK) antibodies, a positive response to a short-acting acetylcholinesterase inhibitor (Tensilon test) and abnormalities on repetitive stimulation with NCS and EMG. Muscle biopsy is not necessary. In some patients myasthenia gravis is associated with either enlargement (hyperplasia) or a tumour of the thymus gland. Other myasthenic syndromes are rare.

Peripheral nerves

Damage to the peripheral nerves will generally give both sensory and motor symptoms and signs. However, the peripheral motor nerve can be preferentially involved in some neuropathies as well as in conditions such as *poliomyelitis* and *motor neurone disease*, which target the actual motor neurone cell body in the ventral horn of the spinal cord and/or brainstem. The typical features of damage to the peripheral motor nerve are weakness, wasting, fasciculation and loss of reflexes – a lower motor neurone (LMN) lesion. Investigation of LMN syndromes involves excluding nerve entrapment as it exits the spinal cord by MRI imaging, along with NCS and EMG – the latter showing features of denervation with spontaneous motor discharges from the muscle that has lost its normal innervation.

Spinal cord

The involvement of spinal cord pathways gives a variety of motor syndromes (see Chapters 37 and 54). In rare cases there is involvement of spinal cord interneurones, leading to continuous motor unit activity (CMUA) and *stiff man* syndrome (see Chapters 35 and 36). Involvement of descending motor pathways from the brain in the spinal cord causes an upper motor neurone (UMN) syndrome of weakness, spasticity, increased reflexes, and clonus and extensor plantars. It is unusual for this pathway to be selectively involved in spinal cord pathology and when it does happen, the patient often also has LMN signs and has a form of motor neurone disease called *amyotrophic lateral sclerosis* or *Lou Gehrig disease*. However, if only UMN signs are seen then the patient is said to have *primary lateral sclerosis*. Structural lesions of the spinal cord typically produce a combination of motor and sensory signs and symptoms. Investigation involves MRI, with cerebrospinal fluid (CSF) examination if an inflammatory aetiology is suspected and in some cases neurophysiological testing with EMG, NCS and central motor conduction time (CMCT).

Brain

Damage to supraspinal structures can produce a variety of motor signs and symptoms. Involvement is most commonly seen in *cerebrovascular accidents* (*CVAs*) with involvement of all the descending motor pathways from the cortex to the brainstem and spinal cord. This gives rise to contralateral hemiparesis with UMN signs. If the left hemisphere is involved there is typically major disturbance in speech. Occasionally, damage is restricted to the motor cortex, when the patient may present with focal motor seizures such as *Jacksonian epilepsy* (see Chapters 39 and 61). The mainstay of investigation of supraspinal motor abnormalities is MRI and/or computed tomography (CT), and CSF examination if an inflammatory aetiology is suspected. In some cases genetic testing is helpful.

Other sites commonly involved in disease processes

Basal ganglia

This produces either a slowness of movement such as in *Parkinson's disease*; an abnormality of limb posture and movement (*dystonia*) or the development of uncontrollable involuntary movements such as *chorea* and *hemiballismus* (see Chapter 42).

Cerebellum

This produces incoordination of movement with slurred speech and abnormal eye movements (see Chapter 40). The disease processes that typically affect this part of the CNS are *multiple sclerosis*, drugs such as anticonvulsants and alcohol along with a series of rare genetic conditions called the *spinocerebellar ataxias* (*SCAs*) (see Chapter 63). It can also be involved by tumour growth in which case the situation may be complicated by the development of *hydrocephalus* through compression of the fourth ventricle and its outflow foramina (see Chapter 5).

Did you know?

The longest paper ever published in the famous neurology journal *Brain* was by Kinnier Wilson in 1912 and described Wilson's disease. It was 212 pages long!

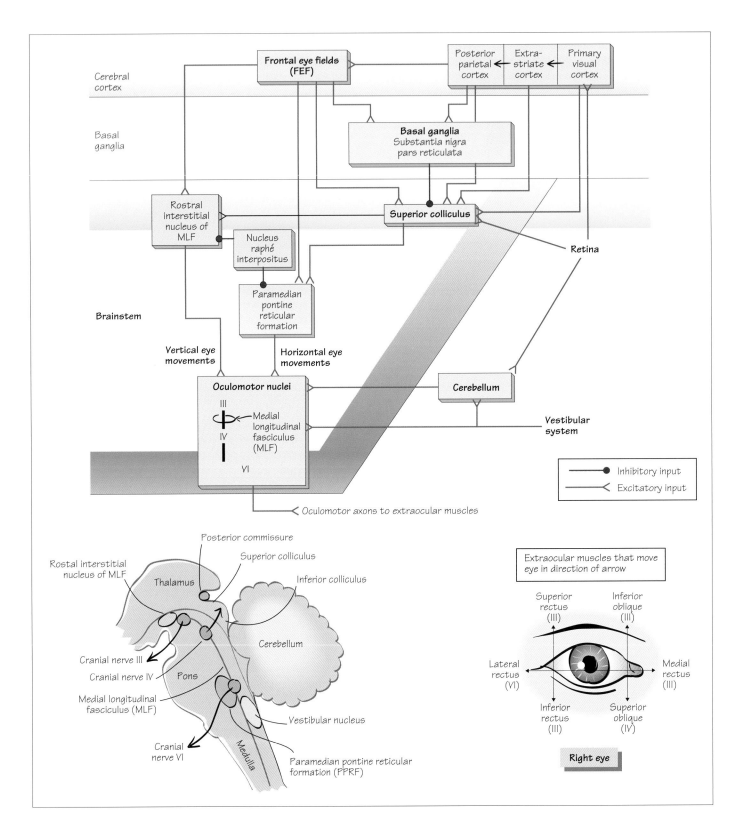

Neuroanatomy and Neuroscience at a Glance, Fourth Edition. Roger A. Barker, Francesca Cicchetti, Michael J. Neal.

The accurate **control of eye movements** involves a number of different structures, from the extraocular muscles to the frontal cortex, and failure to achieve this control results symptomatically in either double vision (diplopia), blurred vision or oscillopsia (perception of an oscillating image or environmental movement). In clinical practice, disruption of the final pathway from the oculomotor nuclei (third, fourth and sixth cranial nerves) to the extraocular muscle represents one of the major causes of diplopia (e.g. *myasthenia gravis*; see Chapter 16), as does inflammation (e.g. *multiple sclerosis*) in the medial longitudinal fasciculus (MLF) pathway linking the oculomotor nuclei.

Types of eye movement

There are three major types of eye movement.
• **Smooth pursuit** or the following of a target accurately – which is controlled primarily by posterior parts of the cortex in conjunction with the cerebellum.
• **Saccadic eye movements** – where there is a sudden shift of the eyes to a new target and which are controlled by more anterior cortical areas, the basal ganglia and superior colliculi in the midbrain.
• **Sustained gaze** – where the eyes are fixed in one direction and which is primarily a function of the brainstem (especially the paramedian pontine reticular formation [PPRF] and rostral interstitial nucleus of the MLF).

Eye movements, like the motor system in general, can be either **voluntary** (when the command comes from the frontal eye field) or **reflex** (when the command originates from subcortical structures and posterior parietal cortex).

Manifestations of disordered eye movement include a loss of conjugate movements; broken pursuit movements; inaccurate saccades; gaze palsies; and nystagmus. **Nystagmus** is defined as a biphasic ocular oscillation containing an abnormal slow and corrective fast phase, the latter defining the direction of the nystagmus.

Anatomy and physiology of central nervous system control of eye movements

• The **frontal eye fields** (FEF; predominantly Brodmann's area 8) are found anterior to the premotor cortex (PMC; see Chapter 38). Stimulation of this structure produces eye movements, typically saccades, to the contralateral side, and may be seen clinically in some epileptic patients.

Damage to this area reduces the ability to look to the contralateral side so the patient tends to look towards the side of the lesion. The FEF primarily receives from the posterior parietal cortex and projects to the superior colliculus, other brainstem centres and the basal ganglia.
• The **posterior parietal cortex** (corresponds to Brodmann's area 7 in monkeys) contains a large number of neurones responsive to complex visual stimuli, as well as coding for some visually guided eye movements (see Chapter 34). It is especially important in the generation of saccades to objects of visual significance via its connections with the FEF and superior colliculus.

Damage to this area, in addition to causing deficiencies in visual attention and saccades to objects in the contralateral hemifield, can impair smooth pursuit eye movements as evidenced by loss of the **optokinetic reflex**. This is a reflex in which the eyes fixate by a series of rapid movements on a moving target, such as a rotating drum, with vertical lines as fixation targets.
• The **primary visual cortex and its associated extrastriate areas** are involved in both saccadic and smooth pursuit eye movements (see Chapters 25 and 26). Their role in saccadic movements is primarily through the projection of V1 to the superior colliculus, while the role in smooth pursuit is via extrastriate area V5 (see Chapter 26), and projections to the FEF, posterior parietal cortex and pons.

Damage to the striate and extrastriate areas, in addition to producing field defects and specific deficiencies of visual function (see Chapters 25 and 26), can also cause major abnormalities in smooth pursuit eye movements.
• The **basal ganglia** have a major role in the control of saccadic eye movements (see Chapters 41 and 42). The caudate nucleus receives from the FEF and projects via the SNr to the superior colliculus.

Abnormalities in saccadic eye movements are seen clinically in a number of basal ganglia disorders. For example, in *Parkinson's disease* the saccadic eye movements tend to be slightly inaccurate with undershooting to the target (hypometric saccades).
• The **superior colliculus** in the midbrain is important in the accurate execution of saccades (see Chapter 25). The **cerebellum and vestibular nuclei** have important complex inputs into the brainstem oculomotor system and are especially important in the control of pursuit movements, as well as mediating the vestibulo-ocular reflex (see Chapters 29, 40 and 49).

Damage to the cerebellum and vestibular system causes broken pursuit eye movements, inaccurate saccades and nystagmus.
• The **rostral interstitial nucleus of the medial longitudinal fasciculus (riMLF)** is important in the control of vertical saccades and vertical gaze (both up- and downgaze) and receives important inputs from the FEF and superior colliculus while projecting to all the oculomotor nuclei.

Damage to this structure or disruption of its afferent inputs therefore produces deficiencies in both these eye movements, and this can occur in a number of conditions including some neurodegenerative diseases.
• The **PPRF** receives from the FEF, superior colliculus and cerebellum and is responsible for horizontal saccades and gaze. It is thought that this structure may work in conjunction with another pontine nucleus, the **nucleus raphé interpositus**. This latter nucleus contains omnipause neurones, which normally exert tonic inhibition on the burst neurones of the PPRF (and riMLF) mediating the saccadic impulse.

Damage to nucleus raphé interpositus results in random chaotic eye movements or *opsoclonus*. In contrast, damage to the PPRF causes deficiencies in saccadic eye movements as well as ipsilateral gaze paresis.
• The **MLF** mediates conjugate eye movements through interconnections between all the oculomotor nuclei and is commonly affected in some diseases of the central nervous system (CNS) such as *multiple sclerosis* (see Chapter 62).

A lesion in this structure causes an *internuclear ophthalmoplegia*, with nystagmus in the abducting eye and slowed or absent adduction in the other eye.

Did you know?

The human eye can make up to 420 saccades per minute or eight per second.

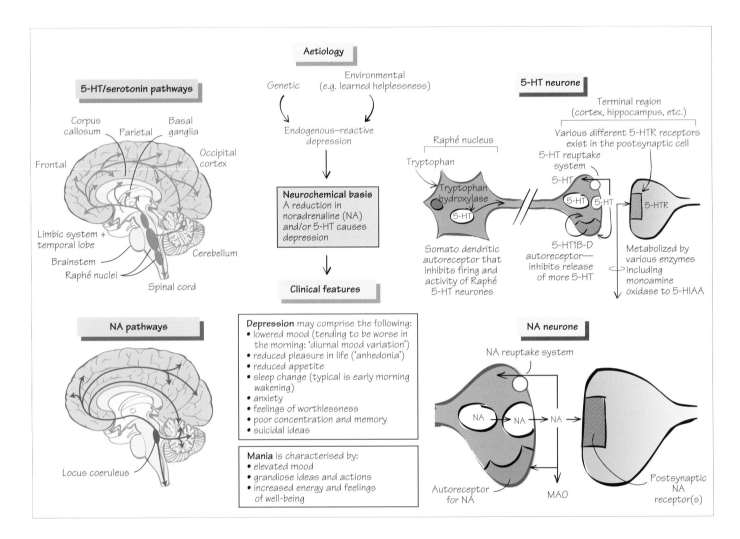

'Affect' refers to mood and affective disorders comprise of both a pathological lowering (***depression***) and elevation (***mania***) of mood. Bipolar affective disorder (manic-depression) refers to an oscillation between depression and mania. These conditions are not simply characterized by mood changes, however, and depression may comprise a number of characteristic features.

Both depression and mania may be accompanied by features of psychosis (delusions and hallucinations; see Chapter 58). The nature of the psychosis tends to be mood-congruent: in depression, the patient may believe that he or she is guilty of something or hear voices that are critical and unpleasant. Mania may be accompanied by grandiose delusions.

Depression
Aetiology
This is a common and mania disorder with a lifetime prevalence that has been estimated to be as high as 15%, with women affected more than men (approximately 2:1). It can occur in response to adverse circumstances (**reactive depression**), as well as for no

apparent circumstantial reason (**endogenous depression**), although often the distinction between these two different types of depression is not that clear-cut. In both cases the depression probably arises through a combination of genetic and environmental factors.
• Genetic: while a number of genes have been implicated in affective disorders, specific genes for depression have not been identified, so it is thought to have a polygenic component – which is maybe more significant in patients with bipolar disorders.
• Environmental and psychological factors are also extremely important. Background personality factors have been implicated as have social stressors, which have been hypothesized to produce depression by inducing in individuals a sense that they have no personal control over events in their lives (akin to **learned helplessness** in rats). This basic psychological model has been extended and superseded by the view that 'depressive cognitions' are fundamental to depression. That is, because an individual holds specific beliefs and attributional styles, he or she may be more vulnerable to the development of a depressive illness. This view is central to the emerging use of cognitive therapies in depression.

Neuroanatomy and Neuroscience at a Glance, Fourth Edition. Roger A. Barker, Francesca Cicchetti, Michael J. Neal.

Neurochemical basis of depression

The **monoamine theory of depression** suggests that the illness is caused by reduced monoamine transmission. It derives from the observation that the tricyclic antidepressants – remarkably effective in the treatment of the illness – upregulate monaminergic transmission. However, the direct evidence for monoamine disturbance in depression is scant and inconsistent.

The **serotonin hypothesis** suggests that depression is linked to reduced serotoninergic function and gains support from the antidepressant efficacy of the newer generation of treatments: the selective serotonin reuptake inhibitors (SSRIs). Furthermore, temporary depletion of tryptophan (a precursor of serotonin) levels causes a transient but profound resurgence of depressive symptoms in people who have been successfully treated with SSRIs and in people with a depressive illness in remission.

Cognition in depression

Depression is associated with impairments or changes in performance on a number of tests of cognitive function. Memory deficits are prominent and occur across memory domains (working memory and episodic memory; see Chapter 46) and across modalities (verbal and visuospatial). Psychomotor retardation is also common with depressed people showing an apparent lack of motivation (see Chapter 47) and marked slowing of speech and motor functions, the latter manifest in generally slowed reaction times. Sustained attention may be poor, as may planning and problem-solving. Interestingly, some of the changes in memory and attention are characterized by an interaction with the emotional nature of test material. For example, patients may preferentially remember or attend to stimuli that have negative connotations. They may also be more likely to perceive neutral stimuli as being emotionally negative.

Treatment

A number of different therapies are employed for the treatment of depression, including **psychotherapy** and **electroconvulsive therapy** (ECT); however, the most commonly used approach is with **antidepressant drugs**. Most of the drugs used in the treatment of depression inhibit the reuptake of noradrenaline (norepinephrine) and/or serotonin (5-hydroxytryptamine [5-HT]). Less commonly used drugs are monoamine oxidase inhibitors (MAOIs). Because both uptake inhibitors and MAOIs increase the amount of noradrenaline and/or 5-HT in the synaptic cleft and so enhance the action of these transmitters, it has been argued that depression resulted from an 'underactivity' of these monoaminergic systems (see above). In mania and bipolar affective disorders lithium has a mood-stabilizing action. **Lithium** salts have a low therapeutic: toxic ratio and adverse effects are common. **Carbamazepine valproate** and **lamotrigine** also have mood-stabilizing actions and can be used in cases of non-response or intolerance to lithium. The mechanisms involved in the mood-stabilizing effects of these drugs are unknown.

Amine uptake inhibitors

Tricyclic antidepressants (e.g. **imipramine**, **amitriptyline**) have proven antidepressant actions but no one drug has greater efficacy. The choice of drug is determined by the most acceptable or desired side effects. For example, some have sedative actions (e.g. **amitriptyline, dosulepin**) and are more useful for agitated and anxious patients (see Chapter 59). Withdrawn and apathetic patients may benefit from less sedative drugs (e.g. **imipramine, lofepramine**). In addition to blocking amine uptake, the tricyclics block muscarinic receptors, α-adrenoreceptors and H1 histamine receptors. These actions frequently cause dry mouth, blurred vision, constipation, urinary retention, tachycardia and postural hypotension. In overdosage, the anticholinergic activity and a quinidine-like action may cause cardiac arrhythmias and sudden death (cardiotoxicity).

Some newer drugs (serotonin-noradrenaline reuptake inhibitors), e.g. **venlafaxine**, inhibit the reuptake of serotonin and noradrenaline but lack the antimuscarinic and sedative effects of the tricyclics.

Drugs that selectively inhibit serotonin re-uptake (SSRIs) (e.g. **fluoxetine**) are less sedative, do not have the troublesome autonomic side effects of the tricyclics and are safer in overdoses. However, they have their own spectrum of adverse effects, the most common being nausea, vomiting, diarrhoea and constipation. They may also cause sexual dysfunction.

Monoamine oxidase inhibitors

The older MAOIs (e.g. phenelzine) are irreversible non-selective inhibitors of monoamine oxidase. Their efficacy is similar to that of the tricyclics. They are rarely used now because of their adverse effects (postural hypotension, dizziness, anticholinergic effects and liver damage). Also there may be potentially serious interactions with sympathomimetic amines (e.g. ephedrine), often present in cough mixtures and decongestive medicines, or food containing tyramine (e.g. game, cheese). Tyramine is normally metabolized by MAO in the liver. If the enzyme is inhibited, the tyramine enters the circulation and displaces noradrenaline from sympathetic nerve terminals. This may cause severe hypertension and even stroke.

Moclobemide is a newer drug that selectively inhibits MAO_A and lacks most of the unwanted effects of non-selective MAOIs.

Atypical antidepressants

These drugs have little, if any, effect on serotonin or noradrenaline reuptake and do not inhibit MAO. Mirtazapine and trazodone are sedative antidepressants but have few autonomic effects. Because they are less cardiotoxic than the tricyclics, they are less dangerous in overdosage.

Did you know?

Winston Churchill used the term 'Black Dog' to describe his bouts of depression.

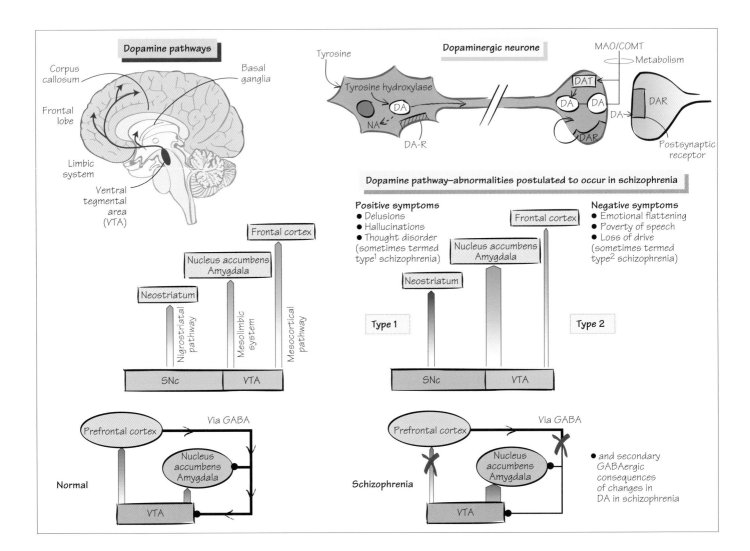

Schizophrenia is a syndrome characterized by specific psychological manifestations, including auditory hallucinations, delusions, thought disorders and behavioural disturbances. It is a common disorder with a lifetime prevalence of 1% and an incidence of 2–4 new cases per year per 10 000 population. It is more common in men and typically presents early in life. Like all psychiatric disorders there is no diagnostic test for this condition, which is defined by the existence of key symptoms.

- *Positive symptoms*:
  - delusions: abnormal or irrational beliefs, held with great conviction and out of keeping with an individual's sociocultural background;
  - hallucinations: perceptions in the absence of stimuli.
- *Negative symptoms*:
  - blunting of mood, apparent apathy, lack of spontaneous speech and action;
  - disordered speech.

Aetiology

A distinction used to be made between type 1 and 2 schizophrenia but this has fallen out of fashion as it may relate more to the length of time that the individual has had the condition. The cause of schizophrenia is unknown but a number of aetiological factors have been suggested:

- Genetic factors: first-degree relatives of people with schizophrenia have a greatly increased risk of developing the disease; around 10% for siblings, 6% for parents and 13% for children. Concordance rates in twins are relatively high with figures varying from 42% to 50% for monozygotic twins and between 0 and 14% for dizygotic twins. Recent Genome Wide Association Studies (GWAS) have also confirmed a genetic basis for the condition.
- Environmental factors: e.g. infections during pregnancy also may have a role, with adoption studies demonstrating the importance of both genetic and environmental factors. In these studies gene–environment interactions have been demonstrated in chil-

Neuroanatomy and Neuroscience at a Glance, Fourth Edition. Roger A. Barker, Francesca Cicchetti, Michael J. Neal.

dren of schizophrenic parents adopted into good versus disturbed adoptive families. In this latter respect one influential theory relating to a family cause appeals to high levels of 'expressed emotion' (hostility, lack of emotional warmth, over-involvement) as a risk for relapse.

The dopamine hypothesis of schizophrenia

Basic model

Simply stated, this embodies the idea that schizophrenia is caused by up-regulation of activity in the mesolimbic dopamine system. The evidence for this theory comes from:
- Dopamine-blocking drugs show an antipsychotic effect.
- Drugs that up-regulate dopamine can produce positive symptoms of psychosis (e.g. amphetamines).
- Some neuroimaging studies in patients have found evidence of dopamine up-regulation.

The dopamine hypothesis has been criticized for the lack of direct evidence in its favour and for certain inconsistencies:
- Dopamine agonists do not produce all of the symptoms of schizophrenia (notably, they do not produce negative symptoms);
- Dopamine-blocking drugs do not act immediately – there may be a long period before symptoms begin to resolve.

Revised model

The above inconsistencies led to the revision that both dopamine up-regulation and down-regulation must be invoked to account for the core features of schizophrenia, with the positive symptoms arising from up-regulation of mesolimbic dopamine function and the negative symptoms from down-regulation of mesocortical function.

However, many still think this as an inadequate explanation of such a complex disorder, and there is a view that schizophrenia is associated with **N-methyl-D-aspartate (NMDA) (glutamate) receptor hypofunction**. This arose from observations that NMDA blockers such as phencyclidine ('Angel Dust') and ketamine (widely used in anaesthesia) produce a psychotic state (including negative symptoms) that is held to be more strongly redolent of schizophrenia than the psychosis produced by dopaminergic agents. Therefore, it has been proposed that glutamate hypofunction may account for both up-regulation of the mesolimbic dopamine system, from a diminished excitatory drive of GABAergic inhibition (i.e. an attenuation of the 'brake' system), and down-regulation of the mesocortical system because of diminished direct drive (the 'activating' system).

Cognition in schizophrenia

Whilst schizophrenia is traditionally described in terms of psychotic symptoms, there is increasing evidence of cognitive deficits, particularly in the memory domain, that may accompany (and perhaps precede) the onset of these symptoms.

Treatment

The mainstay of therapy in schizophrenia remains the use of drugs that block dopamine receptors, of which there are at least five subtypes in the brain (D1–D5 receptors; see Chapter 19). These agents (e.g. chlorpromazine) are called antipsychotics or neuroleptics. Most neuroleptics block D1 receptors but there is a close correlation between the clinical dose of antipsychotic drugs and their affinity for D2 receptors, suggesting that blockade of this receptor subtype may be particularly important. D2 receptors are found in the limbic system and in the basal ganglia, and D3 and D4 receptors are found mainly in the limbic areas.

Antipsychotic drugs (eg chlorpromazine, haloperidol) require several weeks to control the symptoms of schizophrenia and most patients require maintenance treatment for many years. Relapses are common even in drug-maintained patients. Unfortunately, neuroleptics also block dopamine D2 receptors in the basal ganglia, often producing distressing and disabling movement disorders (e.g. parkinsonism, acute dystonic reactions, akathisia [motor restlessness] and tardive dyskinesia [orofacial and trunk movements]) which may be irreversible; see Chapter 42). Blockade of D2 receptors in the pituitary gland causes an increase in prolactin release and endocrine effects (e.g. gynaecomastia, galactorrhoea; see Chapter 11). Many neuroleptics also block muscarinic receptors (causing dry mouth, blurred vision, constipation), α-adrenoceptors (postural hypotension) and histamine H1 receptors (sedation).

Atypical drugs

Some newer drugs have a reduced tendency to cause movement disorders and are referred to as atypical agents (e.g. **clozapine, risperidone, olanzapine, quetiapine**). With the possible exception of clozapine, these drugs are not more efficacious than the older antipsychotic drugs. Clozapine is restricted to patients resistant to other drugs because it causes neutropenia or agranulocytosis in about 4% of patients. Risperidone and other newer atypical agents are increasingly used in the treatment of schizophrenia because they are more acceptable to patients.

It is not clear why some neuroleptics are 'atypical'. Clozapine may be atypical because in addition to being a dopamine D2 antagonist it is a potent blocker of 5-HT2 receptors.

Did you know?

There is great debate as to whether Joan of Arc had schizophrenia, given her hallucinations and obstinate belief and the age at which this started in her.

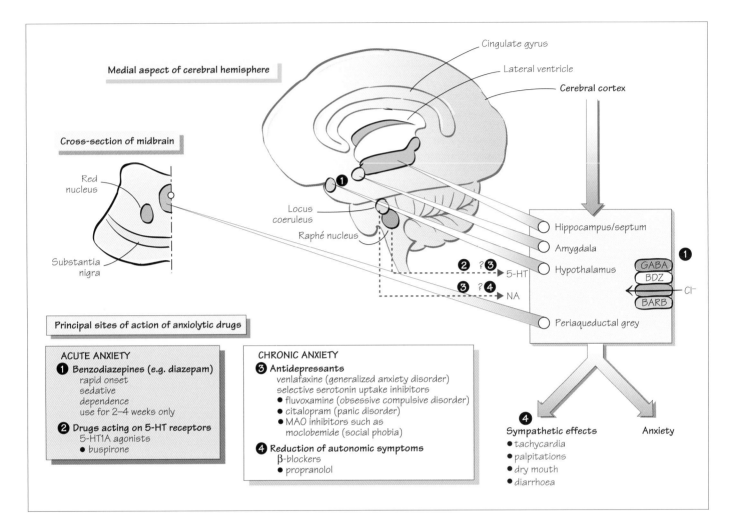

Anxiety is a normal emotional reaction to threatening or potentially threatening situations, and is accompanied by sympathetic overactivity. In *anxiety disorders* the patient experiences anxiety that is disproportionate to the stimulus, and sometimes in the absence of any obvious stimulus. There is no organic basis for anxiety disorders, the symptoms resulting from overactivity of the brain areas involved in 'normal' anxiety. Psychiatric disorders that occur without any known brain pathology are called *neuroses*.

Anxiety disorders are subdivided into four main types: *generalized anxiety disorder*, *panic disorder*, *stress reactions* and *phobias*. Many transmitters seem to be involved in the neural mechanisms of anxiety, the evidence being especially strong for **γ-aminobutyric acid (GABA)** and **5-hydroxytryptamine (5-HT)**. Because intravenous injections of **cholecystokinin (CCK₄)** into humans cause the symptoms of panic it has been suggested that abnormalities in different transmitter systems might be involved in particular types of anxiety disorder. This remains to be seen.

There is some evidence for decreased GABA binding in the left temporal pole, an area concerned with experiencing and controlling fear and anxiety.

There may be disturbances of serotoninergic and noradrenergic transmission in anxiety. Thus, chlorophenylpiperazine (a nonspecific 5-HT1 and 5-HT2 agonist) increased anxiety in patients with a generalized anxiety disorder. These patients also show a reduced growth hormone response to clonidine (an α_2-receptor agonist) suggesting a decrease in α_2-receptor sensitivity. This response is also seen in patients with major depression. This is perhaps not surprising because genetic studies suggest that generalized anxiety disorder and major depression may have a common genetic basis and both disorders benefit from the administration of antidepressant drugs.

Treatment of mild anxiety disorders may only require simple *supportive psychotherapy*, but in severe anxiety anxiolytic drugs given for a short period are useful. The **benzodiazepines** (e.g. *diazepam*) produce their effects by enhancing GABA-mediated inhibition in many of the brain areas involved in anxiety, including the raphé nucleus. Some **antidepressants** (e.g. *amitriptyline, paroxetine*) have anxiolytic activity and they are used for the long-term treatment of anxiety disorders. Their mechanism of action in anxiety is unclear. **β-adrenoceptor antagonists** have a limited use in the treatment of

Neuroanatomy and Neuroscience at a Glance, Fourth Edition. Roger A. Barker, Francesca Cicchetti, Michael J. Neal.

situational anxiety (e.g. in musicians) where palpitations and tremor are the main symptoms. Efforts to discover non-sedative anxiolytics have led to the trial of several drugs that act on specific 5-HT receptors but only one, **buspirone**, has been introduced.

Anxiety disorders

• *Generalized anxiety disorders* have both psychological and physical symptoms. The psychological symptoms include a feeling of fearful anticipation, difficulty in concentrating, irritability and repetitive worrying thoughts that are often linked to awareness of sympathetic overactivity.

• *Phobic anxiety disorders* have the same core symptoms as generalized anxiety disorders but occur only under certain circumstances, e.g. the appearance of a spider (arachnophobia).

• In contrast, *panic attacks* are episodic attacks of anxiety in which physical symptoms predominate (e.g. choking, palpitations, chest pain, sweating, trembling).

Treatment

Benzodiazepines

Benzodiazepines (e.g. diazepam) are orally active central depressants that induce sleep when given in high doses at night (see Chapter 43) and provide sedation and reduce anxiety when given in divided doses during the day. They also have anticonvulsant activity (see Chapter 61), are muscle relaxants and produce amnesia. All these actions are brought about by the potentiation of the action of GABA on the GABA$_A$ receptor, which consists of five subunits.

Benzodiazepines enhance the action of synaptically released GABA by binding to a benzodiazepine receptor site on the GABA$_A$ receptor complex. This causes a conformational change to the GABA binding site, increasing its affinity for GABA.

The main adverse effects of the benzodiazepines are drowsiness, impaired alertness, agitation and ataxia. In anxiety disorders, benzodiazepines should only be given for a maximum of 2–3 weeks because longer treatment risks the development of **dependence**. If this occurs, stopping the drug frequently leads to a **withdrawal syndrome** characterized by anxiety, tremor, sweating and insomnia – symptoms similar to the original complaint.

Sites of action of benzodiazepines in the brain

In general, limbic and brainstem structures seem important in mediating the anxiolytic actions of these drugs. In humans, cerebral blood flow and glucose metabolism studies using positron emission tomography (PET) have not revealed consistent differences in anxious and non-anxious subjects.

Buspirone

Serotonin (5-HT) cell bodies are located in the raphé nucleus of the midbrain and project to many areas of the brain including those thought to be important in anxiety (hippocampus, amygdala, frontal cortex; see Chapter 19). In rats, lesions of the raphé nucleus produce anxiolytic effects, while stimulation of 5-HT1A autoreceptors with agonists such as 8-hydroxy-DPAT produce anxiogenic effects. A role for 5-HT in anxiety was strengthened when it was found that benzodiazepines reduce the turnover of 5-HT in the brain and, when microinjected into the raphé nucleus, reduce the rate of neuronal firing and produce an anxiolytic effect. However, stimulation of postsynaptic 5-HT1A receptors in limbic areas has anxiogenic effects. These opposing pre- and postsynaptic actions may explain why **buspirone**, a 5-HT1A partial agonist, has limited efficacy and works only after several weeks.

β-blockers

The evidence for the role of noradrenaline (norepinephrine) in anxiety is much less compelling than that for GABA and 5-HT. Nevertheless, β-adrenoceptor antagonists (e.g. **propranolol**) have a limited use in the treatment of patients with mild or transient anxiety and where autonomic symptoms such as palpitations and tremor are the most troublesome symptoms. The beneficial effects of β-blockers in these patients may result from a peripheral action because those (e.g. practolol) that do not pass the blood–brain barrier are equally effective.

Peptides and anxiety

Several neuropeptides have been implicated in anxiety. The strongest evidence is for the anxiogenic effect of **corticotrophin-releasing hormone** (CRH), and CRH has also been implicated in depression. This raises the theoretical possibility that a CRH receptor-1 antagonist may have anxiolytic actions and such drugs are under development. **Substance P** may also have anxiogenic effects and an NK1 receptor antagonist is in clinical trials for anxiety and depression. **Cholecystokinin (CCK)** is a gut peptide that is also present in many areas of the brainstem and midbrain and is involved in emotion, mood and arousal. Because CCK$_4$ is one of the few agents (CO$_2$ is another) that elicits genuine panic-like attacks, it was hoped that CCK antagonists would be useful anxiolytics. Unfortunately, clinical trials revealed that non-peptide CCK antagonists are ineffective in anxiety disorders.

Did you know?

Nitrous oxide can alleviate anxiety and carbon dioxide provokes it.

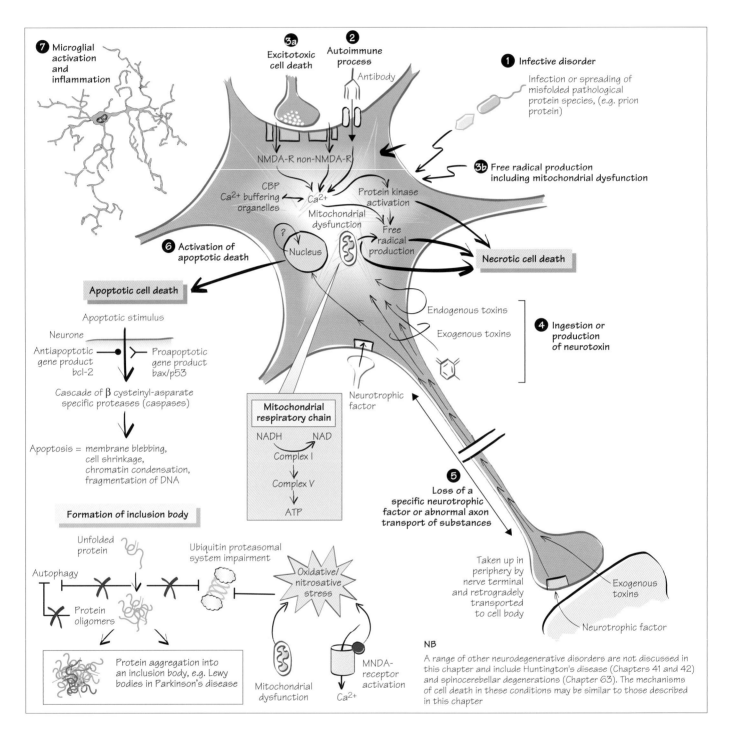

7 Microglial activation and inflammation

3a Excitotoxic cell death

2 Autoimmune process
Antibody

1 Infective disorder
Infection or spreading of misfolded pathological protein species, (e.g. prion protein)

NMDA-R non-NMDA-R

3b Free radical production including mitochondrial dysfunction

CBP
Ca^{2+} buffering organelles
Ca^{2+}
Protein kinase activation
Mitochondrial dysfunction
Free radical production

6 Activation of apoptotic death

?
Nucleus

Necrotic cell death

Apoptotic cell death

Apoptotic stimulus

Neurone

Antiapoptotic gene product bcl-2 ⟶ • ⊣ Proapoptotic gene product bax/p53

Cascade of β cysteinyl-asparate specific proteases (caspases)

Apoptosis = membrane blebbing, cell shrinkage, chromatin condensation, fragmentation of DNA

Endogenous toxins
Exogenous toxins

4 Ingestion or production of neurotoxin

Neurotrophic factor

Mitochondrial respiratory chain
NADH ⟶ NAD
↓
Complex I
↓
Complex V
↓
ATP

5 Loss of a specific neurotrophic factor or abnormal axon transport of substances

Formation of inclusion body

Unfolded protein
Autophagy
Protein oligomers
Ubiquitin proteasomal system impairment

Oxidative/ nitrosative stress

Protein aggregation into an inclusion body, e.g. Lewy bodies in Parkinson's disease

Mitochondrial dysfunction

MNDA- receptor activation
Ca^{2+}

Taken up in periphery by nerve terminal and retrogradely transported to cell body

Exogenous toxins

Neurotrophic factor

NB

A range of other neurodegenerative disorders are not discussed in this chapter and include Huntington's disease (Chapters 41 and 42) and spinocerebellar degenerations (Chapter 63). The mechanisms of cell death in these conditions may be similar to those described in this chapter

Neurodegenerative disorders are those conditions in which the primary pathological event is a progressive loss of populations of CNS neurones over time. However, it is increasingly being recognized that most neurodegenerative disorders have an inflammatory component to them, and that inflammatory diseases of the central nervous system (CNS) (such as **multiple sclerosis**, see Chapter 62) will cause neuronal loss and degeneration.

Aetiology

There are a number of theories on the aetiology of neurodegenerative disorders, which may not be mutually exclusive. Of late there has been much work looking at the genetic risk factors for developing these disorders (see Chapter 63), and some common sets of genes are being found for them, e.g. genes involved with inflammation and immunity.

Neuroanatomy and Neuroscience at a Glance, Fourth Edition. Roger A. Barker, Francesca Cicchetti, Michael J. Neal.

An infective disorder

Neuronal death with a glial reaction (gliosis) is commonly seen in infective disorders (typically viral) with inflammation in the CNS. However, in neurodegenerative disorders such a reaction is not seen, although the observation that *human immunodeficiency virus* (*HIV*) *infection* can cause a dementia has raised the possibility that some neurodegenerative disorders may be caused by a retroviral infection. Furthermore, the development of dementia with spongiform changes throughout the brain in response to the proliferation of abnormal prion proteins as occurs in *Creutzfeldt–Jakob disease* has further fuelled the debate on an infective aetiology in some neurodegenerative disorders (eg α-synuclein in PD).

An autoimmune process

Autoantibodies have been described in some neurodegenerative conditions, e.g. antibodies to calcium channels in *motor neurone disease* (*MND*). However, the absence of an inflammatory response would argue against this hypothesis, although neuronal degeneration with a minimal inflammatory infiltrate can be seen in the *paraneoplastic syndromes* (see Chapter 62) as well as the more recently described autoimmune disorders targeting ion channels and receptors.

The result of excitotoxic cell death and free radical production

Excitatory amino acids are found throughout the CNS (see Chapter 19) and act on a range of receptors that serve to depolarize the neurone and allow Ca^{2+} to influx into the cell. On entering the neurone, calcium is normally quickly buffered; if the level of excitation is great then there may be an excessive influx of Ca^{2+}, which can lead to the production of toxic free radicals and cell death.

Indeed it may even be that the problem lies within the glia and their failure to buffer glutamate. This has been postulated to occur in MND. Furthermore in some cases of *familial MND* there is a loss of one of the free radical scavenger molecules – superoxide dismutase and in *Parkinson's disease*, deficiency in complex I activity of the mitochondrial respiratory chain in the substantia nigra, both of which may lead to the overproduction of free radicals.

The ingestion or production of a neurotoxin

Many toxins can induce degenerative conditions (e.g. parkinsonism with manganese poisoning) but no such exogenous compound has consistently been found to cause any of the major neurodegenerative disorders.

Dementia of the Alzheimer type (*DAT*), is associated with the development of neurofibrillary tangles (NFTs) and senile neuritic plaques (SNPs) in the parahippocampal and parietotemporal cortical areas. The density of NFTs correlates well with the cognitive state of the patient. NFTs contain paired helical filaments made up of an abnormal form of the microtubule-associated protein tau – a protein that normally serves to maintain the neuronal cytoskeleton and maintain normal axonal transport (see Chapter 12). Thus, abnormalities in axonal transport may underlie some neurodegenerative conditions, either as a direct consequence of abnormalities in tau or proteins associated with it. In contrast, SNPs contain abnormal forms of the protein β-amyloid, derived from the ubiquitously expressed membrane-bound glycoprotein amyloid precursor protein (APP).

The reason as to why these abnormal proteins are produced and in what order is not clear – certainly some of the rare familial forms of *DAT* have genetic defects that influence the production of the amyloid protein (although there are rare forms of frontotemporal dementia with parkinsonism that also result from tau mutations). Whatever the reason for the development of these abnormal proteins, the result is cortical cell death. This leads to a secondary loss in the cholinergic innervation of the cortex with an associated atrophy of the cholinergic neurones in the basal forebrain, which has prompted clinical studies in the use of drugs that potentiate CNS cholinergic transmission (**donepezil, rivastigmine** and **galantamine**). These drugs are inhibitors of acetylcholinesterase in the brain. They have been shown in clinical trials to be of some limited benefit.

Most neurodegenerative conditions have now been found to contain intracellular inclusions of abnormal protein (e.g. huntingtin in *Huntington's disease*, tau in some *complex parkinsonian conditions*, α-synuclein in *Parkinson's disease* and *multiple system atrophy*), and may all induce disruption of the ubiquitin–proteosome system (UPS) or the autophagic lysosomal degradation pathway. These systems normally serve to package up and get rid of proteins, and as such their dysfunction will affect the processing and removal of intracellular proteins and the formation of inclusion bodies.

The loss of a specific neurotrophic factor
(Or abnormal axonal transport of substances – see above.)

Neurones are maintained by the production of a specific growth or neurotrophic factor (see Chapters 48 and 49), and the loss of one or some of these factors may underlie the development of the various neurodegenerative disorders. Clinical trials using neurotrophic factors in patients with neurodegenerative disorders have been undertaken with some disputed success with glial cell line-derived neurotrophic factor (GDNF) in Parkinson's disease.

The activation of programmed cell death (apoptosis)

The loss of cells in most conditions (e.g. inflammation) is by a process of necrotic cell death but all cells contain the necessary machinery to initiate their own death: programmed cell death or apoptosis. It is therefore possible that neurodegenerative disorders are caused by an inappropriate activation of this programme, possibly secondary to the loss of a neurotrophic factor.

The role of inflammation

There is increasing interest in the possibility that neurodegenerative processes in the CNS may be enhanced by local inflammatory responses, especially the microglia.

Did you know?

The novelist Iris Murdoch developed Alzheimer's disease and one of the earliest features of this was her reduced use of vocabulary in her books, which had become apparent 10 years before she was diagnosed.

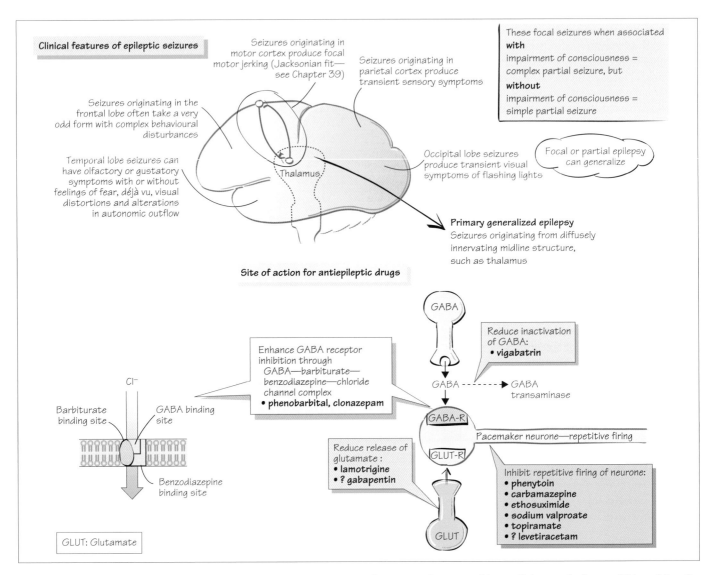

Definition and classification of epilepsy

Epilepsy represents a transitory disturbance of the functions of the brain that develops suddenly, ceases spontaneously and can be induced by a number of different provocations. It is the most prevalent serious neurological conditions, with a peak incidence in early childhood and in the elderly.

Patients may be classified according to whether:
• the fit is *generalized or partial (focal)*, i.e. remains within one small CNS site, e.g. temporal lobe;
• there is an impairment of consciousness (if there is then it is termed *complex*);
• the partial seizure causes secondary generalization.

Overall, 60–70% of all epileptics have no obvious cause for their seizures, and about two-thirds of all patients stop having seizures within 2–5 years of their onset, usually in the context of taking medication.

Pathogenesis of epilepsy

The **aetiology of epilepsy** is largely unknown, but much of the therapy used to treat this condition works by modifying either the balance between the inhibitory γ-aminobutyric acid (GABA) and excitatory glutamatergic networks within the brain or the repetitive firing potential of neurones.

The recording of the electroencephalograph (EEG; see Chapters 43 and 52) reveals that **epileptic fits** (ictal events) are associated with either generalized synchronous or focal spike and wave discharges, although abnormalities can be seen transiently at other times without overt evidence of a seizure (**interictal activity**).

A generalized epileptic fit can take several forms but classically consists of a tonic (muscles go stiff) – clonic (jerking of limbs and body) phase followed by a period of unconsciousness. This used to be termed a grand mal seizure, but is now classified as a generalized tonic–clonic seizure. Petit mal epilepsy is now reclassified as a form of primary generalized epilepsy.

A model for the generation of an epileptic discharge is that:
1. the interictal activity corresponds to a depolarizing shift with superimposed action potentials from an assembly of neurones;

Neuroanatomy and Neuroscience at a Glance, Fourth Edition. Roger A. Barker, Francesca Cicchetti, Michael J. Neal.

2. there follows a period of hyperpolarization as these same neurones activate local inhibitory interneurones while becoming inactivated themselves;

3. with repeated interictal spikes the period of hyperpolarization shortens and this activates a range of normally quiescent ion channels in the neurone as well as raising extracellular K^+ concentrations, all of which further depolarizes the neurones;

4. if sufficient neurones are activated (and the inhibition of local GABA interneurones overcome) then synchronous discharges are produced across populations of neurones which leads to a seizure;

5. the seizure or synchronous discharge is then terminated by active processes of inhibition both within the neurone (through ion channels) and within the neuronal network by GABAergic interneuronal activity.

Although this model is useful, it is clear that different forms of epilepsy have different underlying abnormalities.

• *Primary generalized epilepsy*, which is associated with diffuse EEG changes, is thought to result from abnormalities in specific calcium channels in the thalamus.

• Patients with *complex partial seizures of temporal lobe origin* may have a small scar in the mesial temporal lobe corresponding to neuronal loss and gliosis within the hippocampus, secondary to hypoxic or ischaemic insults early in life.

Treatment of epilepsy

For most patients the treatment of epilepsy involves antiepileptic drugs. A small proportion of refractory patients benefit from a surgical approach, especially if an underlying structural lesion is identified. The most common operation is temporal lobe resection, which has a 60–70% chance of making the patient seizure free.

Tonic–clonic and partial seizures are treated mainly with oral **carbamazepine**, **valproate**, **lamotrigine** or **topiramate**. These drugs are of similar effectiveness and a single drug will control the fits in 70–80% of patients with tonic–clonic seizures, but only 30–40% of patients with partial seizures. In these poorly controlled patients, combinations of the above drugs or the addition of a second-line drug, e.g. **clobazam**, **levetiracetam**, may reduce the incidence of seizures.

Absence seizures are treated with **ethosuximide**, **valproate** or **lamotrigine**. Absence epilepsy occasionally continues into adult life.

Status epilepticus is defined as continuous seizures lasting at least 30 minutes or a state in which fits follow each other without consciousness being fully regained. Urgent treatment with **intravenous agents** is necessary, which, if unchecked, result in exhaustion and cerebral damage. **Lorazepam** or diazepam is used initially followed by **phenytoin** if necessary. If the fits are not controlled, the patient is anaesthetized with **propofol** or **thiopental**.

Mechanisms of action of anticonvulsants

Antiepileptic drugs control seizures by mechanisms that usually involve one of the following:

• **enhancement of GABA-mediated inhibition** (benzodiazepines, vigabatrin, phenobarbital, tiagabine)

• **use-dependent blockade of sodium channels** (phenytoin, carbamazepine, valproate, lamotrigine);

• **inhibition of a spike generating Ca^{2+} current** in thalamic neurones (ethosuximide, valproate and lamotrigine).

• **Valproate** also seems to increase GABAergic central inhibition by mechanisms that may involve stimulation of glutamic acid decarboxylase activity and/or inhibition of $GABA_T$ activity.

• **Vigabatrin** is an irreversible inhibitor of $GABA_T$, which increases brain GABA levels and central GABA release.

• **Tiagabine** inhibits the reuptake of synaptically released GABA and therefore increases central inhibition.

• The benzodiazepines (e.g. **clonazepam**) and **phenobarbital** also increase central inhibition, but by enhancing the action of synaptically released GABA at the $GABA_A$ receptor–Cl^- channel complex (see Chapter 59).

• Absence seizures involve oscillatory neuronal activity between the thalamus and cerebral cortex. This oscillation involves (T-type) Ca^{2+} channels in the thalamic neurones, which produce low threshold spikes and allow the cells to fire in bursts. Drugs that control absences (**ethosuximide, valproate** and **lamotrigine**) reduce this Ca^{2+} current.

Carbamazepine, valproate and lamotrigine are widely used because of their efficacy and well-documented but largely tolerable side effects. The advantages of **sodium valproate** are its relative lack of sedative effects, its wide spectrum of activity and the mild nature of its adverse effects (nausea, weight gain, bleeding tendencies, tremor and transient hair loss). The main disadvantage is that occasional idiosyncratic responses cause severe or fatal hepatic toxicity and teratogenicity. For this reason, **carbamazepine** or lamotrigine is often preferred.

• **Lamotrigine** is a relatively new drug with a broad range of efficacy and seems to be relatively safe in pregnancy.

• **Phenytoin** is a difficult drug to use because of its complex metabolism, such that it may take up to 20 days for the serum level to stabilize after changing the dosage. Therefore, the dosage must be increased gradually until fits are prevented, or until signs of *cerebellar disturbance* occur (nystagmus, ataxia, dysarthria). Other unpleasant side effects, including gum hypertrophy, acne, greasy skin, coarsening of the facial features and hirsutism.

• **Phenobarbital** is effective in tonic–clonic and partial seizures but is very sedative. Tolerance occurs and sudden withdrawal may precipitate status epilepticus.

• **Vigabatrin**, **gabapentin**, **topiramate** and **levetiracetam** are newer agents introduced as 'add-on' drugs in patients where epilepsy is not satisfactorily controlled by other antiepileptics.

• **Pregabalin** is a prodrug of gabapentin with greater potency.

• **Ethosuximide** is only effective in the treatment of absences and myoclonic seizures (brief jerky movements without loss of consciousness).

• **Clonazepam** is a potent benzodiazepine anticonvulsant that is effective in absence, tonic–clonic and myoclonic seizures. It is very sedative and tolerance occurs with prolonged oral administration.

Anticonvulsant therapy in pregnancy requires care because of the teratogenic potential of many of these drugs, especially valproate and phenytoin. In addition, there is concern that *in utero* exposure to valproate may damage neuropsychological development even in the absence of physical malformation.

Did you know?

In some patients with epilepsy, changing to a ketogenic diet can help control their seizures because this diet (which is very high in fats and low in carbohydrates) forces the body to burn fat and generate ketones, which the brain then uses for its energy source.

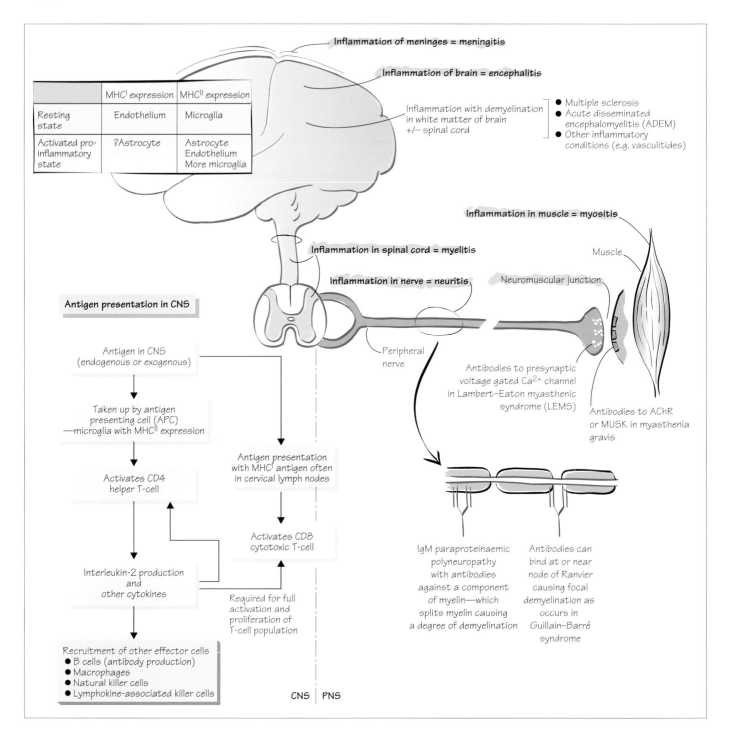

	MHC^I expression	MHC^{II} expression
Resting state	Endothelium	Microglia
Activated pro-inflammatory state	?Astrocyte	Astrocyte Endothelium More microglia

Inflammation of meninges = meningitis

Inflammation of brain = encephalitis

Inflammation with demyelination in white matter of brain +/− spinal cord

- Multiple sclerosis
- Acute disseminated encephalomyelitis (ADEM)
- Other inflammatory conditions (e.g. vasculitides)

Inflammation in muscle = myositis

Inflammation in spinal cord = myelitis

Inflammation in nerve = neuritis

Muscle

Neuromuscular junction

Antigen presentation in CNS

Peripheral nerve

Antibodies to presynaptic voltage gated Ca^{2+} channel in Lambert–Eaton myasthenic syndrome (LEMS)

Antibodies to AChR or MUSK in myasthenia gravis

Antigen in CNS (endogenous or exogenous)

Taken up by antigen presenting cell (APC) —microglia with MHC^{II} expression

Antigen presentation with MHC^I antigen often in cervical lymph nodes

Activates CD4 helper T-cell

Activates CD8 cytotoxic T-cell

Interleukin-2 production and other cytokines

Required for full activation and proliferation of T-cell population

IgM paraproteinaemic polyneuropathy with antibodies against a component of myelin—which splits myelin causing a degree of demyelination

Antibodies can bind at or near node of Ranvier causing focal demyelination as occurs in Guillain–Barré syndrome

Recruitment of other effector cells
- B cells (antibody production)
- Macrophages
- Natural killer cells
- Lymphokine-associated killer cells

CNS | PNS

Central nervous system immunological network

The central nervous system (CNS) has relative **immunological privilege** compared with the peripheral nervous system (PNS) and most other parts of the body. The reasons for this are as follows:

• The **blood–brain barrier** (**BBB**) normally prevents most lymphocytes, macrophages and antibodies from entering the CNS (see Chapters 5 and 13).

• It has a very poorly developed lymphatic drainage system.
• There is only low level expression of major histocompatibility complex (MHC) antigens.
• There are no antigen presenting cells.
However, breakdown of the BBB can greatly alter this situation.

In the resting state some activated T lymphocytes are able to cross the BBB and circulate within the CNS. In addition, **MHC expression** is confined to only a few cells although the situation is

Neuroanatomy and Neuroscience at a Glance, Fourth Edition. Roger A. Barker, Francesca Cicchetti, Michael J. Neal.

different in the inflamed state. Thus, once triggered, an immune response can be amplified and propagated by the secretion of cytokines and induced MHC expression, with the opening up of the BBB. In these circumstances the **microglia** are thought to be important as the **antigen-presenting cells** and their interaction with T-helper lymphocytes is then pivotal in generating a full-blown immunological reaction.

Recently there has been great interest in the possible role of inflammation in neurodegenerative disorders of the CNS and the extent to which this is seen simply as a reaction to the cell degeneration or as a primary contributory factor in causing the loss of these cells (see Chapter 60).

Clinical disorders of the central nervous system with an immunological basis

Multiple sclerosis

Multiple sclerosis is a common neurological disorder in which the patient characteristically presents with episodes of neurological dysfunction secondary to inflammatory lesions within the CNS. Pathologically, these lesions represent small areas of demyelination secondary to an underlying inflammatory (mainly T cell) infiltrate – the trigger and target for which is not clear. The lesions often resolve with remyelination and clinical recovery, although with time a permanent loss of myelin ensues with secondary axonal loss and the development of fixed disabilities.

To date the most successful symptomatic therapy is high-dose steroids which hastens recovery from acute relapses but does not alter the long-term disease process. Of late, though, a number of more aggressive immunotherapies with drugs that target the T cells seem to be more effective, especially if given early on in the course of the disease before there has been significant axonal loss.

Acute disseminated encephalomyelitis

This is a rare inflammatory demyelinating disease of the CNS that occurs as a complication of a number of infections and vaccinations (e.g. measles and rabies vaccination). It is a monophasic illness (unlike multiple sclerosis) characterized by widespread disseminated lesions throughout the CNS that pathologically consists of an intense perivascular infiltrate of lymphocytes and macrophages with demyelination. In some cases it is fatal. This condition resembles **experimental allergic encephalomyelitis**, which is a well-characterized T cell-mediated disorder against a component of myelin (probably myelin basic protein) induced by inoculating animals with a combination of sterile brain tissue and adjuvants. This disorder is often used experimentally to model multiple sclerosis.

Other immunological diseases

A number of other diseases with an immunological basis can affect the CNS and these include those diseases that primarily affect blood vessels (the *vasculitides*).

In addition, there is a rare group of disorders in which there is CNS dysfunction as a remote effect of a cancer, *paraneoplastic syndromes*. In these conditions antibodies to components of the CNS are generated, presumably triggered by the tumour, which then lead to neuronal cell death and the development of a neurological syndrome, e.g. anti-Purkinje cell antibodies cause a profound cerebellar syndrome by the immunological removal of this cell type in the cerebellum. The exact mechanism by which these antibodies exert their effect is not known as antibodies normally do not cross the BBB, but pathologically there is often evidence of a lymphocytic infiltrate in the affected structure which implies that the antibody is capable of inducing an immune-mediated process of neuronal loss.

Finally it has been shown that a number of CNS disorders are caused by antibodies to specific ion channels or receptors – e.g. anti-K+ channel antibodies causing a limbic encephalitis or anti-N-methyl-D-aspartate (NMDA) receptor antibodies causing psychoses, a movement disorder and encephalopathy – many of which are *not* associated with any underlying malignancy but are primary immunological disorders. Indeed there is a growing interest in the possibility that some patients with psychiatric disorders may have an autoimmune disease targeting a receptor/ion channel.

Clinical disorders of the peripheral nervous system with an immunological basis

The PNS has fewer of the protective features of the CNS so it is more susceptible to conventional immune-mediated diseases.

• The **peripheral nerve** is affected by a number of immunological processes, including *Guillain–Barré syndrome*. In this condition there is often a preceding illness (e.g. *Campylobacter jejuni* or cytomegalovirus infection) that induces an immune response which then cross-reacts with components in the peripheral nerve (e.g. certain gangliosides). This then induces focal demyelination in the peripheral nerve, which prevents it from conducting action potentials normally (see Chapter 17). In time the patient usually recovers, although they may require immunotherapy with either plasma exchange or intravenous immunoglobulin. A similar condition is seen in some diseases where abnormal amounts of a component of antibodies are produced (the *paraproteinaemias*).
• The **neuromuscular junction** can be affected by immunological processes as occurs in *myasthenia gravis* and the *Lambert–Eaton myasthenic syndrome* (see Chapter 16).
• **Muscles** can be involved in inflammatory processes. The most common form of this is *polymyositis*, which is a T cell-mediated condition associated with proximal weakness and pain. In contrast, *dermatomyositis* is a B cell-mediated disease centred on blood vessels, which causes a painful proximal muscle weakness in association with a florid skin rash. This latter condition can represent a paraneoplastic syndrome in more elderly patients with tumours in the lung, breast, colon or ovary.

Did you know?

In 1890, Emil von Behring discovered that the blood of animals infected with different diseases contained chemicals that attacked the diseased cells – this observation led to the discovery of antibodies.

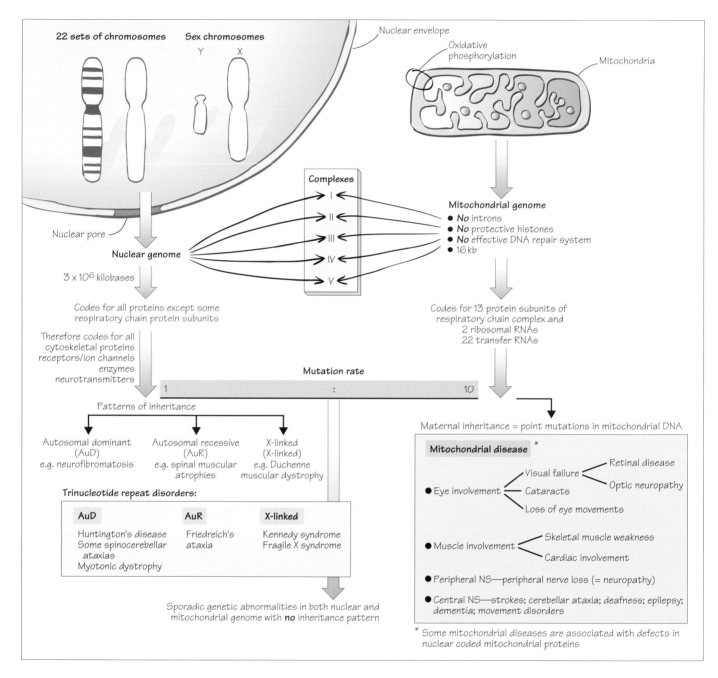

A large number of genetic disorders involve the nervous system, and some of these have pathology confined solely to this system. Recent advances in molecular genetics have meant that many diseases of the nervous system are being redefined by their underlying genetic defect.

Three major new developments have revolutionized the role of genetic factors in the evolution of neurological disease. First, genes encoded in the maternally inherited **mitochondrial genome** can cause neurological disorder; Second, a number of inherited neurological disorders have as their basis an expanded trinucleotide repeat (**triplet repeat disorders**); Third, the ability to use sophisticated genotyping of individual cases (exome sequencing) to find novel mutations is starting to yield new insights into diseases of the nervous system.

Disorders with gene deletions

Many different disorders within the nervous system result from the loss of a single gene or part thereof. For example, *hereditary neuropathy with a liability to pressure palsies*, in which the patient has a tendency to develop recurrent focal entrapment neuropathies

Neuroanatomy and Neuroscience at a Glance, Fourth Edition. Roger A. Barker, Francesca Cicchetti, Michael J. Neal.

in association with a large deletion on chromosome 17, which includes the gene coding for the peripheral myelin protein 22 (PMP 22).

Disorders with gene duplications

The duplication of a gene can, under some circumstances, cause disease. An example of this is in certain types of *hereditary motor and sensory neuropathy*, where the patient develops distal weakness, wasting and sensory loss in the first decades of life. In some of these cases there is duplication of part of chromosome 17, including the gene coding for PMP 22.

Disorders with gene mutations

This is the most common form of genetic defect and in these diseases there is a mutation in the gene coding for a specific enzyme or protein which results in that product failing to work normally. An example of such a situation is found in some familial forms of *motor neurone disease* (see Chapter 60) and *muscular dystrophies* (see Chapter 21) as well as *myotonic syndromes* (see Chapter 14).

Disorders showing genetic imprinting

Genetic imprinting is the differential expression of autosomal genes depending upon their parental origin. Thus, disruption of the maternal gene(s) on a certain part of chromosome 15 (15q11-q13) causes *Prader–Willi syndrome* (mental retardation with obesity, hypogenitalism and short stature) while disruption of the same genes from the father causes *Angelman's syndrome* (a condition of severe mental retardation, cerebellar ataxia, epilepsy and craniofacial abnormalities).

Mitochondrial disorders

Mitochondria contain their own DNA and synthesize a number of the proteins in the respiratory chain responsible for oxidative phosphorylation (see Chapter 60), although the vast majority of mitochondrial proteins are encoded by nuclear DNA.

Thus, mitochondrial disorders (deletions, duplication or point mutations) can result from defects in:
- these nuclear-coded genes;
- the mitochondria genome.

However, mitochondrial DNA mutates more than 10 times as frequently as nuclear DNA and has no introns (non-coding parts of the genome), so that a random mutation will usually strike a coding DNA sequence. As mitochondria are inherited from the fertilized oocyte, disorders with point mutations in the mitochondrially coded DNA show maternal inheritance (always inherited from the mother). However, within each cell there are many mitochondria and so a given cell can contain both normal and mutant mitochondrial DNA, a situation known as **heteroplasmy**, and it is only when a given threshold of mutant mitochondria is reached does the disease result.

The clinical disorders associated with different defects in the mitochondrial genome are legion, and the reason why some areas are targeted in some conditions and not others is not clear.

Trinucleotide repeat disorders

A number of different disorders have now been identified that have as their major genetic defect an expanded triplet repeat, i.e. there is a large and abnormal expansion of three bases in the genome. In normal individuals triplet repeat sequences are not uncommon but once the number of repeats exceeds a certain number the disease will definitely appear.

This pathological triplet (or trinucleotide) repeat either occurs in the coding part of a gene (e.g. *Huntington's disease*; see Chapter 42) or in a non-coding part of the genome (e.g. *Friedreich's ataxia*). The resulting expansion either causes a loss of function (e.g. frataxin in *Friedreich's ataxia*) or a new gain of function in that gene product (e.g. huntingtin in *Huntington's disease*). This latter aspect is of interest as the new protein appears to have a function that is unique to it and which is critical to the evolution of the neurodegenerative process. However, the mechanism by which this protein produces selective neuronal death in specific CNS sites is not known as many of the mutant gene products are widely expressed throughout the brain and body.

The consequence of a large unstable DNA sequence as occurs in these disorders is that the triplet repeat can increase during mitosis and meiosis, resulting in longer triplet repeat sequences (**dynamic mutations**). This means that the most likely time for triplet expansion is during spermatogenesis and subsequent fertilization/embryogenesis, and has two major implications. First, longer repeats tend to occur in the offspring of affected men and, second, longer repeats tend to occur in subsequent generations. This results in patients of subsequent generations presenting with earlier onset and more severe forms of the disorder – a phenomenon known as **genetic anticipation** as longer repeat sequences are associated with younger onset and more severe forms of the disease.

Genome-wide association studies

In recent years the ability to look across the whole genome in populations of patients with diseases of a complex genetic basis has proved possible both technically and financially. The use of a large number of markers to cover the whole genome has identified a number of regions conveying risk in disorders of the central nervous system (CNS), such as Parkinson's and Alzheimer's disease. This is turn will yield new insights into the common sporadic forms of the disease, as hitherto the genetics of these disorders has largely been in the domain of rare mendelian forms of the disease.

Did you know?

The first announcement that the 'secret of life' (i.e. the structure of DNA) had been solved was made by Watson and Crick in the Cambridge pub 'The Eagle' in 1953.

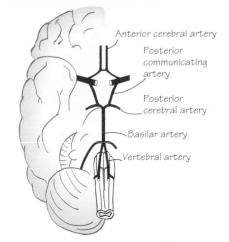

Anterior cerebral artery

Posterior communicating artery

Posterior cerebral artery

Basilar artery

Vertebral artery

The vertebrobasilar system can be affected at any part and produces a wide range of stroke syndromes
- Occlusion of vertebral artery produces variable clinical defects (one classical form is the lateral medullary syndrome).
- Occlusion of the basilar artery causes coma, bilateral signs involve the whole body and often leads to death

Lateral medullary syndrome of Wallenberg
– Occlusion of posterior inferior cerebellar artery (PICA)
– Ipsilateral sensory loss on face (Vth nerve)
– Ipsilateral ataxia (cerebellar peduncle + cerebellum)
– Vertigo/nausea/vomiting (cranial nerve VIII)
– Horners syndrome (descending sympathetic tract)
– Dysphagia/dysarthria (cranial nerves IX, X)

Medulla oblongata

CBM

CBM

Anterior cerebral artery supply (ACA)
- Sensory loss over contralateral leg
- Urinary incontinence
- Frontal signs
  – grasp reflex
  – change in behaviour
  – gegenhalten increase in muscle tone
- Paralysis of contralateral foot/leg

Middle cerebral artery supply (MCA)
- Paralysis of contralateral face/arm/leg
- Contralateral sensory loss
- Speech/aphasia if left hemisphere
- Homonymous hemianopia

Posterior cerebral artery supply (PCA)
- Homonymous hemianopia
- Cognitive/memory defects
- Can involve thalamic/ brainstem involvement in some cases

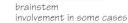

Anterior spinal artery occlusion
- Loss of motor control (UMN + LMN at level of occlusion)
- Loss of pain/temperature
- Preservation of proprioception/vibration perception (see Chapter 54)

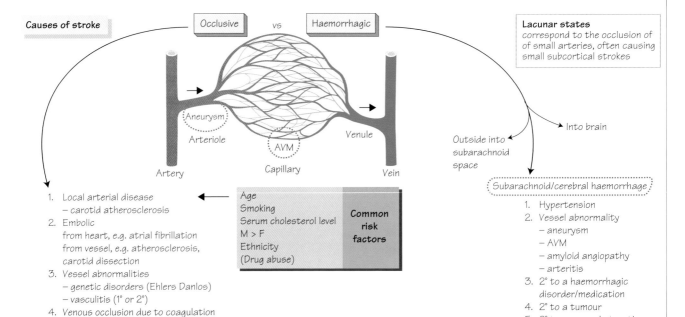

Causes of stroke

Occlusive vs Haemorrhagic

Aneurysm

Arteriole

AVM

Artery

Capillary

Venule

Vein

1. Local arterial disease
   – carotid atherosclerosis
2. Embolic
   from heart, e.g. atrial fibrillation
   from vessel, e.g. atherosclerosis, carotid dissection
3. Vessel abnormalities
   – genetic disorders (Ehlers Danlos)
   – vasculitis (1° or 2°)
4. Venous occlusion due to coagulation abnormalities; tumour, pregnancy, drugs

Age
Smoking
Serum cholesterol level
M > F
Ethnicity
(Drug abuse)

Common risk factors

Lacunar states
correspond to the occlusion of of small arteries, often causing small subcortical strokes

Into brain

Outside into subarachnoid space

Subarachnoid/cerebral haemorrhage

1. Hypertension
2. Vessel abnormality
   – aneurysm
   – AVM
   – amyloid angiopathy
   – arteritis
3. 2° to a haemorrhagic disorder/medication
4. 2° to a tumour
5. 2° to venous obstruction

Neuroanatomy and Neuroscience at a Glance, Fourth Edition. Roger A. Barker, Francesca Cicchetti, Michael J. Neal.

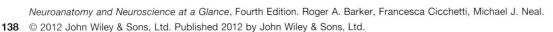

Definition of stroke

A *stroke* or cerebrovascular accident (CVA) is typically an event of sudden onset (although it can occur over hours in some patients where a major vessel is slowly thrombosing). It is due to an *interruption* of blood supply to an area of the central nervous system (CNS) that causes irreversible loss of tissue at the core with a penumbra of compromised tissue around the area that may still be salvageable. If the disturbance in blood flow is temporary it causes a *transient ischaemic attack* or TIA. This is often a harbinger of a stroke. Stroke is common and its consequences depend on the vessel that has been occluded.

Investigation of stroke

- History and examination
- Computed tomography (CT)/magnetic resonance imaging (MRI)
- Blood tests – including full blood count, erythrocyte sedimentation rate, renal function, glucose and lipids
- Electrocardiogram (ECG) which may be repeated and prolonged if a cardiac source for the stroke is suspected

Other investigation may include an ECHOcardiogram and imaging of the blood vessels and/or a CSF examination and this depends on the type of stroke (see Table 64.1).

Rare causes of stroke

The most common causes of stroke are atherosclerosis and embolic disease from the blood vessels to the brain and the heart. The other causes are quite rare. Other syndromes that resemble stroke include *mitochondrial disease* (see Chapter 63), where there can be a sudden onset of neurological deficits due to problems in the mitochondria and *not* in the vasculature. Such events in the brain typically do not obey vascular territories when investigated with MRI for example.

Treatment of stroke

- Consider local thrombolysis if a single major vessel is involved: e.g. basilar artery/venous sinus
- Acutely (if <3–4 hours) and no contraindication thrombolysis
- Treat any risk factors eg stop smoking, lower-cholesterol etc and start aspirin/perindopril/statin
- Heparin if major venous sinus thrombosis
- Surgery, if recognizable lesion causing stroke is identified e.g. >70% carotid artery stenosis/aneurysm
- Rehabilitation therapy

Did you know?

Every year, over 6 million people worldwide die from a stroke.

Table 64.1 Types of stroke and the investigations required

Type of stroke	Investigations
Occlusive or ischaemia	Check any problems in heart with an echocardiogram and ECG and possible a cardiological opinion
	Check no systemic problems with blood tests as above
	May need to image the blood vessels to and in the brain to see the extent of atherosclerotic disease in the vessels
	May need to test the CSF to check presence/absence of inflammatory changes in the blood vessels (i.e. a vasculitis)
Haemorrhagic	Imaging of vessels to see if there is any underlying abnormality
	Blood tests to rule out more general problems with coagulation in the blood (clotting screen)
	Echocardiogram in cases of suspected mycotic/septic aneurysms in the brain, which may have arisen from endocarditis (in cases of suspected mycotic/septic aneurysms secondary to endocarditis)
	May need to test the CSF to check presence/absence of inflammatory changes in the blood vessels (i.e. a vasculitis)

65 Neuroradiological anatomy

The ability to better delineate the anatomy of the central nervous system (CNS) in everyday neurological practice using modern imaging techniques has increased with improvements in technology and its widespread adoption in hospitals throughout the world. The major methods for imaging the nervous system are discussed in Chapter 53, but in general magnetic resonance imaging (MRI) is the best way to look at anatomical structure and its capacity to do this is dependent on the strength of the magnetic field that can be generated with the scanner. Most hospitals use a 1.5 Tesla (T) machine, but increasingly 3T machines are being used and for research purposes 7T scanners have been developed for human use.

While the introduction of more sophisticated MRI and computed tomography (CT) sequences has enabled us to better define the vasculature of the brain, the gold standard is still formal angiography and indeed is the only way to visualize the blood vessels in the spine if this is needed, which is rare.

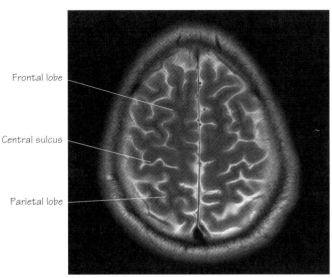

Figure 65.1 The posterior parietal and prefrontal cortex

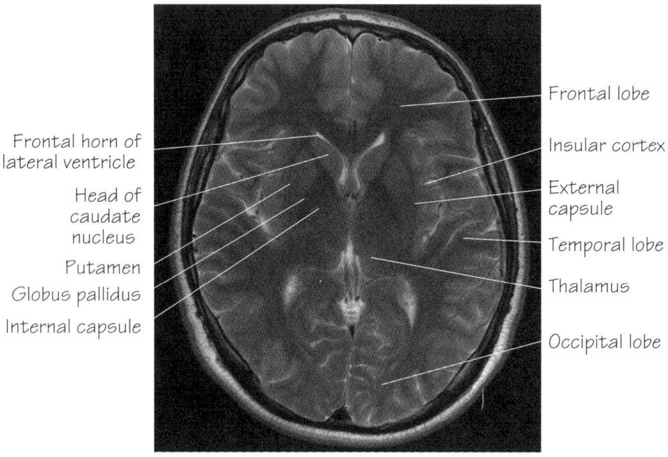

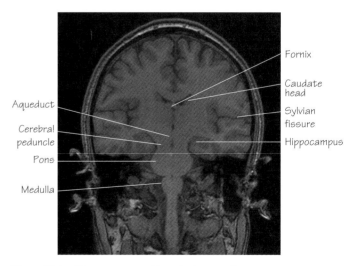

Figure 65.3 The basal ganglia

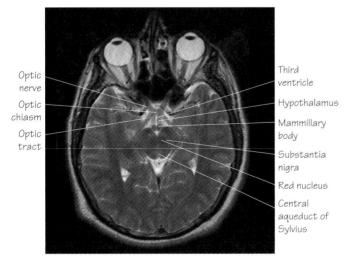

Figure 65.2 *The visual pathways and subcortical visual areas*

Figure 65.4 Hippocampus and its relation to other structures

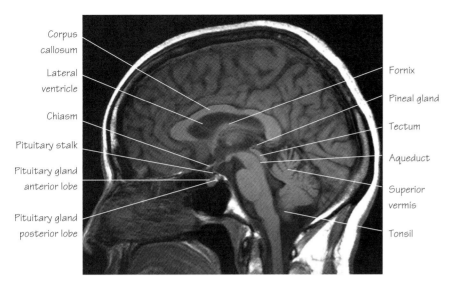

Figure 65.5   The hypothalamus

MRI of the cerebral hemispheres

MRI of the cerebral hemispheres clearly reveals a large number of structures which are illustrated in Figures 65.1 to 65.5. In particular:

• The different lobes of the brain can be clearly seen although the central sulcus in the human brain lies more posteriorly than one would imagine.

• The basal ganglia structures can be seen in terms of the caudate, putamen and globus pallidum. The subthalamic nucleus and substantia nigra are harder to see, although the latter is becoming easier to recognize with newer MRI scanners.

• The thalamus and the integrity of the ventricular system.

• The major pathways running in the internal capsule and the corpus callosum.

• The visual pathways can also be clearly seen up to the optic tracts. The optic radiations cannot be seen using standard imaging paradigms. Getting clear pictures of the optic pathway can be difficult and sometimes special sequences are needed to look at it in detail if there is a high suspicion of pathology.

• Limbic system structures are much harder to see, given their location on the medial aspects of the temporal lobe. The hippoc-

ampi can usually be seen, although if volumetric loss in this structure is being sought (e.g. in cases of possible Alzheimer's disease) then special imaging protocols should be used as it is easy to mistakenly see atrophy in this structure using standard scan sequences.

• The pituitary and its relationship to the visual pathways and hypothalamus can also be seen.

MRI of the posterior fossa

CT scans can be used to look at the gross structure of the brain, but it is unable to give much information on smaller lesions, especially within the posterior fossa. Thus MRI is the modality of choice for delineating the anatomy of the brainstem and cerebellum. MRI of the posterior fossa can reveal a number of structures (Figures 65.4–65.6):

• The major divisions of the brainstem and its connection to the cerebellum and the ventricular system as it passes through the aqueduct to the fourth ventricle.

• The different lobes and parts of the cerebellum especially the cerebellar tonsil and where it lies relative to the foramen magnum (e.g. Arnold–Chiari malformations) (see Chapter 5).

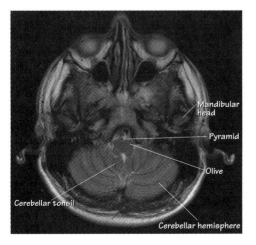
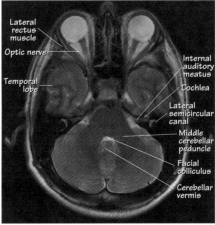
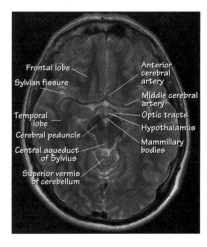

Figure 65.6   The Brainstem

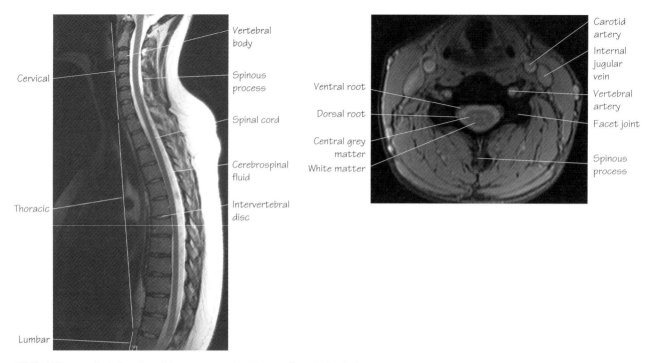

Figure 65.7 MRI scan of whole spine with a cross-sectional image of cervical spine

• Within the brainstem itself a number of structures can normally be seen. On occasions higher-resolution scans can be undertaken to look at specific parts of the brainstem, e.g. acoustic neuromas with high-resolution CT scans through the internal auditory meati.

MRI of the spinal cord (Figure 65.7)

This is typically used to look at the integrity of the spinal cord and the spine around it, to ensure that there is no compression of the spine by lesions extrinsic to it (e.g. disc herniations) or lesions within it, such as tumours.

Vasculature of the brain (Figure 65.8)

Dye can be injected into the circulation followed by the rapid capture of images as the dye moves through the different arterial vessels before draining through the venous system. This is the best way to pick up any vascular abnormalities such as small aneurysms or arteriovenous malformations.

Did you know?

Our brain requires 20% of the entire body's blood flow.

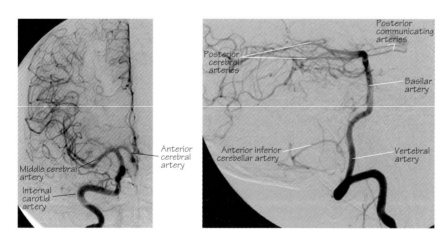

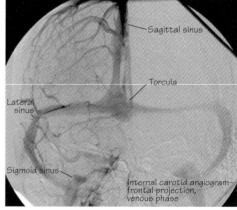

Figure 65.8 Blood supply of the central nervous system

Case studies and questions

Chapter 1

A 44-year-old woman delivers a full-term baby, and on examination it is noticed that he has a opening on his lower back with a membrane covered cyst.

1 *What developmental problem is this?*

Chapter 2

A 24-year-old man falls 4.5 m (15 ft) off a ladder onto a concrete floor and is knocked out. He is taken to hospital by his friends, and when he wakes up 2 days later he discovers he cannot move his legs and arms, but can only shrug his shoulders.

1 *In which nervous system is the lesion?*
2 *What is the likely site of that lesion?*
3 *What is the lesion likely to be?*

Chapter 3

A 67-year-old man presents with a few months history of fainting when standing quickly especially after meals. He has also developed constipation with some nocturnal diarrhoea, urinary retention and impotence. On examination he has a significant drop in blood pressure on standing and feels faint. His pupils respond poorly to light but there are no other abnormalities on examination. As part of his investigations he is found to have no change in his heart rate on electrocardiography (ECG) with exercise. His routine blood tests are all normal.

1 *What is the diagnosis?*
2 *What is the significance of the ECG findings?*

Chapter 4

A baby has major problems with constipation soon after birth. His investigations show that a small part of his large bowel is unable to contract and relax at all.

1 *What is the diagnosis?*
2 *What causes this?*

Chapter 5

A 16-year-old boy comes in with a short history of headache, photophobia and a new petechial rash. On examination he is drowsy with a low blood pressure and neck stiffness.

1 *What is the diagnosis?*
2 *What is the most likely causative agent?*
3 *What is the treatment?*

Chapter 6

A 28-year-old man presents with a stuttering onset of left-sided weakness involving the arm more than the leg and face. He had pain around his right eye at onset that is now settling. On examination he has right-sided Horner's syndrome and left-sided hemiparesis with some sensory loss.

1 *What is the likely diagnosis in this young man?*
2 *How would you prove it?*
3 *Why has he got Horner's syndrome?*

Chapter 7

A 58-year-old woman presents with tinnitus in her left ear that has been getting worse over the past few years. On examination, she has deafness in the left ear, a degree of facial weakness on the left and difficulty in fully abducting her left eye.

1 *Which cranial nerves are involved?*
2 *Where is the lesion?*
3 *What is the likely cause of the syndrome?*

Chapter 8

A 28-year-old woman presents with dizziness, nausea and vomiting that has come on over a week. On examination she has a weak left side of the face, difficulty moving the eyes to the left, a loss of feeling on the left side of the face, and some weakness down the right side of the body with some sensory loss down the same side.

1 *Where is the lesion likely to be and why is the left side of the face involved and the right side of the body?*
2 *How would you investigate her problem?*

Chapter 9

A 43-year-old woman presents with an evolving sensory disturbance in her legs with some weakness. On examination she has sensory loss in her left leg for light touch and proprioception with a sensory level at T10, and in the right leg she has a loss of pain and temperature. She has a slightly stiff left leg with brisk reflexes.

1 *Where is the lesion?*
2 *How would you prove the nature of the problem?*
3 *Do you know what this syndrome is called?*

Chapter 10

A 65-year-old man presents with a 6-month history of a change in personality and behaviour. He has become rather childish and impulsive, and he tends to not be very attentive to what is being said to him but seems quite happy. More recently he has acquired a taste for sweet things to eat.

1 *Where is the problem likely to lie?*
2 *What could be the cause of this syndrome?*

Chapter 11

A 26-year-old woman presents with new-onset amenorrhoea and galactorrhoea. On examination she has a bitemporal visual field defect. She has also noticed that she is passing much more urine that normal and drinking more.

1 *What is the diagnosis?*
2 *Why does she have a visual field defect?*
3 *What is the cause of her polyuria and polydipsia?*

Chapter 12

A 78-year-old man presents with a 6-month history of rapidly progressive cognitive decline with some jerking myoclonic movements of his limbs. On examination he is largely mute with no focal limb or cranial nerve deficits. A computed tomography (CT) scan of his head shows atrophy and all his routine blood tests are normal.

1 *What cells are affected by this disease process?*
2 *What is the likely diagnosis in this man?*

Chapter 13

A 19-year-old woman presents with a 10-day history of an evolving sensory disturbance in her legs that began in her feet and then spread up to involve both legs to the umbilicus bilaterally. She has some slight leg weakness and bladder disturbance. It remains like this for a few days and then improves over the course of a month back to normal.

1 *Which cells in the central nervous system is likely to be mediating the disease process?*
2 *What is causing the neurological disturbance?*
3 *What is the likely diagnosis?*

Chapter 14

A 16-year-old man presents with episodes of weakness after exercise or certain types of heavy meal. During one of these attacks he is unable to move, but can breath normally. He always recovers back to normal.

1 *Where does the problem lie in his nervous system?*
2 *What is that problem likely to be?*

Chapter 15

A 36-year-old man is recovering from acute gastroenteritis when he notices that he is developing tingling and numbness in his hands and feet. Over the next 2 days these sensory symptoms spread up his arms and legs and he also starts to develop weakness in the same distribution. On examination he has mild flaccid weakness of all four limbs with areflexia and a glove and stocking sensory loss.

1 *What part of his nervous system is being affected?*
2 *What is the problem at a pathophysiological level?*
3 *What is the likely diagnosis?*

Chapter 16

A 28-year-old presents with a 3-month history of drooping of her eyelids, more on the right than the left, which occurs mainly in the evening and is associated with some slurring of speech and slight difficulty in swallowing and chewing.

1 *Where is the problem in her nervous system?*
2 *What is significant about when she gets her symptoms?*
3 *What is the likely diagnosis?*

Chapter 17

A 41-year-old man presents with increasing back pain and stiffness in his legs. He is known to have type 1 diabetes mellitus. On examination he has a very arched back (hyperlordosis) and very stiff legs which are not spastic, but are stiff especially when walking. He is found to have high levels of glutamic acid decarboxylase (GAD) antibodies in his blood and diagnosed as having stiff man syndrome.

1 *What type of synapse is primarily affected in this condition?*
2 *Why are his legs stiff?*

Chapter 18

A 78-year-old woman presents with a 6-month history of slowing up, with rigidity, a mask-like face and a slight tremor. She was recently diagnosed as having Ménière's disease and started on metoclopramide 7 months ago.

1 *What is the cause of her parkinsonism?*
2 *Why has she developed this condition?*
3 *Is it reversible?*

Chapter 19

A 27-year-old man presents with a history with unilateral headaches with nausea, vomiting, photophobia and visual distortions. He has had these attacks on and off for many years and they typically last up to a day.

1 *What is the diagnosis?*
2 *What neurotransmitter system is thought to underlie this condition?*

Chapter 20

A 25-year-old man presents with a slowly progressive non-painful weakness of his shoulders and upper legs, such that he is having difficulty getting up stairs and getting out of chairs and taking things down from high shelves. On examination he has some wasting of his proximal muscles with weakness but no loss of reflexes, sensory loss or fasciculation.

1 *What type of disorder does he have?*
2 *What question would you ask him?*
3 *How would you investigate him?*

Chapter 21

A 23-year-old man presents with episodes of weakness that are typically provoked by certain types of meals and exercise. During one of these attacks he has no movement in any of the muscles, but his breathing is maintained normally and he has no sensory loss.

1 *What is this condition known as?*
2 *What is its basis?*

Chapter 22

A 45-year-old businessman has a few weeks' history of loss of dexterity in his hands and an unstable gait. On examination he cannot feel light touch or pin prick to the wrists and ankles bilaterally and he also has bilaterally impaired proprioception in the fingers and toes. Power seems normal and his reflexes are depressed or absent.

1 *Where is the problem?*
2 *Why has he lost dexterity and has an unstable gait?*
3 *When would his symptoms be worse?*

Chapter 23

A 36-year-old architect comes to clinic saying he is having increasing problems driving home from work at night and he has also noticed that he is bumping into things more often when he goes to bed. On examination he has constricted visual fields with some speckling of the peripheral retina on fundoscopy.

1 *What condition does he have?*
2 *What is the problem in this condition?*
3 *Why does he have these symptoms?*

Chapter 24

An 81-year-old woman gives a 2-year history of difficulty reading and watching television. She has no real problems with walking around and has no history of any other medical or neurological problems. On examination she has early cataracts and visual acuities bilaterally of 6/48.

1 *What is the most likely diagnosis?*
2 *Why is she having difficulty reading and watching TV?*

Chapter 25

A 23-year-old woman presents with a 10-day history of pain on moving the right eye with a loss of central visual acuity. On examination she had reduced visual acuity in the right eye with normal eye movements and fundoscopy. She has reduced colour vision in her right eye with a right relative afferent pupillary defect.

1 *What is the most likely diagnosis?*
2 *What will happen to the pupil in the right eye when a light is shone first in the left eye and then the right? Why?*

Chapter 26

A 54-year-old man notices that following a stroke he cannot see colours properly.

1 *What is the diagnosis?*
2 *Where is the lesion?*

Chapter 27

A 6-year-old boy is found to be failing at school. He is inattentive, his speech is poor and he is lagging behind his peers. He often complains of earache and there is no family history of any problems. On examination he appears not to pay much attention, but otherwise there are no obvious neurological deficits.

1 *What may be the problem in this child?*
2 *How would you investigate this?*
3 *How would you treat this?*

Chapter 28: (a) Auditory pathways

A 44-year-old woman presents with left-sided tinnitus; also, every time a loud noise is heard she develops left-sided facial twitching. On examination she has left-sided sensorineural deafness with a slight left-sided lower motor neurone lesion.

1 *Where is the lesion?*
2 *What could the lesion be?*
3 *Would her sound localization be abnormal?*

Chapter 28: (b) Language

A 63-year-old woman presents with a 3-week history of progressive difficulties talking and some clumsiness of the right hand. On examination she has a subtle right upper motor neurone seventh nerve palsy and a non-fluent aphasia with preserved comprehension and writing.

1 *Where is the lesion?*
2 *What is the lesion likely to be?*
3 *How would you investigate her?*

Chapter 29

A 43-year-old woman has an acute episode of profound dizziness with nausea and vomiting such that she has to go to bed and cannot get up for several days. She slowly recovers, but then presents with brief episodes of profound dizziness and nausea when she turns over in bed at night or when she turns her head suddenly during the day.

1 *What is the original diagnosis?*

2 *What has she now developed?*
3 *How would you prove and treat the latter?*

Chapter 30

A 26-year-old man presents with a 1-year history of intermittent episodes of 'feeling odd'. He described attacks where he would suddenly feel panicky with butterflies in his stomach and a perception of an odd smell of burning rubber with a strange metallic taste in his mouth. These attacks would last about 20–30 seconds and on occasions, others had reported that he looked slightly blank with some lip smacking. These latter attacks would last at most a minute and the patient would be back to normal straight after the events.

1 *What is being described?*
2 *Where are the abnormalities originating from?*
3 *What investigations would be helpful?*

Chapter 31

A 36-year-old vegan presents with a 6-month history of unsteadiness of gait, visual problems and numbness of the hands and feet. On examination, she looks pale and has slight loss of pallor of the optic nerve head on fundoscopy. She has pseudoathetoid movement of her hands with sensory loss that includes proprioception. In the lower limbs she is ataxic with a similar pattern of sensory loss, but slightly brisk knee jerks and extensor plantar responses.

1 *What is the most likely diagnosis?*
2 *Why does she has pseudoathetoid movements of the hands?*
3 *What test would you do to prove the diagnosis?*

Chapter 32

A 20-year-old woman fractured her right ankle while skiing 3 years ago. She now presents with a chronically painful right foot that she cannot walk on. On examination, she will not let you touch her elevated right foot because it is so painful. The foot is red, hairless and the skin has a shiny appearance. She has come to see you because she would like to have the foot amputated.

1 *What is the most likely diagnosis?*
2 *Would you recommend amputation?*

Chapter 33

A 74-year-old man presents with a pain over his forehead on the left. Two months previously he had had vesicular rash that had then scabbed over and had affected the first division of the trigeminal nerve on the left. He has no other complaints and there is nothing to find on examination.

1 *What is the most likely diagnosis?*
2 *How would you treat it?*

Chapter 34

A 62-year-old man is brought to the memory clinic by his relatives. He feels there are no major problems but his wife says that for the last year he has become more forgetful, he often cannot remember where he has left things and often behaves inappropriately. He has developed a great passion for desserts and has put on some weight. He has no significant previous medical history. On examination he has poor attention, a pout and grasp reflexes.

1 *What is the most likely diagnosis?*
2 *Why is his memory poor?*
3 *What tests would you do?*

Chapter 35

A 31-year-old woman with multiple sclerosis has a relapse with new lesions in her lower cervical spinal cord and cerebellum bilaterally.

1 *What motor features will she exhibit?*

Chapter 36

A 77-year-old man presents with a 6-month history of weakness of his left hand. He has no significant previous medical history. On examination he has normal cranial nerves apart from a wasted, fasciculating tongue. In the upper limbs he has widespread wasting, more on the left than the right with extensive fasciculations. He has weakness of left elbow extension and flexion as well as in the hand. In the lower limbs he has widespread fasciculations with some wasting and relatively well-preserved power. He has brisk reflexes in his arms and legs.

1 *What is the most likely diagnosis?*
2 *How would you prove this?*

Chapter 37

A 58-year-old man presents with a 20-year history of a slowly evolving spastic gait without any other problems. He has a family history of this condition. On examination he has greatly increased tone in the legs with relatively well-preserved power. He has bilaterally brisk lower limb reflexes with extensor plantars and clonus and a normal sensory examination. He had normal upper limb and cranial nerve examination, with normal spinal and brain imaging.

1 *What type of motor lesion does he have affecting the legs?*
2 *What is the likely diagnosis?*

Chapter 38

A 72-year-old man presents with sudden onset left-sided weakness.

1 *What is the problem?*
2 *Where is the lesion?*
3 *Why is he weak?*

Chapter 39

A 65-year-old man presents with intermittent episodes of abnormal movement involving his right hand. These episodes can last for a few minutes and the abnormal jerking movements can spread to involve the whole arm and face with loss of speech.

1 *What is being described?*
2 *Where is the lesion?*
3 *What is the lesion likely to be?*

Chapter 40

A 42-year-old woman presents with a 10-year history of slurred speech, unsteadiness of gait with falls and clumsiness of the hands. There is a strong family history with several members having similar problems with motor control, including one of her sisters, her father and uncle.

1 *What would you expect to find on examination?*
2 *What is the likely diagnosis?*

Chapter 41

A 46-year-old man presents with a 2-year history of abnormal movements. There is a family history of a movement disorder complicated by major psychiatric and cognitive problems. On examination, the patient has widespread involuntary dance-like movements of all four limbs as well as the face, mouth and trunk.

1 *What movement disorder is being described?*
2 *What is the most likely diagnosis?*

Chapter 42

A 72-year-old man has had Ménière's disease for many years but it has got worse of late. As a result he has been started on the antiemetic metoclopramide. For the past few months he has noticed that he has difficulty keeping up with his wife when walking, that he has become rather stooped and his voice has got quieter, and he has an occasional tremor of his right hand.

1 *What syndrome is he suffering from?*
2 *What would you find on examination?*
3 *What is the most likely diagnosis?*

Chapter 43

A 49-year-old lorry driver is referred by the police to you following a recent road traffic accident. The driver had no recollection of what happened but a witness said they saw him asleep at the wheel at the time of the accident which was at around 2 pm. To direct questioning he said he slept well, but often felt tired when he got up in the morning. On examination, he weighs 127 kg (20 stone) and has some ankle oedema and plethoric facies.

1 *What tests would you do?*
2 *What do you think the diagnosis could be?*
3 *What treatment would you recommend, if any?*

Chapter 44

A 23-year-old man is involved in a major road traffic accident and is brought into hospital unconscious. He is intubated, ventilated and placed on the intensive care unit where over the course of the next few weeks he improves to the point that he can self-ventilate but he shows no obvious movements to command. His MRI shows that he sustained a major injury to his upper brainstem, and with this he now has some slight degree of brain atrophy. You are asked whether it is worth pursuing active treatment in this man, given his poor level of consciousness and responsiveness.

1 *What would you recommend?*
2 *What is the likely diagnosis?*

Chapter 45

A 35-year-old woman presents with a few year history of episodes of sudden intense fear. She describes these attacks as occurring for no obvious reason and consist of her feeling intensely frightened as though something awful is about to happen to her. These last a few seconds and then she is left rather shaken. On examination there are no abnormal findings.

1 *What is being described?*
2 *What would you do to prove this?*

Chapter 46

A 68-year-old woman presents to the memory clinic with a 1–2-year history of being more forgetful. Her family complains that she is getting more absent minded, loses things around the house and tends to get confused quite easily, especially when she is placed into a new environment, such as when they go on holiday. On examination she has no abnormal neurological signs, but her 5-minute recall of a name and address is one out of seven. She is

able to name objects normally as well as copy complex figures. She is talkative, however, and enjoys telling you about her school days.
1 *What type of memory deficit does she have?*
2 *What is the likely diagnosis?*

Chapter 47

A 43-year-old man has recently had a very unusual stroke that has left him with bilateral caudate infarcts. His general practitioner (GP) sends him back to you saying that he has become depressed but he is not really responding to antidepressants. On examination he has a rather flat affect and is reluctant to engage in any activities either in the clinic or on subsequent neuropsychological testing.
1 *What would you do and why?*

Chapter 48

A 43-year-old man has a left leg deep vein thrombosis that has propagated from the superficial veins in his lower leg. A decision is made to explore the venous system with the hope of removing the clot that is extending into the deep veins of the leg behind the knee. On coming round from the operation he is aware of numbness down the back of the foot and calf.
1 *What has happened?*
2 *Will it recover?*

Chapter 49

A 1-year-old child is referred with problems of a squint. On examination he has a major divergent squint.
1 *What needs to be done?*
2 *Why should this be done?*
Note: There are no case studies for Chapters 50–55.

Chapter 56

A 28-year-old woman presents with a 1-week history of diplopia, with some facial numbness and weakness. She has no previous medical or neurological history of note. On examination she has an internuclear ophthalmoplegia with numbness over the left side of the face and facial weakness involving both the upper and lower facial musculature on the left. She also has brisk reflexes throughout with extensor plantars.
1 *Where is the lesion causing her diplopia?*
2 *What is the likely diagnosis?*
3 *What test would you arrange for her at this consultation?*

Chapter 57

A 23-year-old woman presents with early morning wakening, poor appetite, reduced libido and a sense of helplessness. On examination she is rather tearful with some odd slightly paranoid, ideation. She has a facial rash, some arthralgia with joint swelling and very slight proximal limb weakness. Routine blood tests show she is anaemic with a raised erythrocyte sedimentation rate (ESR) and a degree of renal failure.
1 *What is the diagnosis?*
2 *What treatment would you offer?*

Chapter 58

A 19-year-old man is referred by his university course tutor as he has not been turning up for lectures. On meeting him, he avoids looking at you and talks about the fact that he cannot go out as he is now aware that everyone is watching him and talking about him. This he finds very disturbing, especially as these same people are also trying to steal his thoughts, all of which he knows is true, because he hears his flat-mate talking about it to some others at night.
1 *What action would you take?*
2 *Does he require any treatment?*

Chapter 59

A 63-year-old man presents with a 2-year history of episodes of panic. They occur for no good reason and he suddenly feels incredibly anxious with palpitations, sweating and an intense headache. During these attacks, which typically last for a few minutes at a time, his blood pressure and hear rate are very high and he feels very sweaty.
1 *What is the diagnosis?*
2 *How would you prove it?*

Chapter 60

A 71-year-old woman presents with a 4-month history of rapidly evolving dementia. She has no significant previous medical history. Her condition began with her becoming confused and wandering off at night, with a tendency to sleep during the day. On examination she is very thin, mute and unresponsive with widespread myoclonic jerks.
1 *What is the differential diagnosis?*

Chapter 61

A 17-year-old girl presents with episodes of going blank. She has no memory for these events but her friends say that during these attacks she suddenly stops doing whatever she is doing, then talks gibberish, smacks her lips and fiddles with her hands. On coming round 20–30 seconds later she carries on as normal.
1 *What is the diagnosis?*
2 *What would you say to her?*

Chapter 62

A 42-year-old man presents with a recent onset of odd behaviour, amnesia and seizures. He is initially taken to a psychiatric ward where he is seen to have odd attacks, and he is then referred to the neurologist. On examination, he appears to be having complex partial seizures and on magnetic resonance imaging (MRI) there are bilateral high signal changes in the hippocampi.
1 *What is the diagnosis?*
2 *How would you treat him?*

Chapter 63

A 25-year-old woman is referred up with weakness in her hands and feet. She is found to have symmetrical sensory loss and mild weakness with marked wasting of her hand and feet muscles. Her father has a similar condition, but there is no real family history outside this, although her younger sister has had a number of orthopaedic procedures on her feet as she has pes cavus.
1 *What may be the diagnosis?*
2 *How would you prove this?*

Chapter 64

A 79-year-old woman presents with a 1-hour history of sudden onset right-sided weakness and aphasia.
1 *What is the likely diagnosis and why?*
2 *What tests would you do and why?*
3 *What treatment, if any, would you offer?*
Note: There is no case study for Chapter 65.

Answers

Chapter 1

1 This is case of spinal bifida and the abnormality is either a meningocoele or meningomyelocoele.

Chapter 2

1 Central nervous system.
2 Mid-lower cervical spine.
3 A fracture of the spine secondary to the fall. In all similar cases the spine should be stabilized before the patient is moved at the time and scene of the accident.

Chapter 3

1 The man is developing autonomic failure.
2 In the normal situation, the Valsalva manoeuvre should cause a change in heart rate that is most easily seen on a prolonged ECG recording. However, in this case the man has a generalized autonomic failure and this includes the innervation of the heart which is under direct autonomic control, so there is no change in his heart rate rate when he exercises.

Chapter 4

1 Hirschsprung's disease.
2 It is a developmental problem in which there is no development of the enteric nervous system in a part of the colon.

Chapter 5

1 Meningococcal meningitis and septicaemia. The rash with the low blood pressure means that the patient has a systemic infection as well as a meningitis – the latter giving him the headache and stiff neck.
2 The likely organism is *Meningococcus* – this characteristically gives rise to the rash with signs of septicaemia and meningitis.
3 Antibiotics should be administered immediately with supportive therapy ahead of any investigations. This is because meningococcal septicaemia is associated with high mortality and it has been shown that the earlier the antibiotics are given (usually penicillin) the better the clinical outcome.

Chapter 6

1 He has had a right hemispheric stroke as he has a left-sided hemiparesis of relatively abrupt onset.
2 The stroke is likely to be due to a carotid dissection as he is young, the onset was stuttering with periorbital pain and he has right-sided Horner's syndrome. The best way to prove all this is to do an MRI scan of his brain to show the stroke and a T_2 fat-suppressed MRI of his neck to look for the dissection.
3 The sympathetic fibres innervating the eyelid and eye pass along the carotid artery and thus can be affected when there is damage to the vessel itself, such as in a dissection with blood tracking into the vessel wall.

Chapter 7

1 The eighth cranial nerve (deafness), seventh cranial nerve (facial weakness) and sixth (failure of abduction) on the left.

2 The lesion is likely to be where all these three nerves share a common pathway, which is at the cerebellopontine angle.
3 The commonest lesion at this site is a vestibular nerve schwannoma, but it is unusual for it to cause other cranial nerve palsies prior to surgical resection. Other lesions that arise at this site are meningiomas and dermoid/epidermoid cysts.

Chapter 8

1 The lesion is likely to be in the left side of the pons affecting the paramedian pontine reticular formation (PPRF), which controls horizontal eye movements and the trigeminal sensory pathway. The descending motor tracts and ascending sensory pathways also pass through this part of the brainstem but they decussate below this level and hence they cause features contralateral to the brainstem lesion.
2 An image of the brainstem is needed and this should be an MRI, given the need for a high-resolution scan which cannot be achieved with CT.

Chapter 9

1 In the spinal cord on the left at the level of T10 or above. The reason why the lesion could be higher is that it is possible for lesions further up the spinal cord to give rise to similar features because of the topographical organization of the spinal cord. However, in this case the absence of any signs in the arms means the lesion is likely to be within the thoracic spinal cord.
2 A scan of the cervicothoracic cord is needed to discover the nature of the lesion causing the syndrome.
3 A Brown–Sequard syndrome.

Chapter 10

1 He is developing a frontal lobe syndrome.
2 It is always important to exclude a mass lesion in the frontal lobe as a cause of this, such as a meningioma, but the likely cause in a man of this age is the development of a dementing process such as frontal variant frontotemporal dementia.

Chapter 11

1 A pituitary tumour that is producing excessive amounts of prolactin – a prolactinoma.
2 The tumour has extended beyond the pituitary fossa and is compressing the optic chiasm, giving the characteristic field defect as it compresses the crossing fibres.
3 Diabetes insipidus is due to disruption of the pathway from the hypothalamus to the posterior pituitary containing vasopressin or antidiuretic hormone.

Chapter 12

1 Central nervous system neurones.
2 A dementing illness such as Alzheimer's disease or, given the speed of progression, rarer disorders such as Creutzfeldt–Jakob disease.

Neuroanatomy and Neuroscience at a Glance, Fourth Edition. Roger A. Barker, Francesca Cicchetti, Michael J. Neal.

Chapter 13

1 Oligodendrocytes.

2 Demyelination of the axons in the spinal cord around the nodes of Ranvier causes disturbances of nerve conduction in the sensory and motor pathways to the legs and bladder.

3 As a young woman with an episode of spinal cord demyelination, she is likely to have or go onto develop multiple sclerosis.

Chapter 14

1 In the ion channels in his skeletal muscles.

2 An inherited channelopathy causing a type of periodic paralysis.

Chapter 15

1 Peripheral nervous system.

2 Demyelination of his peripheral motor and sensory nerves with conduction slowing and block, typically around the nodes of Ranvier.

3 Guillain–Barré syndrome.

Chapter 16

1 At the neuromuscular junction.

2 This suggests fatigability, with the symptoms being worse at the end of the day.

3 Myasthenia gravis.

Chapter 17

1 Inhibitory γ-aminobutyric acid (GABA)ergic synapses in his spinal cord.

2 Because he has lost some inhibition of the motor neurones, such that they have become overactive and so send excessive impulses to the muscles, causing them to be permanently active.

Chapter 18

1 She may have idiopathic Parkinson's disease (PD), but it is more likely that it is drug induced secondary to the introduction of metoclopramide.

2 Metoclopramide is a dopamine receptor blocker and so will mimic PD by virtue of the fact that it will block the dopaminergic nigrostriatal pathway.

3 Yes, assuming she truly only has drug-induced parkinsonism and not preclinical/prodromal PD which has been brought out by the drug.

Chapter 19

1 Migraine.

2 The 5-hydroxytryptamine (5-HT) or serotonin system.

Chapter 20

1 He has a proximal myopathy.

2 One should ask to see if there is a family history of muscle disease and whether he has any weakness around the face and autonomic problems, as rarely myasthenia gravis and the Lambert–Eaton myasthenic syndrome can present in this way.

3 Creatine kinase (CK), electromyography (EMG), genetics for known limb girdle muscular dystrophy, possibly a muscle biopsy, and it may also be worthwhile doing antibody tests for AChR/muscle specific kinase (MUSK)/voltage-gated calcium channels.

Chapter 21

1 Periodic paralysis.

2 It is due to an inherited abnormality in a muscle ion channel and this is typically either the sodium or chloride channels.

Chapter 22

1 In the peripheral nervous system with the symmetrical loss of sensation in both feet and hands.

2 The loss of sensation and proprioception means that he cannot coordinate his movements properly and as such he is clumsy and unstable.

3 At night, when he cannot compensate using visual cues.

Chapter 23

1 Retinitis pigmentosa.

2 There is a progressive loss of rods due to an inherited problem in the proteins that form the rods.

3 He is losing his night sight as the rods are the main cells that are responsible for this form of sight (see Chapter 24)

Chapter 24

1 Macular degeneration of the elderly.

2 She has loss of the cells in the macula, which includes the fovea, as such she is slowly losing the capacity to see detail in the centre of her vision. She is fine walking around because for this she simply needs her peripheral vision, which is unaffected in this condition.

Chapter 25

1 Optic neuritis.

2 It will dilate. This is because the initial constriction in the right eye is driven by the visual information that passes down the optic nerve from the normal left eye. However, on swinging the light to the right eye, the midbrain will receive a reduced input due to the demyelinating lesion in the right optic nerve so the pupil will dilate.

Chapter 26

1 Central achromatopsia.

2 Area V4.

Chapter 27

1 Chronic otitis media causing a conductive hearing loss, which means that he cannot hear what is being asked of him, nor the speech of others.

2 The simplest way to do this would be to look in the ear and conduct hearing tests to confirm the presence of chronic otitis media or glue ear.

3 The important management issues are to treat the chronic otitis media and to alert the school about the problem so that his teachers can better manage the issue, rather than keep excluding him for bad behaviour. The treatment of chronic otitis media often involves the insertion of grommets in the tympanic membrane to drain the fluid and prevent a recurrence of the problem.

Chapter 28 (a)

1 Left cerebellopontine angle.

2 An irritative space-occupying lesion such as a meningioma, dermoid or epidermoid cyst.

3 Probably not, as the development of a slowly growing lesion leads to compensation within the central auditory pathways.

Chapter 28 (b)

1 A left frontal lesion involving Broca's area and the motor cortical areas of the face and hand.
2 Given the 3-week progressive history, the lesion is likely to a space-occupying mass, so either a primary glioma or metastases.
3 Imaging of the brain with CT or preferably MRI.

Chapter 29

1 Viral labyrinthitis.
2 Benign paroxysmal positional vertigo (BPPV).
3 Hallpike manoeuvre, and then treat with Epley's manoeuvre.

Chapter 30

1 Simple (no impairment of consciousness) and complex (impaired consciousness) partial seizures.
2 Temporal lobe.
3 EEG may help localize the site of the epilepsy, although the history is highly suggestive of the lesion site. MRI would be useful to see if there is a selective lesion in the temporal lobe underlying this epilepsy, whether it be a scar or a space-occupying lesion.

Chapter 31

1 Subacute combined degeneration of the spinal cord. This causes dorsal column loss, spinocerebellar tract involvement, optic nerve demyelination as well as peripheral neuropathy with some involvement of the descending motor pathways.
2 The major loss of proprioception means that the patient does not know where their hands/fingers are in space so they move involuntarily as a result.
3 A serum B_{12} level with a blood picture in keeping with a megaloblastic anaemia (which in this case is likely to be dietary in origin). MRI of the spine may show demyelination in the posterior regions of the spinal cord and nerve conduction studies will show a neuropathy. In addition she will have prolonged visual evoked responses.

Chapter 32

1 Complex regional pain syndrome.
2 No. The complex regional pain syndrome is due as much to maladaptive central nervous system pathology and peripheral nerve damage/dysfunction. While the latter may be making a contribution, it is more likely that there are changes within the central nervous system (CNS) that underpin much of her pain syndrome. As such, amputation will offer no pain relief.

Chapter 33

1 Post-herpetic neuralgia.
2 Topical capsaicin.

Chapter 34

1 A frontal lobe syndrome.
2 This is because he has poor attentive skills, and so he does not take in the relevant information to remember.
3 In the first instance a scan to exclude a frontal lesion, such as a slow-growing meningioma.

Chapter 35

1 She will have a combination of motor problems, She will have a disturbance of descending motor pathways to the legs so she will have upper motor neurone lesions with increased tone, weakness, increased reflexes, clonus and extensor plantar responses. In addition she will have bilateral ataxia with upper limb incoordination with an intention tremor, dysdiadochokinesis and an unsteady ataxic gait.

Chapter 36

1 Motor neurone disease (MND). The widespread lower motor neurone features with brisk reflexes is only really compatible with MND in this age group.
2 The clinical diagnosis is sufficient. However, one could do an MRI of brain and spinal cord with cerebrospinal fluid (CSF) analysis to exclude a meningitic process and an EMG to show widespread denervation, although this is obvious from the clinical features. Nerve conduction studies should show normal sensory conduction with or without reduced motor responses.

Chapter 37

1 An upper motor neurone lesion of the legs.
2 The spastic paraparesis with a strong family history and normal imaging makes this likely to be a case of hereditary spastic paraparesis. Typically these patients have a long history of an evolving spastic paraparesis with normal investigations and relatively well-preserved power in the face of marked spasticity.

Chapter 38

1 A stroke, given the acute onset in a man of this age.
2 Right hemisphere; it is likely to be a right middle cerebral artery infarct.
3 He has infarction of his motor cortical areas and the descending pathways from these areas.

Chapter 39

1 A jacksonian epileptic seizure taking its origin in the hand region of the motor homunculus and spreading laterally to involve the arm, face and the speech area.
2 Left motor cortex.
3 An irritative lesion in the region of the left primary motor cortex. Such a lesion could be a tumour such as a meningioma, or a small cortical venous infarct.

Chapter 40

1 One would expect to see nystagmus, dysarthria, past pointing with an intention tremor, gait ataxia and heel-shin incoordination.
2 An autosomal dominant spinocerebellar ataxia of which there are many different types. Several of these can be tested for genetically, as they are a form of triplet repeat disorders (see Chapter 63).

Chapter 41

1 The widespread dance-like movements are characteristic of chorea, and are typically seen in patients with basal ganglia disorders.
2 Given the family history, age and the type of movement disorder, the most likely diagnosis is Huntington's disease.

Chapter 42

1 He has a parkinsonian condition.

2 Mask-like face, possibly drooling, quiet hypophonic speech, arm rigidity with a rest tremor, and bradykinesia. On standing he would have a stooped gait with a festinant walk and reduced arm swing, and possibly impaired postural reflexes.

3 It is not clear whether he has drug-induced parkinsonism secondary to the metoclopramide, or whether the use of this drug has simply unmasked his latent idiopathic PD. The best way to find out is to (i) stop the medication and see if he returns to normal and/or (ii) undertake a DAT scan to see if he has an intact nigrostriatal dopaminergic pathway.

Chapter 43

1 The differential diagnosis is between a cardiac dysrhythmia, epilepsy or sleep apnoea causing him to fall asleep. Thus the investigations would include: ECG monitoring for cardiac dysrhythmias; EEG monitoring; and a sleep study.

2 Given his size and some evidence of right heart failure with the history of feeling tired in the morning despite a good night's sleep, the most likely diagnosis is obstructive sleep apnoea (OSA).

3 If the diagnosis of OSA is confirmed, he should lose weight and if necessary given appropriate ventilator support at night to keep his airway open (so called nocturnal continuous positive airway pressure [CPAP] therapy). He should then be retested to ensure that his condition is being adequately treated.

Chapter 44

1 He is still in the acute stages of his recovery, and is young with a relatively well-circumscribed lesion. As such there is a high probability that he will continue to improve and thus active measures should be pursued at this stage.

2 It is imperative that this man is investigated or assessed for locked-in syndrome, given the site of his lesion. This can be done by paying careful attention to his responses to simple commands along with neurophysiological and functional imaging to assess the extent to which he can activate his cortex to peripheral stimuli.

Chapter 45

1 It is highly likely that she is describing short (simple partial seizures) epileptic seizures that originate and remain localized to the amygdala.

2 Ideally one needs to capture an attack by recording one of her episodes while an EEG recording from her brain is being made. However, this is not always possible or necessary as a routine EEG may reveal abnormal discharges over the temporal lobe, and abnormalities within the amygdala may also be apparent on high-resolution MRI.

Chapter 46

1 She has an anterograde memory deficit, assuming she could take in the name and address normally. Typically patients are given a name and address and asked to repeat it back, until such time as they have taken it in and then asked 5 minutes later to say what it was. She has normal visuospatial function and has no major language problems as far as one can tell.

2 The history and deficit on anterograde memory is typical of Alzheimer's disease.

Chapter 47

He is likely to have a state of abulia secondary to his unusual strokes. Typically patients with lesions of the caudate nucleus have a state of reduced motivation as well as problems of set shifting, so they superficially appear depressed and easily confused. This having been said there is no treatment of abulia, so excluding an underlying depression is a necessary part of the work-up of such patients. However, if he has had two decent courses of antidepressants, they should be stopped and he should be referred for rehabilitation – which may help some aspects of his condition, especially the problems of set shifting.

Chapter 48

1 During the surgical procedure the sural nerve has been damaged and as such there is sensory loss secondary to this.

2 It is impossible at this stage to know the extent to which it will recover as the nerve may have been accidentally severed, or more likely just bruised. In either case some recovery will occur as the nerve recovers and regenerates. Thus, he will probably make an almost complete recovery from this local nerve injury.

Chapter 49

1 The squint needs to be corrected and the good eye patched.

2 Failure to do this will lead to functional blindness in the eye with the squint, as it will fail to compete with the good eye for cortical space. Thus, the earlier the abnormality is detected and corrected the better, otherwise if it is left beyond the critical period, the deficit will become permanent.

Note: There are no case studies for Chapters 50–55.

Chapter 56

1 She has Internuclear ophthalmoplegia (INO), so the lesion will be in her medial longitudinal fasciculus.

2 The presentation in a young woman of an evolving brainstem syndrome is most likely to represent the first demyelinating episode of multiple sclerosis.

3 A brain MRI to confirm that she has demyelinating lesions to account for her presentation and to exclude any other lesion involving the pons.

Chapter 57

1 While she presents with a history of depression, it is likely that this is secondary to some underlying medical problem and given the clinical findings and investigation results, she is likely to have systemic lupus erythematosus (SLE).

2 The diagnosis of SLE needs to be confirmed and treated. Although she may require antidepressant therapy, this is not the first-line treatment here as her affective state is secondary to her underlying medical condition.

Chapter 58

1 The features are all those of schizophrenia, with the paranoid ideation and auditory hallucinations talking about him in the third person. However, it is important to get opinions from other people who know him, and also to exclude other causes such as drug abuse and, although less likely, chronic untreated temporal lobe epilepsy.

2 Yes. He is failing in his degree, so his behavioural abnormalities are interfering with his normal life.

Chapter 59

1 He could be having panic attacks, but they appear not to occur in any specific context and they are associated with features of intense sympathetic hyperactivity. Thus it is important that phaeochromocytoma is excluded (a tumour of the chromaffin cells of the adrenal medulla).

2 To prove he has this tumour, urine samples are required to look for excessive catecholamine secretion. If these are positive, imaging will be required. These tumours are typically found in the adrenal area, although not uncommonly they can occur at a number of other extraadrenal sites, due to their embryological origin with migration of the sympathetic precursor cells into the developing adrenal medulla.

Chapter 60

1 There are relatively few conditions that cause rapidly evolving dementia. It is always important to exclude severe depression, as such patients can become mute, catatonic and cachexic, in which electroconvulsive therapy (ECT) may be the treatment of choice (see Chapter 57). However, in this case the likely diagnosis is Creutzfeldt–Jakob disease, given her early circadian rhythm abnormalities and myoclonic jerks with rapid clinical course, although these can also be seen in some cases of Alzheimer's disease. One should also consider paraneoplastic encephalitis, cerebral vasculitis and angiocentric lymphoma. The latter two conditions cause abnormalities on MRI, while the paraneoplastic encephalitides can be investigated by looking for certain specific antibodies.

Chapter 61

1 The history is typical for temporal lobe seizures, which are a form of complex (as there is an impairment of consciousness) partial (as they only affect a part of the brain) seizures.

2 She requires investigation with an EEG and MRI to help prove the clinical diagnosis and exclude an underlying aetiological lesion that requires a different treatment from standard antiepileptic therapy. She should then be started on an appropriate antiepileptic agent, given her age and sex. She should be told about the driving regulations and issues to do with anticonvulsants, the oral contraceptive and pregnancy. It is important that she is followed up and supported because of the problems of dealing with such a diagnosis at this particular age. This may also involve a discussion about the risk of SUDEP (SUDden unExPected death), to ensure that she takes the tablets and tries to adopt a sensible lifestyle to reduce the risk of more seizures.

Chapter 62

1 He has a limbic encephalitis that is either paraneoplastic in nature or due to a potassium channel antibody. He should therefore be investigated with blood tests for the relevant antibodies and tests for an underlying malignancy.

2 If he has a primary autoimmune limbic encephalitis, he requires immunotherapy that involves plasma exchange and the introduction of steroids and other immunosuppressants such as azathioprine. If he has an underlying malignancy driving the limbic encephalitis, the tumour needs to be found and treated.

Chapter 63

1 The development of slight weakness in the presence of marked wasting at this age with a family history (albeit very limited) is suggestive of a hereditary motor and sensory neuropathy (HMSN).

2 Nerve conduction studies are often markedly abnormal and worse than the clinical signs and may be found to also be abnormal in 'unaffected' family members. Genetic testing can now be undertaken for a number of different HMSNs and this can therefore be offered to the patient (although many HMSNs have still to be defined genetically).

Chapter 64

1 Occlusion of the left middle cerebral artery with infarction of the left hemisphere, including motor sensory and language areas in the frontal, parietal and temporal lobes.

2 Urgent CT scan to exclude haemorrhage.

3 If the history is accurate and there are no other contraindications, this patient would be suitable for thrombolysis.

Note: There is no case study for Chapter 65.

Index

Page numbers in *italics* represent figures

A delta fibres *72*, 73
acalculia 77
acetylcholine 15, *14*, *16*, 45, 47, 50–1
    receptors 48, 50–1
acoustic neuroma 23, 142
actin *48*, 49, *50*, 50–1
action potential *38*, 39
    propagation 42
activation hypothesis 105
acute disseminated encephalomyelitis 135
adaptation 53
adenosine triphosphate (ATP) *16*, 17, 47, 49, 51, 55
adrenal gland *14*
adrenocorticotrophic hormone (ACTH) 31
adult neurogenesis 11
affective disorders *124*, 124–5
afferent sensory nerves *52*, 53
agraphia 77
akinetic mutism 101
alar plate *10*, 11
alcohol 15, 97
alexia 77
allodynia 73, 74
all-or-nothing phenomenon 39
alpha-motor neurones (α-MNs) *80*, 80–1, 82, 107
Alzheimer's disease 45, 47, 101, 103, 131
amacrine cells 57
amine uptake inhibitors 125
amino acids 19, 45, 47, 131
amitriptyline 75, 125, 128
amphetamines *104*, 127
amplitude (or loudness) 63
ampullae 67
amygdala *30*, 100, 101, 104–5
amyloidosis 15
amyotrophic lateral sclerosis 121
analgesia *74*, 74
anencephaly 11
Angelman's syndrome 137
angiography 115, *116*, 116–17, *140*, *142*
anosmia 23, 69
antagonist muscle 81
anterior cerebral arteries *20*, 21
anterior cingulate cortex 84
anterior nucleus *28*, 29
anterior (or ventral) root *12*, 13, *14*, 26
anterior spinal arteries *20*, 21
anterior spinal artery syndrome *118*, 119
anterograde memory 113
anticonvulsants 133
antidepressants 11, 75, 95, 97, 125, *128*, 128–9
antidiuretic hormone (ADH; vasopressin) *30*, 31
antiepileptics *132*, 132–3
antigen-presenting cells 135
antihistamines 97
antimuscarinic drugs 95
antiparkinsonian drugs 95
antipsychotics 127
anxiety 47, *128*, 128–9
aphasia *65*, 65

apoptosis 131
aqueduct of Sylvius *18*, 19, 25
arachnoid granulations *18*, 19
arachnoid mater *18*, 18
arachnoid membrane *12*, 13
archeocerebellum 90
ascending nociceptive pathways 73
ascending reticular activating system 97
ascending sensory pathways 13, *26*, 27, 53
aspirin 75
association areas 53
association cortices *76*, 76–7
astereognosis 77
astigmatism 57
astrocytes *34*, 34–5, 73
astrocytomas 35
asynergy 90
ataxia 90
attention 98, 113
atypical facial pain *110*
auditory system 52, 55, *62*, 63, *64*, 65
auditory transduction 55, 63
Auerbach's plexus *16*, 17
autism 98–9
autonomic nervous system 11, *12*, 13, *14*, 15, 47
    hypothalamus 30
axoaxonic synapse *32*, 33
axodendritic synapse *32*, 33
axolemma *32*, 33
axon collaterals *32*, 33
axon hillock *32*, 33
axons 13, *32*, 33
    unmyelinated 42–3
axoplasm 33
axoplasmic flow 33
axosomatic synapse *32*, 33

balance 52, 55, *66*, 67
ballismus 79, 95
barbiturates *104*
basal forebrain *10*, 46
basal ganglia *12*, 13, *92*, 92–3, *140*, 141
    development *10*
    diseases *94*, 94–5
    eye movements *122*, 123
    disorders *120*, 120–1
    motor systems *78*, 79
basal plate *10*, 11
basilar artery *20*, 21
basilar membrane *62*, 63, 65
Becker's muscular dystrophy 49
Bell's palsy 23
benign paroxysmal positional vertigo (BPPV) 67
benzodiazepines 97, *128*, 129, 133
berry aneurysms 21
beta-adrenoceptor antagonists 129
beta-blockers 95, 129
bipolar cells 57
bitter taste *68*, 69
blackouts 111
bladder *14*, 15
blindsight 61, 98, 99
blind spot 57

blobs 61
blood-brain barrier (BBB) 19, *34*, 35, 134
blood tests *114*, 114
bone morphogenic proteins (BMPs) *10*, 11
botulinum toxin 15, *40*, 41
bouton 33
bowel *14*, 15
brain 119, 121
    biopsy 115
    blood supply 21, 142
    development *10*, 11
    see also individual parts
brainstem *12*, 13, 61, *84*, 84–5, *141*
    anatomy 24, 25
Broca's areas *20*, 64, 65
Brodmann's areas 29, 59, *60*, 61, 76–7, 84–5
Brodmann's map *28*, 29
bronchial tree *14*
Brown-Séquard syndrome *118*, 119
bulbar palsy 23
buprenorphine 75
buspirone 129
butyrophenones 127

C fibres 73, 75
caloric testing 67
capsaicin 75
carbamazepine 75, 125, *132*, 133
carpal tunnel syndrome 81, 118
cataplexy 97
cataracts 57
cauda equine *26*, 26
caudate *20*, *92*, 93
cell membrane 33
central aqueduct stenosis 19
central canal *10*, 11
central motor conduction time 115
central nervous system (CNS) 11, *12*, 13, *108*, 108–9, 142
    blood supply *20*, 21
    eye movements 123
    imaging *116*, 116–17
    immunological network 134–5
    main neurotransmitters *46*, 47
    regenerative capacity 109
central pattern generators *82*, 82–3
central sulcus *28*
central vestibular pathway disorders 67
centre surround receptive field 57, 61
cerebellar peduncles 13, *24*, 25
cerebellum *10*, *24*, 85, *88*, 89–91
    disorders 90, *120*, 120–1
    eye movements *122*, 123
    motor systems *78*, 79, 89
    organization *12*, 13, *88*, 89
cerebral cortex *12*, 13, *28*, 29
    development *10*
cerebral hemispheres *12*, 13, *20*, *28*, 84, 86
    dominance *13*
    MRI 141
cerebral peduncles 25
cerebrospinal fluid (CSF) 13, *18*, 18–19
    analysis 115

cerebrovascular accidents (CVAs) see strokes
cerebrovascular disease *138*, 139
chemical synapses 33, 40–1
chemotransduction *54*, 55
chocolate 47
cholecystokinin 128, 129
chorda tympani 69
chorea 79, 95, 121
choreoathetoid cerebral palsy 95
choroid plexus *18*, 19
choroid plexus papilloma 35
chronic pain 73, 75
chronic tension headache *110*
cingulate gyrus *100*, 100–1
circle of Willis *20*, 21
circular symmetric receptive field 61
cisterna magna 18
cleft substance *40*
clobazam 133
clomipramine 97
clonazepam 133
closed-loop movement 78
clozapine 127
cluster headache *110*
cocaine *104*
coccygeal nerve *12*, 13
cochlea *62*, 63
cochlear nucleus *24*, *64*, 65
codeine 75
cognition 125, 127
cognitive examination *112*, 112
colour blindness 57
columnar hypothesis 29
complex cells 61
complex regional pain syndrome 15, 73, 74
computed tomography (CT) *114*, 115, 140
   central nervous system 116–17
concentration 113
conditioning 103
conductance 37
conduction block 43, 95
conductive deafness 63
cones 57
consciousness *98*, 98–9
convergence of input 27
co-ordination 79, 113
cortical columns 87
cortical dysplasia 11
cortical motor areas *84*, 84–5
cortical plate 29
corticobulbar tracts 84
cortico-cortical connections *28*
corticospinal tract (CoST) *20*, *24*, 27, 71, 83,
   84–5
corticotrophin-releasing hormone 129
cotransmission 43
cranial nerves 13, *22*, 23, 25, 113
   I (olfactory) 13, *22*, 23, 25, 69, 113
   II (optic) 13, *22*, 23, 25, 113
   III (oculomotor) *14*, *22*, 23, 25, 113
   IV (trochlear) *22*, 23, 25, 113
   V (trigeminal) *22*, 23, *25*, 113
   VI (abducens) *22*, 23, *24*, 25, 113
   VII (facial) *14*, *22*, 23, 69, 113
   VIII (vestibulocochlear) *22*, 23, *24*, 63, 65, 113
   IX (glossopharyngeal) *14*, *22*, 23, *24*, 25, 69,
      113
   X (vagus) *14*, *22*, 23, 25, 69, 113

   XI (spinal accessory) *22*, 23, 113
   XII (hypoglossal) *22*, 23, 113
craving 105
Creutzfeldt-Jakob disease 131
cribriform plate *68*, 69
critical firing threshold *38*, 39
crossbridging 49, *50*, 50–1
curare 41
current 37
cyclic adenosine monophosphate (cAMP) *54*, 55,
   69
cyclo-oxygenase inhibitors 75

deafness 63
decerebrate posture 83
decussation 27
dementia of Alzheimer type 45, 47, 101, 103,
   131
demyelinating neuropathy 35, 43, 115, *134*, 135
dendrites *32*, 32–3
dendritic spines 33
dentate gyrus 11, 100
dependence 129
depolarization *38*, 39, *50*, 50, *54*, 55
depot preparations 127
depression 45, 47, 97, *124*, 124
dermatomyositis 49, 135
descending motor pathways 27, *78*, 79, *82*, 83,
   89–91, 121
descending sensory pathways 13
desensitization 45
dextropoxyphene 75
diabetes insipidus 31
diabetes mellitus 15, 17
diamorphine (heroin) 75
diazepam *128*, 129, 133
diencephalon *10*
digit span 102
diplopia 23, *110*, 113, 121
distributed system theory 29
dizziness 111
donepezil 131
dopamine 47, 95, *104*, 105
   schizophrenia *126*, 126–7
dopamine agonists 95
dopamine dysregulation syndrome 105
dopamine replacement therapy 95
dorsal column 27, 53, 71
dorsal column nuclei *24*, 25, 71
dorsal horn 11, 27, *72*, *74*, 75
dorsal/posterior roots 13, *14*, *26*, 26
dorsal root ganglia *10*, 11, *12*, 13, *70*, 71
dorsal spinal nerves *12*, 13
dorsal spinocerebellar tract 83
dosulepin 125
down-regulation 45
drug addiction 47, 93, *104*, 104–5
Duchenne's muscular dystrophy 49
dura mater *12*, 13, *18*, 18
dynamic mutations 137
dysarthria *65*, 90, 133
dysdiadochokinesis 90
dysmetria 90
dysphagia 23
dysphasia *64*, 77
dyspraxia 21, 77, 113
dystonia 41, 79, 95, 109, 121
dystrophin 49

ear *62*, 63
echolocation 65
Edinger-Westphal nucleus *58*, 59
EE cells 65
efferent conducting pathway 15
EI cells 65
electrical synapses 33, 41
electrocardiography 115
electroconvulsive therapy 125
electroencephalography *96*, 96–7, 115, 132
electromyography 115
emotion *104*, 104–5
encephalitis *110*, 115, 117, *134*
end-bulb 33
endocytosis 41
endogenous depression 124
endogenous opioid substances 73
endolymph 67
endoneurial tubes 107
endoplasmic reticulum *32*, 33, *40*, 51
endozapines 47
end-plate potential *40*, 41
enteric nervous system 13, 15, *16*, 17
entacapone 95
entorhinal cortex 100
ependymal cells 34, 35
ependymal layer *10*, 11
ependymomas 35
epilepsy 11, 19, 53, *110*, 132, 132–3
   ion channels 37
   neurotransmitters 45, 47
   primary motor cortex 87
   temporal lobe 69, 101, *132*, 133
   vestibular system 67
episodic memory *102*, 103
Epley's manoeuvre 67
equilibrium potential 39
ethanol *104*
ethosuximide 133
evoked potentials 115
examination 111
   nervous system *112*, 113, *114*, 114–15
excitatory amino acids 45, 47, 131
excitatory postsynaptic potentials 43
excitotoxic cell death 45, 47, *130*, 131
experimental allergic encephalomyelitis 135
explicit memory *102*, 102, 103
external ear (auditory meatus) *62*, 63
extrapyramidal disorders 82
extrastriate areas 59, *60*, 61, 123
eye *14*, 15, 21
   nerves *22*, 23
eye movements 95, *122*, 123
   sleep *96*, 97

F-actin 49
fatigue 111
feature detection 53
feedback inhibition 43
fentanyl 75
fictive locomotion 83
final common pathway 79
firing threshold *38*, 39, 53
flexor reflex afferents 83
fluoxetine 125
focal nerve entrapment *118*, 118
focal peripheral lesions 15
foot drop *118*, 119

foramen magnum *12*, 13, *18*, *24*, 25
foramina of Luscha and Magendie *18*, 19
foramina of Munro *18*, 19
fourth ventricle *10*, *18*, 19, 121, 141
fovea 57, *60*, 61
free radical production *130*, 131
frequency *62*, 63
frequency coding 52
Friedreich's ataxia 137
frontal cortex 61
frontal eye fields 59, 61, 84, *122*, 123
frontal lobe *12*, 13, *30*, 77
    function *112*, 113
frontotemporal dementia (FTD) 77, 103
functional MRI 115, 116, 117

GABA 45, 47, 83, 128–9, *132*, 132–3
GABA-benzodiazepine-barbiturate receptor
    44
gabapentin 75, *132*, 133
galantamine 131
gamma motor neurones (γMNs) *80*, 81, 82
ganglia 13
ganglion cells 57, 59
gate theory of pain 75
gemmules 33
gene deletions 136–7
gene duplications 137
gene mutations 137
general anaesthesia 51, *98*, 98, 117
generalized anxiety disorder 128–9
genetic anticipation 137
genetic imprinting 137
genome-wide association studies 137
GI tract *14*, *16*, 17
giant cell/temporal arteritis *110*
glioma tumour 19
globus pallidus *20*, 21, *92*, 92
glossopharyngeal nerve 69
glutamate 45, 47, 127
glycine 45, 47
Golgi apparatus *32*, 32
Golgi tendon organ 79, 81
grandmother cell 29
granule cells (GrCs) 89
grey matter *12*, 13, *18*
growth cone 11, 109
Guillain-Barré syndrome 15, 17, 37, 43, 135
gustatory receptors 69
gustatory transduction *68*

haemorrhage 21
hair cells *62*, 63, 67
half centres 83
headaches *110*
heart *14*
heavy meromyosin protein 49
hedonia hypothesis 105
helicotrema *62*, 63
hemiballismus 95, 121
hereditary motor and sensory neuropathy 41,
    137
hereditary neuropathy with liability to pressure
    palsies 136
heroin 75
herpes encephalitis 117
heteroplasmy 137
hierarchy 29

high-threshold mechanoreceptor (HTM) 73
hippocampi complex 100, 102
hippocampus *10*, *12*, *20*, *30*, *100*
Hirschsprung's disease 17
history taking 111, 114–15
HIV 131
homonymous hemianopia with macular sparing
    21
homonymous muscle 81
horizontal cells 57
Horner's syndrome 15
Hubel and Wiesel model *60*, 61
Huntington's disease *94*, 95, 103, 131, 137
hydrocephalus 11, 19, 35, 121
hydrolysis 45
5-hydroxytryptamine *see* serotonin
hyperalgesia 73
hypercolumn 61
hypercomplex (end-stopped) cells 61
hyperekplexia 45, 79
hypermetropia 56
hyperpolarization *38*, 39, *54*
hypersomnia (daytime sleepiness) 97
hypertonia 83
hypocretins *96*, 97
hypothalamus *14*, 15, *30*, 30–1, *141*
    development *10*, 11
    olfaction and taste 69
    visual system 59, 61
hypotonia 83, 90

Ia afferent nerve endings 81
Ia inhibitory interneurones 81, 83
iatrogenic disorders 17
Ib afferent fibres 81, 83
ibuprofen 75
imaging *114*, 115, 140–2
    CNS *116*, 117, 142
imipramine 75, 125
immunological disorders *134*, 135
immunological privilege 19, 134
implicit memory *102*, 102, 103
incentive salience 105
incoordination 90
inferior colliculus *10*, *24*, 25, *64*, 65
inferior olive *24*, 25
inflammation 49, 131
inflammatory myositis 121
inhibitory amino acids 45, 47
inhibitory postsynaptic potentials *42*, 43
inner ear *62*, 63
inotropic receptors 45
input-output coupling 87
insomnia 97
interblobs 61
interictal activity 132–3
intermediate zone *12*, 13
intermediolateral column 27
internal carotid arteries *20*, 21
interneurones (INs) 78, 79, *80*, 81, 82
    pain 73, *74*, 75
internuclear ophthalmoplegia 123
intracranial pressure 19, 21, 23, *110*, 110
intralaminar nuclei *28*, 29
investigations 111
ion channels *36*, 36–7, 44, 53
irritable bowel syndrome 17
Isaac's syndrome 41

Jacksonian epilepsy 121, *132*
Jacksonian march 87
joint position sense 113

keratitis 57
Klüver-Bucy syndrome *104*, 104
Korsakoff's syndrome 31

labyrinth *66*, 67
labyrinthitis 67
lacrimal and salivary glands *14*, 23
lacunar infarcts 21
Lambert-Eaton myasthenia syndrome 15, 37, *40*,
    41, *134*, 135
laminae of Rexed *26*, 27
lamotrigine *132*, 133
language 21, *64*, 65, 65, 113
large intestine *16*, 17
lateral column 13
lateral geniculate nucleus *28*, 29, *108*
    visual system *58*, 59, *60*, 61
lateral inhibition 27, 53
lateral medullary syndrome of Wallenberg 21
lateral motor neurone pool 83
lateral motor system 83
lateral ventricles *10*, 11, *12*
learned helplessness 125
learning hypothesis 105
leucodystrophies 35
levetiracetam *132*, 133
levodopa 95
Lewy bodies 94
ligand grated channels 36
light meromyosin protein 49
limb girdle muscular dystrophy 49, 121
limbic encephalitis 37, 135
limbic system 13, *20*, 69, 79, *100*, 100–1
    function 83, 101
    MRI *140*, 141
Lissauer's tract *26*, 27
lithium 125
local anaesthesia 75
locked-in syndrome 99
locomotion *82*, 82–3
locus coeruleus *46*, 47, 97
lofepramine 125
long-latency reflexes 87
long-sightedness 56
long-term depression 45, 89, 101, 109
long-term memory *102*, 103
long-term modulations of synaptic transmission
    43
long-term potentiation 45, *100*, 101
lorazepam 133
Lou Gehrig disease 121
lower motor neurone lesions 79, 81, 121
lumbar nerves *12*, 13
lumbar puncture *114*

M channels 57, 59, 61
magnetic resonance angiography/venography
    115, 117
magnetic resonance imaging (MRI) *114*, 115,
    140–2
    central nervous system 116–17
major histocompatibility complex (MHC) 134–5
malignant hyperthermia/hyperpyrexia 51
malignant meningitis 19, 115

Index **155**

mania 124–5
mantle layer 11
marginal layer *10*, 11
marijuana 93
mechanoelectrical transduction *54*, 55
medial geniculate nucleus *28, 29*, 65
medial lemniscus *24, 25*, 53, 71
medial longitudinal fasciculus *24, 25*
medulla *10, 12*, 13, *24, 25*
medullary-cervical junction *24*
Meissner's corpuscles 71
Meissner's plexus *16*, 17
membrane enzymes 44
memory 11, 98, 101, *102*, 102–3, 113
memory acquisition 101
meninges 11, *12, 13, 18*, 18–19
meningioma 19, 69
meningitis 19, *110*, 115, *134*
meningocoele 11
meningomyelocoele 11
Merkel's discs 71
mesencephalon *10*, 13
mesolimbic system 105
metabolic myopathies 51
metabotropic receptors 45
metencephalon *10*
methadone 75
microglia 73, 131, 135
microglial cells *34*, 35
microtubules *32*
midbrain *12*, 13, 21, *24, 25*, 59
    development *10*
    dopaminergic projections *46*
middle cerebral arteries *20*, 21
middle ear *62*, 63
midpons *24*
migraine 37, 47, 53, *110*
miniature end-plate potential *40*, 41
minimally conscious state (MCS) 99
mitochondria *32, 32, 48*
mitochondrial cytopathies 95
mitochondrial disorders *136*, 136–7, 139
mitochondrial genome *136, 136*
modality 53
Mollaret triangle 90
monoamine oxidase inhibitors 95, 125
monoamines 45, 47, 125
monocular deprivation 109
morphine 75
motivation *104*, 104–5
motor cell bodies 27
motor homunculus *86*, 87
motor neurone disease (MND) 23, 81, 107, 121,
    131, 137
motor neurones 26, 26–7, 82–3, 120
    lesions 79, 81, 121
    lower 79, *80*, 80–1, 121
motor systems 78, 78–9, *82*, 82–3, 103
    disorders *120*, 120–1
    examination *112*, 113
motor unit *78*, 80
mucosal function *16*, 17
multiple sclerosis 35, 43, *110*, 130, *134*, 134–5
    brainstem 25
    imaging 117
    ion channels 37
    eye movements 123
    investigation 114

motor system 121
    pain 74
    vestibular system 67
multiple system atrophy 15, 131
multipolar neurones 33
muscle activity *16*, 17
muscle biopsy 115
muscle disorders *110*, 121
muscle spindle 79, *80*, 80–1
muscular dystrophies 49, 121
myasthenia gravis *40*, 41, 49, 121, *122*, 123,
    135
myelencephalon *10*
myelinated fibres *42*, 43
myelin sheath 33
myelitis *110, 134*
myelography 115
myelopathy *110*
myenteric plexus *16*, 17
myoclonus 90
myofibrils *48, 48*
myopia 57
myosin *48*, 49, 50–1
myosities 49
myositis 49, *134*
myotonia 37
myotonic dystrophy 121
myotonic syndromes 137

Na⁺–K⁺ exchange pump *38*, 39
naloxone 75
naproxen 75
narcolepsy 97
Nernst equation *38*, 39
nerve biopsy 115
nerve conduction *42*, 42–3
nerve conduction studies *114*, 115
nerve terminal *32*, 33
nervous system *10*, 11, *12*, 13
    examination *112*, 113
    investigation *114*, 114–15
neural crest *10*, 11
neural groove *10*, 11
neural plasticity *106*, 106–7, *108*, 108–9
neural plate *10*, 11
neural stem cells 109
neural tube *10*, 11
neuritis *134*
neuroblasts 11
neurochemical disorders *124*, 124–5, *126*, 126–7,
    128, 128–9
neurodegenerative disorders *110, 130*, 131
neurofibromatosis type I 35
neurofilaments *32*, 33
neurogenesis 11
neurogenetic disorders *136*, 136–7
neuroglial cells *34*, 34–5
neuroimmunological disorders *124*, 124–5
neuromodulation *44*, 45
neuromuscular junction *40*, 40–1, *48*, 135
    disorders 41, 47, 51, *110*, 120, 121
neuromuscular transmission disorders 41
neuromyotonia *40*, 41
neurones 11, 13, *14, 15, 32*, 32–3
    enteric nervous system *16*, 17
neuropathy *110*, 111, *118*, 119
neuropeptides 45, 47, 129
neurophysiological disorders *132*, 132–3

neuroradiology *140*–2, *140*–2
neuroses 128
neurotoxins 131
neurotransmitters *44*, 44–5, *46*, 47
neurotrophic factors 11, *106*, 106–7, *108*, 108–9,
    131
nicotine *104*
night blindness 55
Nissl substance *32*, 33
nitric oxidesynthase *16*
nitrous oxide 129
NMDA receptors 45, 73, 101, 127
nociceptive pathways *72*, 73
nociceptors *72*, 73
nodes of Ranvier 33, 37, 43
noise 53
non-NMDA receptors 45, 101
non-REM sleep 96–7
non-selective cation *40*
non-steroidal anti-inflammatory drugs (NSAIDs)
    75
noradrenaline (norepinephrine) *14, 15, 16*, 47, 75
notochord *10*, 11
nuclear bag and chain fibres 81
nucleus ambiguus *24, 25*
nucleus of lateral lemniscus (NLL) *64*, 65
nucleus raphe interpositus 123
nucleus of the solitary tract *68*, 69
nystagmus 90, 123

obstructive hydrocephalus 19
obstructive sleep apnoea syndrome 97
occipital lobe *12*, 13
occipitoparietal cortex 59
ocular dominance columns *60*, 61, *108*, 109
oestrogens 105
off-centre receptive field 57
olanzapine 127
olfaction 52, *68*, 69
olfactory bulb *10*, 11, *68*, 69
olfactory stimulus 69
olfactory tract *68*, 69
olfactory transduction 55
oligodendrocytes 33, *34*, 34, 35
oligodendroglioma 35
on-surround receptive field *57*
open-loop movement 78
opioids 75, *104*
opsoclonus 123
optic chasm *30, 30*
optic disc 57
optic vesicle *10*
optokinetic reflex 123
orexins 97
organ of Corti 55, 63
orientation 112
orientation selective columns 61
oscillopsia 67
ossicles 63
otis media 63
otolith organs *66*, 67
otosclerosis 63
oval window 63

P channels 57, 59, 61
Pacinian corpuscles 71
pain 15, 71, *72*, 73, *74*, 75, *100*
    peripheral 118

palatal tremor 90
paleocerebellum 90
palinopsia 59
panic disorder 128, 129
paracetamol 75
parahippocampal structures *100*, 100–1
parallel pathways 29
paraneoplastic syndromes 107, 131, 135
paraproteinaemias 135
parasubiculum 100
parasympathetic nervous system 13, *14*, 15
parietal lobe *12*, 13, 113
Parkinson's disease 17, 25, *94*, 94–5, 121, 131
   dopamine 105
   eye movements 123
   memory 103
   motor systems 79, 85
   neurotransmitters 45, 47
paroxetine 128
pars compacta *92*, 93
pars reticulata *92*, 93
pedunculopontine nucleus (PPN) *46*, *82*, *92*, 93
peptides 129
perception *98*
periaqueductal grey matter 15, *24*, 25
periodic paralyses 37, 51
peripheral nerve disorders 121
peripheral nervous system *106*, 106–7, 135
peripheral neuropathies 71, 118
peripheral pain syndrome 119
perirhinal cortex 100
permeability 37
phase 63
phenobarbital 133
phenothiazines 127
phenytoin 133
phobias 128, 129
photopic vision 57
photopigments 57
photoreceptors 57
phototransduction *54*, 55
pia mater *12*, 13, *18*, 18
pin prick 113
pitch 63
pituitary tumours 30
plantar response 113
plexopathy *110*
poliomyelitis 81, 107, 121
polymodal nociceptors (PMNs) 73
polymyositis 49, 135
pons *10*, *12*, 13, *20*, *24*, 25
pontocerebellum 89, 90, 91
positive feedback loop 39
positron emission tomography 115, 116, 117
posterior cerebellar arteries *20*, 21
posterior dorsal roots 13, *14*, *26*, 26
posterior fossa 141–2
posterior parietal cortex 71, *76*, 76–7, 79, 84
   eye movements 123
   imaging *140*
   vestibular system 67
   visual system 61
posterior spinal arteries *20*, 21
postganglionic neurones *14*, 15
postherpetic neuralgia 75
postsubiculum 100
postsynaptic membrane 33, 43
postsynaptic receptor 41

postsynaptic secondary folds *40*
Prader-Willi syndrome 137
prefrontal cortex 30, *76*, 76–7, *78*, *140*
pregabalin 133
preganglionic neurone *14*, 15
premotor cortex *78*, 79, *84*, 84–5
presubiculum 100
presynaptic actin network 41
presynaptic active zones *40*, 40
presynaptic autoreceptors 43, *44*, 44
presynaptic membrane 41, 43
presynaptic vesicles *40*
pretectal structures 59
primary afferent 52
primary auditory cortex (A1) 65
primary generalized epilepsy 133
primary lateral sclerosis 121
primary motor cortex (MsI) *84*, 84, 85, *86*, 87
primary sensory area 53
primary somatosensory cortex (SMI) 66, 67, 69, 71, 73
primary visual cortex (V1) 59, *60*, 61, *108*, 123
priming 103
primitive reflexes 113
propofol 133
propranolol 129
proprioception *70*, 71
propriospinal neurones 83
prosencephalon *10*
pseudobulbar palsy 23
pseudo-unipolar neurones 33
psychosis 124
psychotherapy 125, 128
ptosis 15, 23
pulvinar *28*, 29, 59
pupillary light response 59
pure autonomic failure 15
purinergic neurotransmitters 47
Purkinje cell (PuC) 89, 91
putamen *92*, 93
pyramid *24*, 25
pyramidal (corticospinal) tract 83
pyramidal distributions of weakness 79, 83
pyriform cortex 69

quietiapine 127

radial glial fibres 29
radiculopathies 81
raised intracranial pressure 19, 21, 23, *110*, 110
raphé serotoninergic projections *46*
rasagiline 95
reactive depression 124
receptive fields 53, 57, 61
receptors 37, 43, *44*, 44–5
   sensory *52*, 52–3
recoverin *54*
recruitment 53, 81
red nucleus *20*, *24*, 25
referred pain 73
reflex movement 78
reflex sympathetic dystrophies 15, 73
reflexes *112*, 113
refraction 56
refractory period 39
relative afferent pupillary defect 59
REM sleep *96*, 97
Renshaw cells 83

reproductive organs *14*
resting membrane *38*, 39
reticular formation 15, *96*, 96–7
reticular nuclei *28*, 29
reticulospinal tract 27, 83
retina 30, 30, *56*, 56–7, 59
retinitis pigmentosa 57
reverse suturing 109
Rexed's laminae *26*, 27
rhombencephalon *10*
rigor mortis 51
risperidone 127
rivastigmine 131
rods 57
roof plate *10*
rostral interstitial nucleus of medial longitudinal fasciculus 123
rostral migratory system 11
rubella 11
rubrospinal tract 27, 83
Ruffini endings 71

saccadic eye movements 59, 123
sacculus 67
sacral nerves *12*, 13
salt taste *68*, 69
saltatory conduction 43
sarcoglycan complex 49
sarcoidosis 19
sarcolemma *48*, 48–9
sarcomere 49
sarcoplasmic reticulum *48*, 48, *50*, 50–1
savantism 99
scala media *62*, 63
scala vestibuli *62*, 63
Scarpa's ganglion 67
schizophrenia 45, 47, 94, 99, *126*, 126–7
Schwann cells 33, *34*, 34–5, 107
schwannoma 35
scotopic vision 57
second somatosensory area (SMII) 71, 73
secondary intracellular messenger network 53
secondary sensory areas 53
selegiline 95
semantic memory 103
semicircular canals *66*, 67
sensitivity 53
sensorineural deafness 63
sensory afferent fibres 27
sensory examination *112*, 113
sensory homunculus *70*, 71
sensory pathways *26*, *52*, 52–3
sensory processing 27, 53, *74*, 83
sensory receptors *12*, *52*, 52–3, *70*, 71
sensory symptoms 111, *118*, 118–19
sensory systems *52*, 52
sensory transduction *52*, 52–3, *54*, 55
septal nuclei 100
serotonin *16*, 17, 47, 125, *128*, 128
short-sightedness 57
signal to noise ratio 53
simple cells 61
single photon emission computed tomography (SPECT) 115, 116, 117
sinusitis *110*
size principle 81
skeletal muscle *48*, 48–9
   contraction *50*, 50–1

skin *14*
sleep 47, *96*, 96–7
sliding filament hypothesis 51
small fibre neuropathy 119
small intestine *16*, 17
smooth pursuit eye movements 123
sodium valproate *132*, 133
soma 32
somatic efferent fibres *10*
somatosensory system 52, *70*, 71, 109
sonic hedgehog *10*, 11
sound waves *62*, 63
sour taste *68*, 69
spatial coding 53
spatial summation *42*, 43
specificity 53
spina bifida 11, 19
spinal cord *12*, 13, *26*, 26–7, *142*, 142
    ascending pathways 13, *26*, 27, 53
    autonomic nervous system 15
    blood supply *20*, 21
    descending pathways 13, *26*, 83
    development *10*, 11
    disorders 83, *118*, 119, 121
    locomotion *82*, 82–3
    motor systems 79
spinal motor neurones 11, *26*, 27
spinal nerves *12*, 13
spinocerebellar ataxias (SCAs) 121
spinocerebellar tract *26*, 27, 53
spinocerebellum 89, 90, 91
spinomesencephalic tract 73
spinoreticulothalamic tract 73
spinothalamic tract *26*, 27, 53, 73, 119
startle syndromes 45, 47
status epilepticus 133
stearic block 49
stereocilia 55, 63, 67
stiff person syndrome 79, 83, 121
stomach *16*, 17
stress reactions 128
stretch reflex 79, 81
striosomes 93
strokes 87, 121, *110*, *138*, 139
subacute combined degeneration of the spinal
    cord *118*, 119
subarachnoid space *12*, 13, *18*, 18–19
subcortical visual areas *58*, 59, *140*
subiculum 100
submucosal plexus *16*, 17
substance P *16*, 75, 129
substantia nigra *24*, 25, 59, *92*, 93
subthalamic nucleus *20*, 93
subthalamus 21
subventricular zones 11, 29
superior cervical ganglion *14*
superior colliculus *10*, *24*, 25, 59, *122*, 123
supersensitivity 45
supplementary motor area 78, 79, *84*, 84–5
suprachiasmatic nucleus 59
sustained gaze 123
sweet taste *68*, 69
Sydenham's chorea 95
sympathetic nervous system 13, *14*, 15, 73

symptoms *110*, 111
synapses *32*, 32–3, *40*, 40–1
synaptic cleft 33, *40*, 41
synaptic integration *42*, 42–3
synergistic muscles 81
syringomyelia 73, *118*, 119

taste 52, *68*, 69
tectorial membrane *62*, 63
tectospinal tract 27, 83
telecephalon *10*
temazepam 97
temperature 71, 113
temporal/frequency coding 53
temporal lobe *12*, 13, 113
temporal lobe epilepsy 69, 101, *132*, 133
temporal summation *42*, 43
tendon reflexes 81
thalamus *12*, 13, *28*, 29, 59, 65, 85
    blood supply *20*, 21
    pain *72*, 73, *74*, 75
    ventroposterior nucleus *70*, 71
theory of mind *98*, 98–9
thermal thresholds 115
thick filaments *48*, 49, 50–1
thin filaments *48*, 49, 50–1
thiopental 133
third ventricle *10*, *12*, 30
thoracic nerves *12*, 13
thyrotrophin-releasing hormone (TRH) 31
tiagabine 133
tickling 71
timbre 63
tongue *68*, 69
topiramate *132*, 133
touch *70*, 71, 113
tractus solitarius *24*, 25
tramadol 75
transcortical reflexes 87
transcranial magnetic stimulation (TMS) 85
transcutaneous nerve stimulation (TENS)
    75
transduction 52, 52–3, *54*, 55, 73
transient ischaemic attacks 119, 139
transmembrane pores 37
transverse myelitis 119
transverse tubules *48*, 48–9, 51
travel sickness 67
triads 49, 51
trigeminal neuralgia 75, *110*
trigeminal sensory system 71
trinucleotide repeat disorders *136*, 136, 137
triplet repeat disorders 136
tropomyosin *48*, 49, *50*, 50–1
troponin *48*, 49, *50*, 50–1
tuberculous meningitis 19
tympanic membrane (eardrum) *62*, 63

unmyelinated fibres *42*, 42–3
upper motor neurone lesions 79, 81, 83
up-regulation 45
uptake 45
utricle 67

valdecoxib 75

valproate 125, *132*, 133
vasculitides 135
vasopressin 31
vegetative state *98*, 98, 99
venlafaxine 125
venous drainage 21
ventral/anterior roots *12*, 13, *14*, 26
ventral horns 11
ventral motor nerve *10*
ventral spinocerebellar tract (VSCT) 83
ventricular zones 29
ventroanterior nucleus *28*, 29
ventrolateral nucleus *28*, 29
ventromedial motor neurone pool 82
ventromedial system 83
ventroposterior nucleus *28*, 29, *70*, 71
verbal fluency 113
vertebrae *12*, 13
vertebral arteries *20*, 21
vertebral column 13
vesicle exocytosis *40*
vesicle hypothesis 41
vestibular neuronitis/labyrinthitis 67
vestibular nuclei *24*, 25, 67, 123
vestibular reflexes 67
vestibular system *66*, 67
vestibular transduction 67
vestibulocerebellum 89, 90, 91
vestibulo-ocular reflex 109
vestibulospinal tract 27, 83
vibration perception threshold 113
vigabatrin 133
visceral afferent fibres *10*
visceral efferent fibres *10*, 11
visual acuity 57
visual cortical areas 56, 59, *60*, 61, *108*
visual pathways *58*, 59, *140*, 141
visual systems 21, 53
    cortical areas 56, 59, *60*, 61, *108*
    eye and retina *56*, 56–7
    pathways *58*, 59, *140*, 141
    plasticity *108*, 108–9
visuospatial function 113
vitamin B deficiency 119
volitional movement 78
voltage-dependent calcium ion channels 40
voltage gated channels *36*, 36

Wallerian degeneration 107
waveform 63
Weber–Fechner law *52*, 53
Wernicke's area *20*, *64*, 65
white matter 11, *12*, 13, *18*
white matter tracts *28*, 29
Wilson's disease 95
withdrawal syndrome 129
working memory *102*, 102–3

X-rays *114*, 116
XYW system 57

Z drugs 97
zaleplon 97
zolpidem 97
zopiclone 97

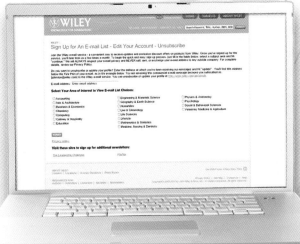
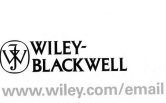
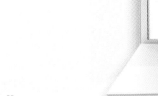

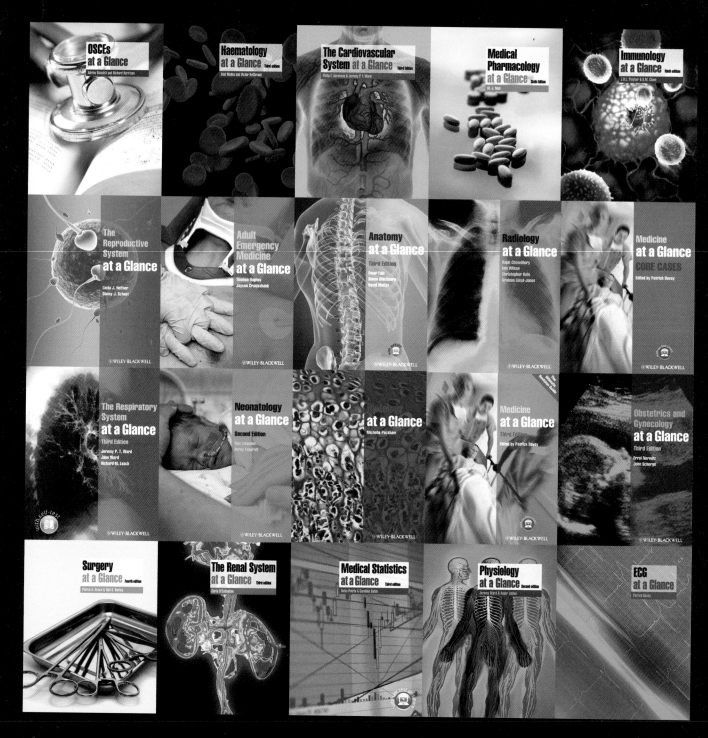

The at a Glance series

Popular double-page spread format • Coverage of core knowledge
Full-colour throughout • Self-assessment to test your knowledge • Expert authors

www.wileymedicaleducation.com

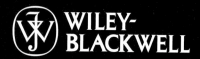